Unveiling the History of Australian Nursing in the First World War

Ruth Rae

Unveiling the History of Australian Nursing in the First World War

Revised 4th edition of

Veiled Lives:
Threading Australian Nursing History into the Fabric of the First World War

Cover Design by Ruth Rae, 2026. Photograph of Ethelda Runnalls Uren, wearing AANS uniform (AWM P10964.01).

First published by The College of Nursing, Burwood, 2009 as *Veiled Live: Threading Australian Nursing History into the Fabric of the First World War (1st& 2nd ed).*

Third edition previously published as book three: *Veiled Live - Threading Australian Nursing History into the Fabric of the First World War (3rd ed)* as part of The History of Australian Nurses in the First World War: An Australian College of Nursing Centenary Commemorative Trilogy (Australian College of Nursing, Canberra, 2015).

EBook 2017 (Amazon.com)

The author would like to acknowledge the Australian Government, Department of Veterans' Affairs, *Saluting Their Service* Commemorative Grants Programme, for support for previous editions.

National Library of Australia Cataloguing-in-Publication entry:

Rae, Ruth 1957 –

ISBN Paperback: 978-1-7640449-3-6 ISBN eBook: 978-1-7640449-2-9

Cover design and formatting: Ruth Rae ©Ruth Rae 2026

1. .Australian Nursing History 2.First Word War History 3. Australian Nurses Biography
4. Australian Colonial History 5. Female Social History

This book is dedicated to civilian and military nurses.

Table of Contents

Abbreviations

AAH	Australian Auxiliary Hospital
AAMC	Australian Army Medical Corps ('Royal' prefix granted 1948)
AANS	Australian Army Nursing Service
ACCS	Australian casualty clearing station/s
ACN	Australian College of Nursing
ADFA	Australian Defence Force Academy
AGH	Australian General Hospital
AIF	Australian Imperial Force
ALH	Australian Light Horse
ANSR	Army Nursing Service Reserve
ANZAC	Australian and New Zealand Army Corps
ARRC	Associate Royal Red Cross (RRC 2nd Class)
ASH	Australian Stationary Hospital
ATNA	Australasian Trained Nurses' Association
AWM	Australian War Memorial
BCCS	British casualty clearing station/s
BEF	British Expeditionary Force
BGH	British General Hospital
BMA	British Medical Association
BSH	British Surgical Hospital
CCS	Casualty clearing station/s
CWGC	Commonwealth War Graves Commission
CXR	Chest x-ray

DGAAMC	Director General Australian Army Medical Corps
DMS	Director of Medical Services
DOE	Date of embarkation
DNA	Deoxyribonucleic acid
EEF	Egyptian Expeditionary Force
GH	General hospital
HMAHS	His Majesty's Australian Hospital Ship
HMAT	His Majesty's Australian Transport
HMHS	His Majesty's Hospital Ship
HQ	Headquarters
HS	Head Sister
IV	Intravenous
KIA	Killed in action
MC	Military Cross
MID	Mentioned in Despatches
MD	Military District
NAA	National Archives of Australia
NME	Non-Military Employment
NRB	Nurses' Registration Board
NSW	New South Wales
NSWANSR	New South Wales Army Nursing Service Reserve
NZANS	New Zealand Army Nursing Service
NZHS	New Zealand Hospital Ship
NZSH	New Zealand Stationary Hospital
PM	Principal Matron

POE	Port of embarkation
POW	Prisoner-of-War
QAIMNS	Queen Alexandra's Imperial Military Nursing Service
QAIMNSR	Queen Alexandra's Imperial Military Nursing Service Reserve
RAAMC	Royal Australian Army Medical Corps
RAANC	Royal Australian Army Nursing Corps
RAANS	Royal Australian Army Nursing Service
RAMC	Royal Army Medical Corps
RBNA	Royal British Nurses' Association
RMS	Royal Mail Ship
RNSH	Royal North Shore Hospital
RPAH	Royal Prince Alfred Hospital
RRC	Royal Red Cross (1st Class)
RTA	Returned to Australia
RVCN	Royal Victorian College of Nursing
RVTNA	Royal Victorian Trained Nurses' Association
SN	Staff Nurse
SS	Steam Ship
TANS	Territorial Army Nursing Service
VAD	Voluntary Aid Detachment
VTNA	Victorian Trained Nurses' Association
WA	Western Australia
WO	War Office
WGH	Welsh General Hospital
WSPU	Women's Social and Political Union

Glossary of Terms

AANS Sister	The first level of promotion within the AANS for civilian qualified ATNA nurses.
Bluebirds	An Australian Red Cross contingent of qualified nurses who were sponsored to serve overseas by community groups. The nurses were often ineligible to join the AANS because they were married.
Bombay	Present-day Mumbai, India.
Dandi	Mode of transport; sedan-like chair used in India, carried by four people.
H1N1	Hemagglutinin 1 Neuraminidase 1: 1919 and 2009 (H1N1 09) influenza virus.
H5N1	Hemagglutinin 5 Neuraminidase 1 (2007 avian influenza virus).
Hepatic	Pertaining to the liver.
Masseuse	Female massage therapist/physical therapist.
Masseur	Male massage therapist/physical therapist.
Matron	The most senior nurse within a civilian hospital or military hospital. The second level of promotion within the AANS for civilian qualified ATNA nurses.
Matron-in-Chief	The most senior nurse in the AANS. There were two appointed during the First World War in 1916. Evelyn Conyers who was responsible for all AANS nurses serving overseas (except those in Salonika), and Ethel Tracy Richardson who was the Australian-based matron-in-chief. The fourth and final level of promotion within the AANS for civilian qualified ATNA nurses.
Military Districts	1 MD - Queensland and Northern Territory; 2 MD - New South Wales (NSW); 3 MD - Victoria; 4 MD - South Australia; 5 MD - Western Australia (WA); 6 MD - Tasmania.
Principal Matron	Most senior nurse responsible for AANS staff who were serving on a particular war front e.g. Salonika or India. The third level of promotion within the AANS for civilian qualified ATNA nurses.

QAIMNS	British nursing service; members were often known as QAs or Regulars. Established March 1902.
QAIMNSR	British nursing service reserve. Established 1908.
Red Crescent	The same humanitarian connotations as the Red Cross.
Staff Nurse	Entry level status in the AANS for civilian qualified ATNA nurses.
Struck of Strength	Removal of a nurse from the roster to be transferred elsewhere
TAB	Vaccine prepared from killed typhoid, paratyphoid A and paratyphoid B bacilli.
TB	Tuberculosis, also known as phthisis or consumption.
Territorial nurse	British nurse who joined the TANS and cared for army patients in civilian, convalescent and territorial hospitals. Similar to home service for Australian nurses.
VAD	Voluntary Aid Detachment - untrained nurse assistant.

List of Tables

Appendices

Author's Note

The reason I have written this book is threefold. The earlier edition was part of a trilogy which is no longer in print. I have re-edited, in some detail, the earlier edition of *Veiled Lives: Threading Australian Nursing History in to the Fabric of the First World War* so that it will be available as a stand alone edition in both electronic and print form.

Secondly, I regret I did not include any reference to the indigenous inhabitants of present day Australia in my earlier books. Indigenous Australians, who have inhabited present day Australia for 60,000 years, were displaced, massacred or stolen during colonisation. In this book I make reference to locations and towns throughout the colonies and later the nation (1901), I respectfully acknowledge the indigenous inhabitants of that same land by including the indigenous country/nation from whence it was taken. I am a white Australian woman of English and Welsh heritage born in Temora; NSW on Wiradjuri country.

Finally, there can be no war without consequences. The Australian nurses who served in the First World War witnessed the consequences and lived with them when peace returned. I have read many histories of this conflict where a nurse is mentioned in passing, usually to demonstrate a love interest of a soldier. If the reader expects this you should put this book down now. The reality is that these women, of all ages, who were professional nurses, risked their lives to save the lives of others. Not always their countrymen, not always soldiers, not always allies. I have included experiences of nurses caring for those who were displaced by the battles which overtook their villages: refugees from their own homes in villages in Greece, France, the Balkans, Russia, and the Middle East. At the end of the war some soldiers wanted to stay, after four years away from their beloved families, they wanted to help rebuild what they had been told to destroy. War doesn't work like that. The nurses saw this first hand. They witnessed the broken bodies. This was difficult enough but the broken spirit of a soldier and a colleague was quite another. This book is a history of Australian nurses who were the witnesses to the consequences of war.

Introduction

Often the history of the First World War is defined in terms of soldiers, battles and casualties. The records of nurses provide a more personal perspective - a more confronting vantage point - that of the female witness who remained strong so that her soldier patients might live. The diaries, letters, narratives and interviews of the nurses, are considered within a wider framework of historical texts, demonstrating that, nurses not only cared for soldiers but also prisoners-of-war and refugees.

The social history of Australia and the women who became qualified nurses in the First World War is an integral aspect of how they coped with the trauma of war. Their early lives often led them to become civilian nurses who were, when qualified with the Australasian Trained Nurses' Association (ATNA), gave them immediate entry into the Australian Army Nursing Service (AANS). The transition from a civilian nurse to a military nurse was confronting and many become physically and psychologically ill. Some endured war wounds while a number died from their war service. This was especially true after war when the influenza pandemic ripped through the world creating global grief within the families of returning servicemen and nurses. The nurse had to once again, put their grief aside and return to civilian nursing.

War brought with it changes in the treatment and management of war wounds including blood transfusions, x-rays and shell-shock. Diseases such as typhoid, dysentery and malaria were not uncommon and vaccinations were in the development stage.

Nurses stationed in France and Belgium in the 1914-18 war had to cope with noise, confusion and even panic as the front-line was constantly changing. Those stationed in the Mediterranean and on transport duty dealt with the ever present risk of drowning when their hospital ships hit mines. Nurses sent to Egypt and India endured the sand, flies and heat while they tended the wounded from Gallipoli and Mesopotamia.

After the war the profession tried to regroup but their contribution was quickly forgotten by those in power and, to a lesser extent, the public. But never the soldiers.

1 Nursing in Australia 1788-1867

I solemnly pledge myself before God and this Assembly to pass my life in purity and in the practice of my profession faithfully – The Nightingale Pledge

The great expanse of the island continent which would ultimately become 'Australia' appeared before the new settlers in 1788 as a blank page on which their history would be written. Initially, it was, for the most part, a male-dominated Anglo-Saxon story built upon the premise that the wild land was tamed and Indigenous people were the beneficiaries of a superior white education. Neither was true.

The first Australian nurses were black but white Australia knows little of their history. Convict women who were transported from Britain also acted as nurses and midwives on the grueling journey to their remote and inhospitable destination in 1788. Nonetheless, it was the Nightingale system of nurse training that had the most profound impact on Australian nursing history. Nightingale established the importance of a non-sectarian, professional nursing workforce during the Crimean War. Australian nurses, who were civilian trained under the Nightingale system, confirmed this during the South African War and the First World War.

Present-day Australia was claimed by a British explorer, Captain James Cook in 1770 and eighteen years later ... *on the afternoon of January 26, 1788, … a fleet of eleven vessels carrying 1,030 people, including 548 male and 188 female convicts … entered Port Jackson or, as it would presently be called, Sydney Harbour.* From a European perspective the land was devoid of civilisation and there appeared to be no infrastructure, no economy, no health service, no society The new arrivals failed to see …*the Aborigines and the fauna around them had possessed the landscape since time immemorial, and no other human eye had seen them. Now the protective glass of distance broke, in an instant, never to be restored.*[1]

The health and well-being of the first-fleeter was not a priority for the British

Government. The tools and equipment brought out from England were of a poor quality and insufficient quantity and with these the convicts, many of whom were untrained or unqualified, were expected to erect shelter. Food supplies and rations were insufficient and the harsh summer climate meant that sheep killed one day were ...*crawling with maggots*... the next.[2] The early years of settlement were indeed cruel for the men and women who colonised Sydney (Gadigal Country), Norfolk Island and Tasmania. Regrettably, many settlers and later explorers made enemies of the Indigenous population, who were in effect in the best position to teach the new arrivals how to survive.[3]

The administrative reforms which saw the country progress from convict colony to a democratic federation by 1901 originated in Sydney. The first public hospital was established at Dawes Point near Sydney, NSW, in 1796. Staffed by convicts, overseers, dressers, wardsmen, gardeners, boatmen and the occasional nurse, who did not receive any pay but were maintained at public expense, the hospital had little to recommend it.

Governor Lachlan Macquarie had the foresight to commission a public works plan which incorporated a general hospital; the plan was dispatched to Viscount Castlereagh, Secretary of State for the Colonies, in March 1810. The wheels of progress were slow and although tenders were called on 17 May 1810, the first public hospital, Sydney Hospital, was not commissioned until 1816. The hospital is located in Macquarie Street, so-named by Governor Macquarie himself. Originally the hospital was staffed by qualified doctors but it was left to convict men and women to act as nurses. Ironically, less than a century later, Macquarie Street was synonymous with medical excellence in NSW.

Initially, the Sydney Infirmary and Dispensary was often referred to as the Rum Hospital by the locals because 45,000 gallons of rum was sold (at 20 shillings per gallon) to provide the necessary revenue of £45,000 to erect the hospital (whose estimated cost was £49,000). On 3 March 1816 the government was notified by the contractors that the Sydney Hospital building was complete, but owing to the number of alterations the building itself was not finally completed until July 1817. It is now known as Sydney Hospital and Sydney Eye Hospital, and henceforth referred to as SHSEH.[4]

Despite the building being quite grand in its day, the nurses of the SHSEH, up until 1869, had not had any training. The first recorded matrons were Mrs Baxter (1845-1851), Mrs Ghost (1852–1866) and Mrs Blake (1867) who were themselves untrained women. Many of their nurses were often intoxicated women with reputations for promiscuous behaviour and believed to be from the convict class.

Given the dearth of quality nursing, the first Catholic bishop in the colony, Dr John Polding, requested the foundress of the Sisters of Charity (Ireland), Mary Aikenhead, to send the services of five Sisters of Charity to attend to the needs of the poor, the infirm and the sick. Following their arrival on 31 December 1838 they initially worked from a house in Parramatta (Dharug Country) and in the following year they moved to Sydney. The need for a free hospital became apparent and in February 1856 the harbour-side residence 'Tarmons' was transferred to the Sisters of Charity. While it is claimed that *...the only criteria for admission to the hospital, called St Vincent's Hospital, were sickness and poverty...* the founding charge sister, Sister Baptist de Lacy, was obliged to leave when it was discovered that she had allowed Protestant bibles into the hospital *...for use by certain patients.*[5] Present day St Vincent's Hospital has a world renowned reputation for medical and nursing excellence.

The origins of nursing

The definition of a nurse is not consistent but the word 'nurse' means *...that nourishes, fosters, and protects...* and is from the Latin *...nutricius.*[6] The Emperor Constantine began to patronise Christianity and the slow Christianisation of Europe began. In 335 CE he closed all military hospitals because he perceived them to be *...pagan institutions.*[7] Deaconesses, who were widowed or unmarried, were, for all intents and purposes, nurses. Deaconesses were ordained by a bishop and it was their calling to care for the poor, the sick and the bereaved. Therefore, when nursing spread to Britain in the 4th century CE, gospel preachings were performed with nursing activities by deaconesses and Christian men; their duties included caring for orphans and the infirm as well as the sick.[8]

In 597 CE, St Augustine, a Benedictine monk, evangelised Christianity in Britain. The Order of the St Augustinian Sisters was founded in 650 CE and is the oldest religious community - of brothers and sisters - devoted solely to nursing. The term 'Sister', which was often used in civilian and military hospitals until the transfer of nurse education to the tertiary sector, originated *...from the monastic tradition when all skilled nursing was done by nuns.*[9] During the latter part of the nineteenth century, nursing was still perceived to be a combination of secular service and religious devotion.[10]

Florence Nightingale (1820-1910) was the maternal granddaughter of William Smith, a politician who championed the weak, the needy and the oppressed; she was to do much the same in her lifetime but with more recognition and more success. Her parents, Fanny and William Edward Nightingale (known as WEN) were wealthy, but WEN had inherited from an uncle and needed to father a son if the fortune was not to pass to his nephew via his sister. However, unlike many Jane Austen characters of the day the family felt secure in the knowledge that WEN owned a property on which a lead mine was discovered and proved to be most lucrative; the family enjoyed a level of financial independence.[11] WEN and Fanny married in 1818, the year Karl Marx was born - it was a time which heralded the early fraying of the social fabric which was underpinned by the English class system.[12]

Their first child was a daughter, Parthenope, who was born at the place of that name near Naples, Italy, in 1819 and on 12 May the following year their second daughter and last child, Florence, was also born in her name place.[13] Florence Nightingale enjoyed an extensive education through travel; a soldier in the Crimea much admired her and asked *...is it not beautiful ... to hear her speak Italian?*[14] She may have benefited from the material wealth of her parents but she inherited the egalitarian principles of her grandfather, a character trait that neither of her parents shared. Despite being devoutly religious, this inherent egalitarianism may explain why Florence Nightingale became a staunch proponent of secular nursing.

When faced with his daughter's failure to settle into the social duties required of a young Victorian woman, her father *...suggested that a husband might be advisable...* but she steadfastly resisted this ongoing social pressure despite serious offers of marriage.[15] A vocation in nursing would give her independence from marriage and when she declined a good prospect of a suitor because she ...*could not bear his life ... to be nailed to a continuation, an exaggeration of my present life without hope of another would be intolerable to me – that voluntarily to put it out of my power ever to be able to seize the chance of forming for myself a true and rich life would seem like suicide...* her parents lost their patience.[16]

Florence Nightingale had attempted to nurse at Salisbury Infirmary when she was twenty-five years old but her family forbade it.[17] When she was thirty her parents sent her on a trip to Egypt and Europe in the vain hope she might realise her social responsibilities and settle down. However, her chaperones enabled her to visit the Kaiserswerth Institute for two weeks and from the moment of her arrival on 31 July 1850 her commitment to becoming a nurse was absolute – as was her family's opposition.[18]

Gradually nursing was being accepted by some physicians and members of the public as an important vocation. Dr Johann Karl Ernst Dieffenbach (1811-1855), a German medical doctor, reputedly published the first book on nursing in 1832.[19] Around the same time, Amalie Sieveking (1794-1859), a resident of Hamburg, demonstrated remarkable courage when she volunteered to assist residents during a cholera epidemic in 1831. Her commitment to improving the social welfare system in her community was matched by a determination to involve women in humanitarian networks, including nursing.[20]

One of the nurses Sieveking taught was Caroline Bertheau (1811-92), who was the superintendent of a hospital in Hamburg and later became the second wife of Pastor Theodore Fliedner. Theodore Fliedner (1800-1864) and his first wife, Friedericke, were instrumental in reforming the Deaconess system of nurse training when they founded the Kaiserswerth Deaconess Institute situated on the Rhine near Düsseldorf, Germany.[21] Initially, in 1833, they focused on reforms in the care and treatment of female prisoners, along the same lines as the improvements introduced by Elizabeth Fry (1780-1845) at Newgate Prison and on convict transports.[22] By 1851, when Nightingale returned to undertake 'training', the institute included a 100 bed hospital, infant school, orphan asylum, penitentiary and training school for schoolmistresses.[23]

The atmosphere at Kaiserswerth was one of religious service and *...prayer accompanied every incident.* Nightingale later recalled that *...we were all encouraged to pray aloud extempore before the whole community.*[24] Nightingale benefited from a brief three month period of training which included the observation of surgical procedures and lectures delivered by visiting physicians. Exposure to surgical procedures was considered to be outside the realm of respectability for women at this time but Nightingale relished the opportunity to learn all she could about the human body.[25]

On her return to England her parents once again put barriers in place to prevent her from realising her ambition. Nightingale started to consider the limitations that her Protestantism placed upon her as a prospective nurse. In 1852 she sought solace in good deeds and met *...a child of fourteen who was being forced into prostitution, tried to rescue the girl, but found no organisation in the Church of England would receive her.* The child was an Irish Catholic, and a friend of Nightingale's, a Catholic priest, helped the child by placing her in the Convent of the Good Shepherd.[26] Nightingale was impressed and developed *...Catholic yearnings...* and saw an opportunity to push through the barriers which prevented her from becoming a nurse. She wrote unrestrainedly*...what a home the Catholic Church would be to me! ... all that I want I should find in her. All my difficulties would be removed. I have to laboriously pick up here and there, crumbs by which to live. She would give me daily bread. The daughters of St Vincent would open their arms to me. They have already done so, and what should I find there. My work already laid out for me instead of seeking it to and fro and finding none; my home, sympathy, human and divine.*[27]

In October 1852 Nightingale finally had an opportunity to escape her home to nurse in a hospital with the Sisters of Charity in Paris, but once again a family emergency caused her to cancel her plans. While in London, Nightingale became aware that 'The Institution for the care of Sick Gentlewomen in Distressed Circumstances' needed the assistance of an able superintendent and she was appointed to the position in April 1853.[28]

The hospital was located at 1 Upper Harley Street, London, and an incident during the first week of Nightingale's appointment speaks to the importance of secular egalitarianism for Nightingale nurses. Her committee wanted the institution to admit only patients who belonged to the Church of England but Nightingale insisted it be non-sectarian. Given that she had for many years sought an opportunity to manage a hospital, she did not lack courage in fighting the committee over this issue. On 20 August 1853 she recorded the situation in a letter to a friend. She wrote ... *My committee refused me to take in Catholic patients, whereupon I wished them good morning, unless I might take in Jews and their Rabbis to attend them. So now it is settled, and in print that we are to take in all denominations whatever, and allow them to be visited by their respective priests and Muftis, provided I will receive (in any case whatsoever that is not of the Church of England) the obnoxious animal at the door, take him upstairs myself, remain while he is conferring with his patient, make myself responsible that he not speak to, or look at anyone else, and bring him downstairs again in a noose, and out into the street. And to this I have agreed! And this is in print! Amen.*[29]

The clinical skills Nightingale needed to nurse so-called gentlewomen were quickly augmented in 1854 when she went to the Middlesex Hospital during the Broad Street pump cholera epidemic. Here she cared for the prostitutes and drunks who frequented the undrained slums with the same care and compassion as she had showed her gentlewomen.[30]

The Crimean War (1854-56)

The Crimean War answered the professional aspirations of Florence Nightingale; she was recognised as a patriot and a nurse.[31] When Nightingale was requested to lead a contingent of forty non-sectarian nurses to the Crimea, she selected twenty-four from religious institutions, ten Roman Catholics, consisting of five Norwood and five Bermondsey nuns, eight nurses from Miss Sellon's Anglican sisterhood, who were known as Sellonites, and six nurses from St John's House, which was a High Church sisterhood. The remaining fourteen were hospital nurses of ...*no particular religion*... and reputedly of no particular moral character.[32] Only thirty-eight women were found suitable but the religious nurses brought the most nursing expertise because they had undergone a degree of training. Nonetheless, religion complicated the implementation of Nightingale's reforms in the Crimea.

Nightingale and her nurses in the Crimea were not too distant from where the Australian soldiers and their nurses would make a name for themselves in 1915. In essence, the strategic importance of the Dardanelles was apparent to all players and during the Crimean War the British and French joined the Ottomans to prevent Russia annexing Ottoman territory.[33]

On agreeing to go to the Crimea, one of the Sellonite sisters, Sarah Anne Terrot (1822-1902), recounted her meeting with Sidney Herbert, the Secretary of War and a close personal friend of Nightingale's, on 21 October 1854. On receiving their papers of agreement he *...spoke of our duties – of modesty and propriety, of enduring hardness, and of carefully avoiding religious proselytising.*[34] This last point caused consternation on a number of occasions; once Sister Sarah Anne *...stood at the foot of a bed on which lay a corpse. An orderly came up and said ... "That young fellow came in a Protestant, but he died a true Catholic"*...she felt compelled to report the incident to Florence Nightingale. The claim was verified by a patient in an adjacent bed who said it *...hurt me to see the nuns get round the poor fellow, and persuade him to join their Church. Poor lad, in his weak state, it was no wonder he should yield. May God forgive them all.* The religion of the said soldier was not stated but when the matter was investigated by Florence Nightingale, the nuns claimed *...his change was of God's free grace, and nothing could be proved.*[35]

While at Scutari, Nightingale was of the opinion that hospital nurses who focused on taking care of the body, as opposed to the soul, were the most useful.[36] This evaluation may be a little unjust because initially the care of the moribund and dying soldiers was often assigned to the nuns and Sellonite sisters, whereas the secular nurses were allocated to those likely to recover.[37] For example, when a dying patient (Church of England) requested someone with whom he could pray, the housekeeper, Mrs Clarke, called on the Sellonite sisters because she thought they were *...more up to that sort of thing than the nurses.*[38]

Those nurses who accompanied Nightingale to the Crimea had to take their nursing orders from her and her alone. This was stipulated so *...a nun or nursing sister ... must take her orders from Miss Nightingale and not her mother superior; and the mother superior must take her orders from Miss Nightingale and not from the Bishop.*[39] This extraordinary concession gave Nightingale a unique position of authority over religious women. Interestingly, the Protestant Institution refused to allow their nurses to be under any authority other than their own committee, so no Protestant nurses accompanied Nightingale.[40]

Nightingale arrived amidst administrative chaos, with additional staff, a great deal of money and the imprimatur of the government of the day. However, she did not have the confidence of the military doctors, who elected to ignore her and decided that the best way to deal with a society do-gooder was to freeze her out. The day after her arrival, Nightingale set up an invalid diet kitchen in the cramped nurses' quarters kitchen and on receiving the permission of the doctors she and her nurses fed the invalid soldiers - but they did not nurse them.[41] The introduction of a diet roll and special meals for the soldiers was in many ways recognition of the importance of nutrition in the recovery phase and a precursor to the specialised field of dietetics. [42] Nightingale was aware, even at this early stage, that nurses would need to take control of diet requisitions from medical officers so that effective and autonomous nursing practices could be introduced so this was achieved before the First World War.[43]

In addition to meal preparation and basic housekeeping, Florence Nightingale offered the nursing services of her staff on arrival but they were refused by the medical officers so she waited. The nurses were alarmed at their inertia while they could hear the cries of the dying men so they felt justified in blaming Nightingale.[44] On 6 November 1854 wounded from Balaclava began to arrive in Scutari and Nightingale could see the military hierarchical system of hospital administration would not be able to withstand the weight of onslaught of many more casualties. Within a week the entire situation was beyond the capacity of the hospital and *…at last the doctors turned to her* [Nightingale].[45]

Florence Nightingale benefited from a revolution in communication during the Crimean War. She had excellent research and writing skills but she presented as modest, even self-effacing, which prompted some men to promote her achievements. William Howard Russell was a convincing communicator and he used the telegraph to keep the British public aware of military developments, both positive and negative, often to the chagrin of the military establishment.[46]

Russell tapped into two key reforms: The improved literacy of the general public and the increasing affordability of information. Both greatly assisted Nightingale's future reforms, not only for military nurses but also for civilian nurses, by highlighting the poor conditions endured by the men and the valuable work of the nurses.[47] On her return from the Crimean War, Nightingale held a unique social position for a woman at this time because she had authority, public respect and a sectarian vocation. As her father was now willing to settle an allowance on her she also enjoyed financial independence. Rather unsurprisingly, she remained unmarried.

Importantly, she harnessed a great deal of political support for her ideas on public health and had access to public revenue via the Nightingale Fund. This came to pass when the outpouring of public emotion and favourable opinion for the work of the nurses in the Crimea was translated into financial support. The revenue from the Nightingale Fund was used to develop a specific nurse training system which formed the basis of the present day secular nursing profession across the United States of America (USA), United Kingdom, Canada and Australia.[48]

The first Nightingale School was opened under the able matronship of Mrs. Wardroper of St Thomas' Hospital, London, on 24 June 1860.[49] The Nightingale system of nurse training incorporated discipline, education, organisation and a vocational commitment. Future Australia desperately needed such a health system.

2 Nightingale Nurses in Australia 1867-1899

... the land and the people are young-hearted together, and the children's spirits not crushed and saddened by the shadow of long years of history – *Ethel Turner*

Sir Henry Parkes, NSW Colonial Secretary (1866-68), was concerned about the filthy and unhygienic practices, corrupt administration, drunkenness and disorderliness of the nurses and other staff who tended the patients at SHSEH. The reputation of Florence Nightingale was by this time well known and she confirmed her position as an expert in nursing and public health throughout her lifetime by publishing seventeen volumes on related topics.[1] An extremely popular book was a nursing text, *Notes on Nursing – What It Is and What It Is Not* (1860), which encompassed the basic principles of clinical care but also outlined the hierarchical hospital system which firmly placed the matron at the top. A matron was unquestionably a woman and it gave her a unique power base rarely afforded to any woman at this time. However, it was the introduction of the Nightingale system of nurse training at St Thomas' Hospital, London, which had an enduring impact on the Nightingale reforms.

The Board of SHSEH was aware of the need for nursing reform but internal power struggles rendered it ineffective in taking appropriate action. In 1866, without reference to the board, Henry Parkes wrote directly to Florence Nightingale and simultaneously instructed the Colonial Agent in London to begin negotiations with her. Nightingale replied the same year, giving her full support to the introduction of trained nurses and the establishment of a training school at SHSEH, which by this time had 190 beds.[2]

This type of request was not uncommon and subsequently there was pressure on St Thomas' Hospital to provide Nightingale trained nurses to communities all over the world. In May 1867 Nightingale, in consultation with Miss Wardroper, drafted a proposal to the President of the SHSEH which included sending Miss Lucy Osburn as lady superintendent (or matron) and five probationers (Mary Barker, Eliza Blundell, Annie Miller, Haldane Turriff and Bessy Chant) to Sydney, primarily to nurse patients and train future nurses.

The negotiations between Nightingale and Parkes ensured the staff would receive board and lodgings and have their passages paid to Sydney. Given the vast distance to the antipodes they would also need to have their return passages to London provided if they desired to end their tenure at the hospital. Miss Osburn as the matron received £150 per annum and each of the probationers received £50 per annum with an expectation of an annual salary increase. Osburn was not only responsible for improving patient welfare in the short term but was to implement a training program so that quality nursing care could spread to all parts of the colonies.[3]

Lucy Osburn (1835-1891)

Lucy Osburn transformed SHSEH from a place which the general public loathed even to visit, let alone stay in, to a hospital steeped in community pride which continues to this day.[4] Her contribution was not confined to Sydney; her implementation of the Nightingale training system had an impact on hospitals throughout the colonies and Australian nurses owe her a great debt as do the communities they served. She had a number of similarities to Florence Nightingale. Born around 1836 in Leeds, she was the youngest daughter of William and Ann; although she came from a privileged family her early ancestry is unclear. From 1856 Lucy Osburn undertook approximately ten years of training, which included visiting Vienna and the Kaiserswerth Hospital, and two years training at St.Thomas' Hospital.[5]

Just over a year after sending his letter to Florence Nightingale, it proved satisfying to Henry Parkes when Miss Lucy Osburn and her nurses arrived in Sydney on the *Dunbar Castle* on 3 December 1867. Despite their agreement there was no provision for accommodation for Osburn or her nurses when they arrived. It was nearly a year before the nurses' accommodation section, the Nightingale Wing, was built and ready for use in September 1868. During the interim the original Mint building, which was unsuitable for such a purpose, accommodated the nurses and a filthy drain situated near Osburn's sitting room caused her to become ill with dysentery. She needed constant nursing care for three weeks but once she recovered she resumed her extensive workload and responsibilities.[6]

An incident occurred soon after Osburn's arrival which confirmed the value of the Nightingale nurses in the minds of the Sydney establishment and the community. During a royal tour of the colonies in 1868, Queen Victoria's second eldest son was shot in the back by Henry James O'Farrell, an Irishman with a sectarian motive.[7] By chance, the assassination attempt failed when the bullet ricocheted off Prince Alfred's ribs and he avoided serious injury. Osburn and her Nightingale nurses went to Government House where they provided immediate nursing care to the Prince. Once he was back to full health the people of Sydney decided to build a hospital as a memorial to his recovery. The process was slow but eventually the Royal Prince Alfred Hospital (RPAH) was commissioned in 1882.[8]

Despite this strangely fortuitous start to her work in Sydney, Osburn constantly had to assert her authority with the male-dominated medical and board members of the hospital.[9] The by-laws stipulated that the lady superintendent had to share her authority with the hospital superintendent; this contravened the Nightingale philosophy, which required *...the whole responsibility of nursing, internal management, for discipline and training (if there be a Training School) of Nurses in the one female head of the nursing staff, whatever she is called.*[10] This was not implemented at SHSEH; Osburn's authority was constantly being undermined, and unfortunately her reforms did not enjoy the support of a majority of the board of directors nor a number of the doctors.

Osburn, although a Protestant, was often accused of trying to create a culture of Catholicism in the hospital. Several minor incidents caused a great deal of public concern during the initial stages of her tenure. To differentiate secular nurses from religious nurses, the most senior secular nurse was referred to as 'Lady

Superintendent'. As a consequence, correspondence intended for Osburn was misdirected to the hospital superintendent and vice versa. Osburn changed her title to 'Lady Superior' to alleviate confusion about the different positions in the lay person's mind. This seemingly innocuous suggestion, coupled with the introduction of the title of 'Sister' for the head nurses, which was an accepted practice at St.Thomas' Hospital, did little to reassure the anti-Catholic faction within the community. In 1869, following another inquiry, it was determined that Osburn should continue to be known as 'Lady Superintendent' and the nurses should be known as head nurses instead of sisters.[11]

During one of the frequent rat infestations at the hospital, Osburn recruited the talents of her beloved pet terrier - a regular pied piper. However, during the culling of the rodents a number of Bibles, amongst other items, were damaged. Osburn ordered the destruction of the damaged items, without particular reference to the Bibles, and consequently a number of Bibles were burnt. The board demanded an inquiry into the burning of Bibles at SHSEH. Sadly and some may suggest spitefully, her dog was not allowed to remain on the hospital grounds, by order of the hospital committee, and as Osburn had to live on-site she was separated from her only loyal companion.[12]

Osburn was criticised for worshiping at the Anglican Christ Church St Laurence by the *Protestant Standard* because it was too High Anglican.[13] She refused to be bullied in this matter and her tenacity endured a number of inquiries into her administration during the first five years. However, in 1873 a Commission of Inquiry into the Public Charities of NSW found that ...*the duties of the nursing staff were discharged in a highly satisfactory manner under the efficient management of Miss Osburn, and that the good effect of the introduction of the Nightingale system was abundantly clear.*[14] Finally, in 1875 Osburn was given full control over the management of the nurses, cooks and hospital servants within the hospital.[15]

Osburn and her nurses set the scene for improvements in nursing care throughout the colonies. Osburn decided to return to England in 1884 to further her education and explore new developments in nursing. Sadly, she developed diabetes, which at this time was not treatable, and she endured sixteen months of pain before dying on

22 December 1891.[16]

Osburn left SHSEH in capable hands. In 1884 Rebecca McKay became the most senior nurse of SHSEH and the following year the title of 'Matron' was introduced.[17] When McKay took over the reins from Osburn there was ever increasing pressure on SHSEH to supply 'trained nurses' for senior positions in country hospitals and twenty additional probationers were hired.[18] McKay was replaced by Nellie Gould, who had completed her training at RPAH.

Julia Ellen (Nellie) Gould (1860-1941)

Always known as Nellie, Gould's early life and education gave her excellent skills for this complex role. She was born in Aberystwyth, Cardiganshire, Wales on 29 March 1860 to Sarah (nee Baker) and Henry Gould. When she was eighteen months old her mother, Henry's second wife, died during childbirth. Her father, an agent, moved the family to Portugal when Nellie was four and arranged home tutoring until she was ten years old. Nellie Gould received a diverse education, attending a Portuguese language school before returning to London, where she attended Midmay Park College and passed the senior Local Cambridge Examination at the age of sixteen. Significantly she became a member of the teaching staff and remained there until 1879. At the tender age of nineteen she moved to Hamburg where she worked as a governess for four years.[19]

Her peripatetic lifestyle and comprehensive education would have given her some significant insights into the social and political life of Europe as Otto Eduard Leopold Bismarck implemented the main tenets of his foreign policies since his realisation of a united German Empire in 1871. Bismarck observed the political changes of countries, near and far, was more important than just geography.[20] Nellie and her step-sister, Emily, decided to visit family who were living in the rural town of Grafton (NSW, Bundjalung Country) in 1884. During this visit RPAH was receiving substantial public attention and Nellie decided to continue her education but this time as a nurse.[21] It was one of the earliest hospitals to be built in the colony and the first designed to teach medical students attached to the University of Sydney. Like SHSEH, it also undertook responsibility for nurse training.[22] When

Gould began her training at RPAH, under the matronship of Miss Elizabeth Leila Murray (1882-85), she was part of the first intake of six probationers. Murray trained at The Kings College Hospital, London and the probationers were fortunate to receive instruction from her as well as benefiting from training in a new, purpose-built hospital.

When Miss Murray resigned from RPAH, Miss Catherine Downs was appointed Matron (1886-91) and indications are that both women were competent and kind role models. Nellie Gould would have learnt a great deal from these two women during her training (1885-87) and afterwards as a trained nurse (1887-89).[23] Gould's first senior nursing position was as Matron of the St Kilda Private Hospital, Woolloomooloo (NSW, Gadigal Country) and then she was appointed the third Matron of the prestigious SHSEH (1891-98).

When RPAH was nearing completion, SHSEH was undergoing protracted redevelopment; this created an unhealthy rivalry, often fuelled by each institution's need for public funding. Gould was matron during the final stages of the building program and the new hospital was ready to accept patients in 1894. However, during the interim the nurses' home known as Nightingale Wing had been used for patients so in 1895 it had to be restored to its original purpose. [24] Gould had the responsibility of administering the nurse training program because matrons had overarching responsibility for nurse training and as one matron claimed *...we took them* [trainees] *in as young girls and sent them out as good women.*[25] It was not until after the First World War that the 'Tutor Sister' position became an integral part of the nursing staff establishment.

There is little doubt that Gould used her skills as a student and an educator to good effect and it was reported that the *...nursing staff, both in training and numbers, has been largely developed.* In 1894 the duration of the nurse training course was lengthened from two to three years and lectures were delivered on a variety of topics by the honorary medical staff. The scope of lecture topics was also extended because the type and number of patients (in-patients and out-patients) dramatically increased once the new hospital was commissioned. The topics covered by the medical officers included elementary anatomy, physiology, invalid cooking and medical and surgical nursing, while Gould and her senior nurses provided practical instruction to the probationers.[26] Since Osburn's time, the SHSEH had been converted from a rat-infested ...*rum hospital*... to one of two leading secular hospitals in the colony of NSW.

Nightingale nurses throughout the colonies

The five trained nurses from St Thomas' Hospital, who accompanied Osburn, were on a three-year contract. Within three years of their arrival, only one, Mary Baker, was still on the staff. Sister Turriff, who had nursed Prince Alfred at Government House when he was shot, married Mr Murray and became Matron of The Alfred in Melbourne (Victoria, Naarm Country). The Alfred was funded along the same lines as RPAH in Sydney.[27] Sister Blundell married Mr Eldrick and became Matron of the Benevolent Society. Miss Bessy Chant married Mr Simpson and continued to do private nursing until her husband's death. She then returned to the profession as matron of Tarban Creek Lunatic Asylum, Gladesville, (NSW, Wallumedegal Country), a leadership position she held for twenty-six years until her retirement in 1908. Miss Annie Miller, the other nurse who cared for Prince Alfred, undertook private nursing in Melbourne for a short period.

Nurse Education

Osburn's role to initiate a nurse training program and educate future nurse leaders was successful. Between 1870 and 1885 no fewer than twelve of her probationary nurses had overall responsibility for nursing services in NSW, Tasmania and South Australia. These nurse leaders included Miss Shorter (Mudgee, NSW, Wiradjuri Nation), Miss Bland (Tarban Creek Lunatic Asylum and later Hobart, Tasmania, Nipaluna Country), Miss Davies (Orange, NSW, Wiradjuri Country), Miss Pearson (Parramatta, NSW), Miss Wilmott (Adelaide, South Australia, Kaurna Country), Miss Gilliam Holden (Children's Hospital, Glebe, Gadigal Country), Miss Windred (Launceston, Tasmania, Kanamaluka Country), Miss Keyes (Bathurst, NSW, Wiradjuri Country), Miss Rucher (Ballarat, Victoria, Wadawurrung Country) and Miss Neyler (Young, NSW, Wiradjuri Country).[28] The geographic breadth covered by the trainees of SHSEH served to perpetuate the honour of Miss Osburn wherever they worked, by training the next generation within the local community.

The Adelaide Hospital

The Adelaide Hospital was the main hospital in the South Australian capital and today it is known as the Royal Adelaide Hospital. The royal prefix was not gazetted until 1939, so it will be referred to as the Adelaide Hospital throughout this book. The Adelaide Hospital adopted a prescribed series of lectures developed by Matron Lückes at London Hospital in 1881.[29] It was most likely introduced in Adelaide by Miss Thaickwaite or her predecessor Miss Banks. Miss A H Gordon became a nurse leader in Western Australia (WA) and trained at the Adelaide Hospital. At the time of her training she was required to undertake three years practical instruction and attend twelve lectures, often given by a doctor. The topics included in the Lückes curriculum were eventually compiled into a text entitled *General Nursing* which was used extensively by nurse leaders; it later became a suggested text for the Australasian Trained Nurses' Association (ATNA).[30]

The subjects covered included two lectures on haemorrhage, fractures, inflammation and repair. Single lectures on antiseptics, preparation for and antiseptic surgery, counter-irrigation, shock, collapse, surgical fever, burns and scalds, pyrexia and nursing cases of acute specific diseases were also included. This curriculum represented a comprehensive education plan for nurses at this time. However, like the SHSEH nurses, the Adelaide Hospital nurses also complained of having inadequate lectures.[31]

District Trained Nursing Society in South Australia

Nurses from Nightingale hospitals in England found the conditions in outback areas of Australia particularly challenging. The District Trained Nursing Society (DTNS) of South Australia was established in 1893 and could be described as the forerunner to community nursing. Unlike the Methodist Wesleyan church in Adelaide, which had a trained nurse visit the sick as an activity of the church, the DTNS was non-sectarian and designed to assist the poor.[32] One future AANS nurse, Mary Ann Latto (known as 'Latto') Bett, born in Dundee, Scotland, daughter to William Cunningham Bett, was a trained nurse and deaconess of the Presbyterian Church.[33]

The Very Reverend John Flynn, a Presbyterian Minister who implemented the Royal Flying Doctor Service in 1928, started his outback service with the development and operation of the Oodnadatta Hospital, South Australia. Sister Bett was only the second nurse to be appointed to Oodnadatta (Ngurabanna Country) or indeed to serve with the Australian Inland Mission in Central Australia in 1912, the year after the hospital was opened.[34] Following more than two years of remote area nursing she enlisted with the AANS and gained three years solid, hard experience as a war nurse.[35] The staff of the early DTNS included veterans of that other war, the South African War, including the much decorated Martha Bidmead.

Transportation was difficult and it was not unusual for a district nurse to utilise the services of bikes, camels, pony and trap, small boats and later motor cars as they battled flooded creeks, fire and drought to get to isolated homesteads. The DTNS in South Australia cared for a populace which endured diseases such as typhoid, influenza (which was often fatal once pneumonia developed), tuberculosis and malignant diseases. Emergency and first aid services were needed to deal with the high level of occupational accidents, especially in the mines and farming areas.[36]

Western Australia

The colony of Western Australia was established in 1825, but the railway from Port Augusta, South Australia (Nukunu Country) to Kalgoorlie, WA (Wongatha Country) did not link up until 1917 - four years after work commenced. Sea transport was preferable to travelling overland until the railway was established.

In 1894, legislation was passed during the second sitting of the Western Australian Parliament that any place could be proclaimed a public hospital. The Perth Public Hospital (1896) and the following year the Fremantle Hospital (Nyoongar Country) were the first two public hospitals to introduce a nurse training program in WA.[37] A prerequisite for a training hospital in WA was a matron who had experience working in a hospital which had had a nurse training school. Miss A H Gordon, who completed her training at the Adelaide Hospital in 1893, was appointed the first matron of Perth Public Hospital.[38]

Lady Rachel Dudley and the Bush Nursing Association

Lady Rachel Dudley was the wife of the Governor-General of Australia (1908-11). Born Rachel Gurney (1867-1920) she was a strong, resourceful and intelligent woman who became Lady Rachel, Countess of Dudley, on her marriage to William Humble Ward Dudley, 2nd Earl, in 1891. As the wife of the Governor-General and mother of seven children, she was concerned that Australians who lived in the outback were ... *so isolated: the old people, the women expecting a baby, the mothers, the children, all need some nursing support.* She then asked the pertinent question ...*What can be done to help them?* From this kernel of an idea a federal scheme to provide nursing support to those who lived in outback Australia was instigated and was later replaced with a number of state-based programs. Her Excellency the Countess of Dudley was Life Patroness of the first Central Council; a precursor to the Bush Nursing Association.[39]

3 Australasian Trained Nurses' Association (ATNA) 1899

The list of candidates for employment and training are overflowing-Nellie Gould

Nurse leaders dealt with differences in the vocational skills of the colonial nursing workforce by forming the Australasian Trained Nurses' Association (ATNA) in December 1899. It has been claimed that *...since the 1860s the status of nursing as a profession for women had improved steadily in Australia, although probably not to the same extent as it had in Britain.*[1] The transformation of the nursing profession from when ATNA was formed until the Great Depression in the 1930s is unprecedented; this was a golden age for Australian nurses. The diligence and outstanding political awareness of a number of remarkable Australian nurse leaders created this watershed.

The need for an association of trained nurses in Sydney was mooted as early as 1892, but it was not until 21 July 1899 that the NSW Trained Nurses' Association came into existence. The association was formed in response to a well-attended public meeting two months previously where it had been decided that *...some scheme should be formulated whereby medical men and the public may be able to procure nurses when they need them and by which they may be able to distinguish the trained from the untrained amongst the many so-called trained nurses.*[2] Rose Creal was the Matron and Superintendent of the training school of SHSEH and she was in attendance at the first and subsequent meetings.

After a number of successful meetings of the association, Miss Nellie Gould, also a founding member, reported that *...the list of candidates for employment and training are overflowing...* in the city hospitals.[3] A growing interest by nurses in their own professional development necessitated a name change to ATNA and the aims were also expanded to include *...a curriculum necessary for the education and training of* *nurses.*[4] The new name reflected the expanding role of the organisation and ATNA came into effect at the meeting of 1 December 1899.[104] Victoria formed a sister organisation, the Royal Victorian Trained Nurses' Association (RVTNA), but the standards required for inclusion on either register were comparable.[5]

Like Nightingale, the Australian nurse leaders harnessed the support of sympathetic and powerful medical leaders like Dr Norton Manning, a mental health reformer, who was convinced trained nurses were an advantage to the health and welfare of his patients.[6] He was the first president and it took another thirty years before a nurse leader, Maud Kellett, was finally appointed to the position in 1929.[7] The original ATNA Register included the names of 598 nurses *...from all states of Australia, New Zealand and Fiji...* and included information about their hospital training and occasionally their family history.

Despite it being a period of religious intolerance in the community, especially between Catholics and Protestants, the religion of the nurses was not included, which was in keeping with the Nightingale ethos of non-sectarianism.[8] For example, Letitia Moreton was born at Brim, near Ballarat (1891) and was educated at the convent school, Daylesford (Victoria, Dja Dja Wurrung Country).[9] She commenced a four-year nurse training course at Bethesda Hospital, Richmond (1909-1914). Bethesda Hospital was the first non-public nurse training hospital in Australia, a Salvation Army hospital, designed to provide care for the poor of Richmond and Collingwood (Wurundjeri Country). Importantly, in the 1940s the hospital provided training opportunities for indigenous nurses as not all nursing schools accepted their admission. Despite an early Catholic education and nurse training with the Salvation Army, she was listed as a Presbyterian on her AANS attestation papers, suggesting Letitia Moreton had an ecumenical disposition.[10]

Nursing reforms in the colony of South Australia moved at a different pace and were ably promoted by Margaret Graham of the Adelaide Hospital. The practice of partially trained nurses charging private patients small fees for care was intolerable so *...with Miss Graham, the sisters got together and the South Australian Branch of the R.B.N. Association was formed, which would ensure the public of having fully-qualified nurses for private work.*[11] The South Australia branch of the Royal British Nurses'

Association (RBNA) was established at a meeting at the Adelaide Hospital in August 1900 and Margaret Graham was the Lady Consul.[12]

There was one important difference between the RBNA and ATNA/RVTNA; the RBNA Registration Board required trainee nurses to complete a period of not less than three years in a hospital recognised by the RBNA Registration Board. The RBNA gained a royal charter in 1895 but the South Australia Branch did not establish its goal of an official register. The main barrier was a logistical one because in 1900 the RBNA only recognised training schools attached to hospitals *...which had a daily average of forty or more occupied beds...* and given that the Adelaide Hospital was the only hospital in South Australia to meet this stipulation there was not widespread support for the RBNA outside Adelaide.

The ATNA and RVTNA sought to create one register which included all hospitals throughout the colonies. The demography of the rural and regional areas meant that smaller hospitals had low daily averages of patients but there was a diversity of patients which created excellent experience for trainee nurses. Therefore, the smaller hospitals in South Australia, which effectively trained nurses but were not recognised by the RBNA, found the ATNA guidelines more appealing.

By 1906 the ATNA had a standard syllabus for nurse training schools which was adopted throughout Australia. However, Margaret Graham continued to have a strong alliance to the RBNA so when the Board of the Adelaide Hospital sought approval to become a registered ATNA Training School it was denied because their matron was not a member. This was rectified within twelve months and Margaret Graham was recognised for her valuable assistance as an ATNA examiner during her professional life.[13]

The impact of ATNA

ATNA was concerned with the establishment of minimum standards of training for nurses; recognising certain hospitals as appropriate training hospitals; approving the nomination of matrons to hospitals that received a Government subsidy and scrutinising the qualifications of applicants who would be placed on a register of trained nurses.[14] Once the ATNA examination was passed the nurse was required to pay 10/6d annually to remain on the ATNA register. This was not a small sum but nurse training was not the only benefit introduced by ATNA because salaries and conditions also improved.

By 1873 Osburn retained only one of her nurses from England, so the staff of SHSEH came from the colonies.[15] Initially, Osburn's full complement of nursing staff consisted of four head nurses, seventeen nurses, seven probationary nurses and one housekeeper. The salaries accorded to each group are telling, especially when the housekeeper and head nurse both received £40 per annum. The probationary (trainee) nurses received £20, while the other nurses had a salary range of £26-£30 per annum. Considering the salaries of her counterparts who were matrons of much larger hospitals more than twenty years later, Miss Osburn received a sizable sum of £250 per annum.[16] By comparison, in 1892 the matron of the Coast Hospital (renamed Prince Henry Hospital, 1934) located at Little Bay (NSW, Kamaygal Country) was responsible for forty-four staff and the training of thirty nurses; she was paid £245 per annum. The cost of her quarters was assessed at £120 per annum, compared to other matrons who only had to pay £56 per annum for board and lodgings.[17]

While it may be claimed that the economic depression of the 1890s was responsible for a general decline in all salaries throughout the colonies, it is interesting to note that a head nurse at the Coast Hospital (NSW, Bidjigal and Gadigal Country) had been paid £85 per annum since 1885. This represents more than a 100 per cent increase over the rates of the SHSEH nurses in 1873. Matrons from rural hospitals often only had a staff of four and their pay scale was dramatically lower than their city counterparts. For example, the matron at Bowral Hospital (NSW, Dharawal Country) received a salary of only £60 per annum in 1902 (it can be assumed this is net of accommodation costs) and in 1908 the matron of the Western Suburbs Cottage Hospital (Sydney) was paid £100 per annum.[18]

Although ATNA established salary guidelines for nurses, this did not ensure consistency of salaries. Following their training in a recognised ATNA training hospital, many nurses worked in private practice caring for people within their homes. In 1908 ATNA resolved that private nurses should charge £3.3 per week to nurse ordinary cases and 10/6d for 12 hour day or night shifts. The standardisation of the pay rates for private nursing was occasionally resented by the nurses. They wanted the autonomy to gauge whether their patients could afford the fee and waive it if they considered the cost would result in financial hardship. However, they were obliged to notify ATNA if this occurred and risked being viewed in a negative light by the ATNA Council.

In 1877 a telegraph line between the eastern colonies and Perth was completed and the news of Lucy Osburn and her nurses became known. In 1896 a two-year nurse training program (later approved by ATNA in 1900) was introduced and Miss Annie Kirkham was the first nurse to gain an ATNA certificate at (Royal) Perth Public Hospital.[19] A general improvement in the standard of nurse education was not translated into other conditions of employment.[20] The accommodation provided to the nursing staff in all the colonies was often sub-standard and lacked privacy.[21] In the 1870s the staff of RPAH had to endure the inconvenience of the nurses' and sisters' sleeping quarters being adjacent to the patients' wards which proved to be an effective method of eliminating the need for night staff. [22]

Elizabeth Glover, a trainee at Perth Public Hospital in 1906, was allocated her accommodation in *...a partitioned section of an old disused ward commanding a view of the morgue and the laundry*. This situation was remedied by the erection of a new one hundred bed nurses' home which was completed in 1909. The Perth Public Hospital Nurses' Home was typical of the quality and style of accommodation provided to nurses during the twentieth century and was still in use until nurse education was transferred to the tertiary sector in the 1970s. Each nurse had her own bed-sitting room and furniture, a communal lounge/recreation room and kitchen amenities. Block ablution facilities were usually provided on each floor.

The Perth Public Hospitals Nurses' Home was appropriately named Kirkham House, in honour of Annie Kirkham. [23] Nurses throughout Australia longed for a 'nurses' home' similar to Kirkham House, but it was not until after the First World War that this became a reality in most Australian hospitals.[24] The requirement to 'live in' was not always interpreted as a burden at this time because it enabled women to leave home without having to be married. The cloistered environment of the nurses' home also liberated these women from the expectations of, and obligations to, their immediate family.

Given that women were often not afforded access to rudimentary education in the colonies, the opportunity to undergo vocational training as a nurse was highly valued. The training program was basically determined by the matron of the hospital. Initially Lucy Osburn introduced a series of lectures relating to anatomy and physiology twice a week. If a patient was admitted with a particular disease she would conduct a lecture with reference to the nursing management of that disease. Therefore, nurse training was initially implemented as a quasi-apprenticeship system. However, it was not long before the pressure of work prevented the nurses from attending the lectures and the theory program lapsed for a few years. Each colony and each hospital, depending on its size and the type of patients admitted, had a different training program.[25]

ATNA standardised nurse training and trainee nurses were rotated between clinical wards to ensure they were exposed to a variety of medical and surgical cases. They were also required to nurse a cross-section of patients including paediatric, geriatric and gynaecological patients. Clinical experience on its own was not sufficient to ensure the nurses had adequate training so a prescribed course of lectures was given by the matron and doctors, who were the acknowledged leaders of their profession.[26]

Prior to ATNA training, hospitals determined whether examinations would be set during the nurse training period. The introduction of the ATNA training program included a stringent set of examinations which had to be successfully completed by the trainee. For example, a hospital with a four-year training program required the trainee to sit four examinations in first year including anatomy, physiology, general and practical nursing. Second year included examinations in medical, surgical and ophthalmic nursing, while third year was devoted to invalid cooking.

Given her experiences at Scutari, Florence Nightingale was duty-bound to write an entire chapter on the subject of invalid cooking.[26] The skilful acquisition of food and creation of a decent meal proved to be particularly useful during the First World War. Nurses competently dealt with an unexpected influx of casualties and limited rations by making meals stretch, often by forgoing their own rations to feed their soldier patients.[27]

The fourth and final year was focused on the hospital or 'House Finals' which, once successfully completed, entitled the student to sit for the ATNA finals. If successful, she was issued with the much coveted ATNA certificate which was occasionally referred to as the *Able To Nurse Anything* certificate.[28] Once ATNA was established there was an exponential growth in confidence in the competence of trained nurses. To be ATNA or RVTNA registered was a pre-requisite for entry into the AANS during the First World War.

When reviewing the ATNA examination questions devised for nurses who had completed four years of training in an ATNA approved hospital, it is easy to forget that the topics covered were once not available for study by women. The 1911 mental nurses' examination included the question ...*what is the brain? Describe its function and structure.*[29] Any attempt to answer this question today would require an encyclopaedic knowledge, excellent memory and more than two hours to write the answer.

Nonetheless, the ATNA training did afford this select group of women a chance to become educated in areas of study which were on the cutting edge of biology, anatomy and physiology. It was possible, though difficult, to become a female doctor, but it was not socially acceptable because gender was a serious barrier to science-based education at this time.

Although ATNA did attempt to standardise nurse education there were variations from hospital to hospital depending on the availability of resources, both human and material. For example, nurses at Perth Public Hospital received lectures from the matron and doctors but the nearby Fremantle Hospital nurses received their tuition from their matron only. The Melbourne Hospital resisted introducing the Nightingale system of nurse training until 1890 despite The Alfred, also located in Melbourne, successfully introducing the much improved system in 1880.

In 1940 Monica Dickens, the great-grand-daughter of Charles Dickens (who created the fictitious nurse 'Sairey Gamp'), commenced her nurse training at King Edward VII Hospital, London. She left soon after and wrote a damning appraisal of the brutalisation of student nurses in a well-received book *'One Pair of Feet'*.[30] A similar incident occurred at the Melbourne Hospital with the infiltration of an unnamed journalist onto the nursing staff. This resulted in a *'behind the screens'* exposé of the activities which resulted in a public outcry. Public pressure ultimately forced the board of the Melbourne Hospital to appoint Isabella Rathie as matron with a view to implementing the Nightingale system of training and getting rid of the Dickensian 'gamps'.[31]

Although Florence Nightingale introduced a system of training at St Thomas' she was not in favour of standardising the program to the same extent as ATNA and other similar organisations around the world. She objected to qualifying as a nurse by examination alone because, she believed, theoretical knowledge failed to consider *...the qualities of character...* of the nurse which were as important *...as the acquisition of technical skill.*[32] Her opposition resulted in a serious division within the embryonic profession which prompted a number of Nightingale-trained nurses in the colonies to stand by the principles of ATNA and openly defy Nightingale. These civilian nurse leaders included Nellie Gould, Jane Bell (1873-1959), Rose Creal, Adelaide (Maud) Kellett (1873-1945) and Grace Wilson; all of whom later became leaders during the 1914-18 war.[33]

Nursing in Australasia

The geographic isolation of Australia and New Zealand from Britain gave the two countries an early affinity which can be traced through the development of their respective nursing professions. In 1901 New Zealand addressed the need for the standardisation of nurse training with the introduction of the Nurses' Registration Act.[34]

Hester Maclean (1863-1932) was a member of both ATNA and RVTNA before she migrated to New Zealand and became influential in founding the New Zealand Trained Nurses' Association. Maclean was born in Sofala, (NSW, Wiradjuri Country) and her early life was marked by the death of her mother. She was educated at an exclusive private school in Sydney but it was not until her father died in 1889 that she was inspired by his nurse to commence her training at RPAH from 1890 to 1893.

Maclean was still training by the time Gould was matron of SHSEH and, while there is no evidence that they knew each other personally, their paths crossed a number of times throughout their respective careers.

While Maclean agreed with Nightingale about the need for nurses to be well-versed in practical as opposed to theoretical knowledge, she found that the benefits of having a well-qualified pool of nurses, as well as the increased interest in the profession that registration brought, outweighed the displeasure of Miss Nightingale. When Maclean was the Assistant Inspector of Hospitals in New Zealand, a nursing shortage in 1909 prompted the introduction of a four-year training program which she agreed to, on the condition the hospital boards offered *...worthwhile additional instruction for their extra year of service.*[35]

Changes to the social landscape

When the Australian writer Ethel Turner penned the children's book *Seven Little Australians* in 1894, she claimed that Australian children differed from their American, English and European counterparts because of their upbringing. Her description of the naughty seven children who made up the brood of Captain Woolcot and his second wife, Esther, leaves the reader with an impression of domestic chaos as opposed to military precision which you might expect in a family with a military father as the head of the household. Turner claimed one of the reasons that *...the miasmas of naughtiness...* were permitted to develop within Australian households at this time was due *...to the sunny brilliancy of our atmosphere.* However, her astute observation that for white settlers *...the land and the people are young-hearted together, and the children's spirits not crushed and saddened by the shadow of long years of history...* encapsulates the truth that future nurses and soldiers who faced the brutality of the South African and First World Wars, grew up within an atmosphere of optimism.[36] The early lives of Rose Creal and Kate Porter offer examples of the diversity enjoyed by and adversity imposed on, young Australians who later became nurse leaders.[37]

Rose Creal and Kate Porter: daughters of Lambing Flats

Rose Creal was the fourth Matron of SHSEH and a prominent Protestant. Ironically, she was of Irish-Catholic heritage and was born in a notorious gold mining area of NSW known as 'Lambing Flats' located on the outskirts of Young. In February 1851 when Edward Hargraves pushed away some dirt to discover gold near Bathurst, he changed the future of the small colony of NSW because the rich mineral resources of Australia were exposed for the first time.[38] Gold brought an influx of people from around the world. It also brought greed and racism to the outback. For example, in 1857, the Buckland River digging near Beechworth (Victoria, Pallanganmiddang Nation) was the scene of an ordered movement, which deteriorated into a brutal uprising, by predominantly American miners against the Chinese *...barbarians*. In fact, the Chinese worked long and hard which often resulted in more success on the fields than those of European and American background.[39]

On 31 March 1862 the young Anne Brady married John Creal at the Catholic Church in Young and they later had a daughter Rose, a few years after the Lambing Flat Riots. Anne's parents John Brady and Bridgett (nee McCloud) were residing in the area when the concentration of five hundred Chinese gold diggers and 1200 Europeans resulted in several clashes between December 1860 and August 1861. The NSW Premier, Charles Cowper, agreed to meet the European miners in an attempt to address some of their concerns but he was unsettled by the visit and subsequent meeting. The miners were left with the impression that the Premier would introduce a Chinese Immigration Restriction Act, but instead, he decided to send troops of the Twelfth Regiment to establish the supremacy of the law. The miners viewed this as a provocative act and their response was one of anger. This anger manifested itself on 30 June 1861 with an assembly of 3,000 people carrying English, Irish and American flags at Lambing Flats. They moved into the Chinese area where they began to destroy property, seize goods and in the words of Manning Clark *...civilised men were converted into brutes*.[40] Eventually the rule of law prevailed, but for the Chinese settlers justice did not. Rose was born a few years later.

When John Porter, builder and stairwright, migrated to Australia from England in 1860-61 he brought with him much needed trade skills, but the discovery of gold held an intoxicating promise for many migrants and he went to Lambing Flats to try his hand at prospecting. However, like many prospectors, John left Lambing Flats with an empty gold pan and settled elsewhere. He found a little piece of heaven on the south coast of NSW near the present day township of Milton (Yuin Country) but his land selection was slightly north-west and was known as *Duck Hole*. In 1870 he married a beautiful woman, Mary Guthrie, and they proceeded to have numerous children. Mary was the daughter of an Irish-Catholic migrant, Thomas Guthrie, who held the nearby area known as *Guthrie's Camp*. The couple lived at a number of locations in the district as their land holdings increased over time and John made a good living *...crafting much cedar furniture and staircases...* in the homes and public buildings of Milton. Ironically their firstborn, John, discovered the Poseidon Gold Mine in November 1906 which was the same day the racehorse *Poseidon* won the Melbourne Cup.[41]

Following John's birth another eleven children were born to the couple and their sixth child, Katherine Agnes Lawrence Porter, was known as 'Kitty' by her family and Kate by her nursing colleagues. In a few decades John Porter's daughter Kate would train under the capable leadership of Rose Creal; two remarkable First World War nurse leaders who were the daughters of Lambing Flats prospectors.[42] Kate Porter was born at Little Forest near Milton in about 1883, a picturesque spot but in those days some distance from SHSEH where she trained. She completed her four-year training course in November 1913 and registered with ATNA in January the following year. Like many SHSEH trainees and notable nurse leaders, Kate Porter enlisted in the AANS during the early stages of the war, but was not called up to join the Australian Imperial Force (AIF) until 20 March 1915 when she was 29 years old.[43]

It is interesting to note that three pairs of AANS nurses shared uncommon names including Ruby Dickinson, Jean Walker and Katherine Porter. Katherine Porter not only shared her first name and surname with another nurse, Katherine Minnie Porter (known as Minnie Kate by her nursing colleagues), they both trained together at SHSEH. Kate Porter from Milton will henceforth be differentiated from Minnie Kate Porter.[44]

The Australian nursing profession came of age during the South African War and the First World War but it was the introduction of the Nightingale system of training and later the implementation of ATNA which provided the groundwork for the profession. Globally, the Nightingale reforms were maximised during times of war because they were initiated during wartime. The discipline and rigour of nurse training in civilian hospitals was easily transferable into the military paradigm. Nursing, like all academic disciplines, has a history and a social context. Initially, nursing was a bridging profession because it developed, in an ad hoc manner, from the ordinary duties of women. The transformation of the perceived amateur duties of domestic care-giving to a skilled vocation which involved the teaching of specialised knowledge was furthered during times of war. The Nightingale system of nurse training was introduced at an opportune time because it educated women during a time of great scientific advancement. Nightingale also created the precedent that military nurses would originate from a pool of civilian trained nurses.

4 A Short Clinical History of Nursing and Medicine

... wore their oldest frock coats ... coats that were stiffly encrusted with the dried blood and pus of previous patients– Guy Williams

Discoveries and improvements in health occurred at a rapid rate in the seventeenth and eighteenth centuries. This was a time when one of Florence Nightingale's nurses became ill with Crimea Fever, leeches were applied to her head to release humors and promote healing - a practice which originated in Egypt centuries before.[1] Basic medical equipment like the hypodermic syringe (with hollow-pointed needle) was not invented until 1853 by Dr Alexander Wood.

Typhoid, chest infections and phthisis (tuberculosis) were common in the colony when Nellie Gould was training at RPAH. Knowledge about immunity was rudimentary and consequently, epidemics were not uncommon ...*between 1879 and 1883, an outbreak of typhoid fever caused 1,616 deaths in Sydney.*[2] *Morbus cordis* (chronic heart disease) and pericarditis (inflammation of the outer lining of the heart) were common conditions. Hydatid cyst was prevalent and most likely symptomatic of unhygienic food handling practices. The high incidence of 'Bright's disease' suggests it was most likely a generic term used at RPAH to describe kidney failure.[3]

Typhoid

The most prevalent disease was typhoid and the nursing management was onerous for the nurse and unpleasant for the patient. The warm bath treatment for typhoid was introduced by Dr Francis Washington Everard Hare. Fever wards were often filled during typhoid epidemics at the end of the nineteenth century and the Hare typhoid bath was used to reduce a patient's temperature. A heavy bath, lined with galvanised iron, was filled with tepid water and taken to the bedside. The patient was sponged with iced water then lowered into the bath for ten minutes and the procedure was repeated until the patient's temperature dropped. Unsurprisingly,...*many typhoid patients developed a "nervous dread of the bath" and had to be coaxed with morphia or brandy to submit to treatment.*[4]

The transfusion of blood

In the early 1600s, when William Harvey discovered that blood circulated around the body by way of the heart, which acts as a pump, he extinguished the notion that the heart was the seat of the human soul.[5] In 1666 Richard Lower ...*transferred blood directly from the artery of one dog to the vein of another...* which prompted experiments into the transfusion of blood between humans. However, the scientific curiosity surrounding blood transfusions was quickly quenched when deaths and subsequent lawsuits began.

The 1800s witnessed significant advances in the technical barriers to transfusions from human to human. In 1818 Dr James Blundell successfully transfused about twelve ounces of blood from a number of donors by way of a syringe into a seriously ill recipient. Blundell later developed a 'gravitator' which used gravitational force to push blood into the vein of a patient. Despite having no knowledge of clotting mechanisms, blood grouping or sterilising techniques he, by chance, had some success. Further experiments were devised to overcome the problem of blood clotting within the transfusing apparatus. Dr (Sir) Thomas Smith successfully defibrinated the blood by painstakingly removing clots via a hair-sieve in 1873. This system was in common usage but the addition of an anti-clotting (anticoagulant) agent was actively sought and Dr Braxton Hicks (obstetrician) unsuccessfully used phosphate of sodium as an anticoagulant in 1883-4. It was not until 1914 that L.Agote (Buenos Aires) and Richard Lewisohn (New York) simultaneously proved that the addition of sodium citrate (not in excess of five grams) was an effective and safe anticoagulant. The problem of blood incompatibility had already been eliminated in 1907 when the four blood groups were identified by J.Jansky in Prague.[6]

Soldiers and medical personnel who served in the South African War did not have the benefit of these advances. A Casualty Clearing Station (CCS) refers to a system of triage (evaluation) and emergency first aid close to the battle.[7] The inclusion of female nurses in the personnel of CCS was initially controversial but their expertise, especially in the operating theatres, made their presence invaluable. During the early stages of the First World War, soldiers were at risk of death from hypovolaemic (low fluid volume) shock. Blood was often taken from someone in the operating theatre (OT) or even on the battlefield and transfused directly into the bleeding soldier (referred to as 'on the hoof'). Although *...by 1917, the citrate method was being widely used in casualty clearing stations and military hospitals in France...*, Elsie Tranter,AANS, observed in January 1918 a blood transfusion in an American hospital in France.[8] She noted the *...donor was a most cheerful youth and both boys were very good during the operation.*[9] Dr Oswald Hope Robertson (USA) revolutionised the storage of blood in glass in 1917. One drawback of bottled blood (Robertson's Bottle) was that the blood needed to be stored in ice.

The dissemination of knowledge to hospitals 'back home' was slower because there was an overwhelming sense of urgency on the battlefield which, understandably, resulted in medical and surgical risk taking. In contrast to what was occurring in CCSs on the Western Front, *...by the end of the war, blood transfusions were occasionally performed at Fremantle Hospital ... a donor's blood was collected into a bowl and a nurse stood with aching arms, stirring and stirring, to prevent the blood clotting until it was transferred into the recipient.*[10] It did not take long for battlefield discoveries to filter through to the civilian hospitals when the war ended - when doctors and nurses came home and exchanged their military uniforms for civilian ones.

Prior to the 1914-18 war, patients who were ambulant and presented to the local hospital were referred to as 'outdoor' or 'outpatients'. However, from 1917, 'casualty' patients (a term derived from war casualties) were described as anyone who was *...killed, injured or otherwise hurt through mishap, accident or disaster.*[11] The casualty department or 'Cas' was an integral and often stressful part of nurse training until the transfer of nurse education to the tertiary sector. Today the Accident and Emergency Department performs much the same role as the old 'Cas', albeit in a more technical manner.

Anti-sepsis

The ancient Egyptians ...*had expert knowledge of drugs and knew the most effective ways to prepare and deliver them*... but they ...*knew nothing of the need for sterility*.[12] However, the Roman encyclopaedist Varro hypothesised that infection might be caused by the ...*unseen entry into the body of tiny, invisible organisms*. The idea of sepsis (infection) has been known to mankind for centuries but the use of antiseptics was still controversial at the end of the nineteenth century.

An antiseptic inhibits the activity and growth of germs by the use of chemicals which may also have a harmful effect on healthy tissue, whereas a disinfectant will kill germs. The process of sterilisation makes objects aseptic (germ-free) by way of a bactericide such as sunlight, heat or chemical disinfectants. Cross-infection occurs when bacteria are transferred from one patient to another, usually through an intermediary such as a doctor, nurse or relative/visitor during a hospital stay.

At the beginning of the nineteenth century, surgeons were the main carriers of infection in the operating theatres because they ...*wore their oldest frock coats ... coats that were stiffly encrusted with the dried blood and pus of previous patients*.[13] Not until Joseph Lister disseminated his research findings in 1867 did the practitioners of medicine and nursing take antisepsis seriously. Antisepsis has been the cornerstone of the Nightingale system of nurse training: in 1859, the year Joseph Lister was appointed Regius Professor of Surgery at Glasgow, Florence Nightingale wrote that ...*every nurse ought to be careful to wash her hands very frequently during the day*.[14] Lister used the germ theories of Louis Pasteur to develop aseptic techniques which included the introduction of carbolic acid spray and effective hand washing by staff in the operating theatres.[15]

In 1899, theatre nursing was difficult but there was a basic knowledge about the Listerian methods. A WA nurse working in a remote gold mining town recalled that nurses ...*had no special gowns or caps; ... went to the theatres ... dipped hands and arms up to the elbow in strong Condy's fluid till they were nearly black, then scrubbed this off in very strong, hot brine*. Once members of the theatre staff were 'sterilised' they ...*were not to touch anything but the dressings and instruments*. This proved a difficult task in the heat and ...*an unsterilized probationer*... mopped the brow of the sister, held the handkerchief so the doctor could blow his nose and just as importantly, in a sterile field, caught ...*any flies which found their way in (as they always did)*.[16]

Surprisingly, larger teaching hospitals in cities on the other side of the country did not immediately implement aseptic procedures. Listerian methods were not universally accepted because some doctors believed the rigmarole of wearing sterile gowns and hand-washing detracted from their reputation. For example, at the (Royal) Melbourne Hospital, Dr Thomas Naghten Fitzgerald (1838-1908) was considered the ...*most outstanding medical figure in Australia*... in the 1890s but he did not adopt the Listerian principles. Conversely, Dr Tharp Mountain Girdlestone (1823-1899), who practiced earlier than Fitzgerald, ...*adopted Listerian principles, and practiced a strict antiseptic routine*... but he was not considered brilliant, merely...*'capable, slow and safe*.[17] A comparative analysis of their patient morbidity and mortality levels would have proved useful to prospective patients.

The term 'sepsis' often applied to a wound infection. An enterprising Edinburgh surgeon, Dr James Syme (1799-1870), ...*used to leave the long ends of ligatures hanging out*... of the surgical incision ...*so the infective matter in the wounds of his patients would drain out into their dressings*.[18] This idea was a precursor to rubber drainage tubes (round or corrugated) which were used during the First World War for common abdominal surgery such as appendicitis.[19] Keeping the wound dry was imperative if infection was to be minimised, and the drains gave any developing pus an outlet.

Nature has a way of dealing with infection and during wartime help from any quarter was welcome. A moss-like plant, sphagnum, was observed to be useful in treating shrapnel wounds because it had the ability to retain moisture and therefore keep the wound dry, promote healing and reduce the risk of infection. A variation of this plant's properties is widely used today in disposable nappies.[20] Maggots were inadvertently a godsend to the casualties of war because they scavenged the septic debris around the wound and warded off infection. An Australian doctor, R. C. Winn, was attending to the casualties of Pozières and Mouquet Farm in August 1916, where he observed that ...*many wounded were brought in who were out for days before being rescued. Some of their wounds were crawling with maggots but looked surprisingly clean*.[21]

Antibiotics

Even today it is not possible to protect the human body against a viral infection, but the discovery of antibiotics and sulphonamides, which assist the body in fighting off bacterial infections, occurred in the second half of the twentieth century. Matron Gertrude Davis was overwhelmed in India when a ship containing Turkish prisoners-of-war (POWs) came into port and she found ...*there was so much sepsis we fairly wallowed in pus.*[22] Alexander Fleming spent the First World War investigating problems associated with septic wounds, of which there was no short supply, and became interested in the natural antibacterial function of leukocyte-rich pus.

It was not until 1942 that the influential Penicillin Committee was formed, enabling Howard Florey, the Australian pathologist who jointly discovered and later developed the practical benefits of penicillin, to complete his research. His discovery made an immense difference to the morbidity and mortality levels of the world population. It was at the conclusion of the Second World War (1945) that Alexander Fleming, Ernst Chain and Howard Florey (who had, fortunately, been rejected for service in the 1914-18 war through ill-health) were awarded the Nobel Prize for Medicine. Each was involved in separate aspects of research which created an understanding of the usefulness of antibiotics.[23] It is hard to imagine not having access to the rudimentary knowledge which underscored this discovery but this was the case during the 1914-18 war.

A virus of plague proportions – influenza

In 1918 the global population was 1.8 billion and the number of people who reputedly died from the 1918-19 influenza pandemic was twenty million. In 2020 the global population was 7.9 billion and the number of people who died from the Coronavirus Disease (COVID-19) was just over seven million. The difference in the death rates tell a story of technical advancements in health, genetics, communication, epidemiology and the general literacy of today's global populace. Prior to the 1914 war a doctor from The Alfred in Melbourne claimed the term 'influenza' originated from the influence of the stars.[24] The level of knowledge was not much advanced from this statement when the AANS nurses, who had endured years of deprivation from war, had to pull up their sleeves and nurse the general population. Many did not get to enjoy the peace as they quickly succumbed themselves.

At the beginning of the twentieth century it was not uncommon for people to die from the effects of influenza. It was two surface proteins - hemagglutinin and neuraminidase - that defined the identity of the virus. The many strains of influenza are reflected by the number of combinations of these two proteins - in 1918 the combination was H1N1, as was the 2009 'Swine flu' combination and later avian influenza (H5N1) which were considered to be a serious pandemic threat. It wasn't until 1997 when a flu particle, which has eight disconnected gene segments, was recreated by Jeffrey Taubenberger. He recreated the genetic code of the 1918 influenza virus using the polymerase chain reaction (PCR). This was achieved by taking a sample of lung tissue from a First World War soldier who had died from influenza and *...amplifying a signal of DNA in a sample.* In December 2019 the (COVID-19) was identified and the SARS-CoV-2 virus quickly spread throughout the world. The widespread implementation of a vaccine was a game changer and it was through the efforts of scientists using gene therapy that the death rate was not higher. [25]

During the 1918-19 influenza pandemic it was down to basic nursing care. Before being able to effectively nurse a patient, it is essential to ask the question 'How do you feel?' Those suffering from influenza felt as though they were *...breathing through meat.* Not everyone who was infected died but those who did usually succumbed within the first 24 hours of symptoms appearing.[26]

Treatment included regular sponges and the application of poultices (also referred to as 'counter irritants' or 'cataplasm'). The preparation of poultices was complicated as the nurses would, under hospital conditions, heat the prescribed ingredients on the stove and then spread it onto poultice cloths which would then be kept warm on an enamel tray in the oven until needed. The poultices were applied directly onto the skin covering the back and front of both or one of the lungs every four hours; the idea being that the poultice would ease the pain of the congestion caused by the influenza.[27]

Poultices were out of favour with nurses by the 1940s owing to the high risk of burns

...with the possible exception of kaolin... but the preparation of a poultice was still included in the general nursing syllabus. Consequently, editors still included information about the use of poultices in recommended nursing texts. Nonetheless, the removal of poultices from nursing practice was understandable when the classifications included rubefacients (redden the skin); vesicants (blister the skin) and cautery (destroy tissue).[28]

Immunisation

In Scutari, one of Florence Nightingale's Sellonite nurses, Sarah Anne Terrot, developed symptoms which were generically referred to as 'Crimea fever'. She endured '*great pain*' in her head accompanied by '*noise*' followed by temporary deafness. While it was believed that her illness was due to bad air, fatigue and mental anxiety, she noted that *...it was very much like, though worse, than the fever I had five years before after nursing nearly five months in the Cholera Hospitals in Plymouth.*[29] The resilience of nurses at this time was often determined by their immune system. Currently the terms 'vaccination', 'immunisation' and 'inoculation' are interchangeable but during the First World War the term 'vaccination' was used when referring to smallpox (the first vaccine developed) and 'inoculation' referred to the vaccines for all other diseases.[30]

Vaccination against smallpox and inoculation against typhoid were prerequisites for entry into the First AIF; any soldier who managed to evade the procedure at the time of enlistment was immediately discharged if he continued to refuse. Cholera inoculation was ostensibly a matter of choice except during an outbreak of the disease amongst the ranks.[31]

There are various types and levels of immunity; in the case of typhoid, active immunity is triggered when an antigen of inactive disease bacteria is injected into the body. This antigenic substance provokes the body's own defence system to form specific antibodies (proteins) to fight the typhoid antigen.[32] Early in 1915 an English doctor, Professor Georges Dreyer, noticed that soldiers in France were being returned home with typhoid fever even though they had been inoculated against the disease. He found that they were, in fact, suffering from paratyphoid. Captain

Archibald, RAMC, served on the recently ceded Greek island of Lemnos, where he treated Gallipoli casualties and confirmed Dreyer's hypothesis. Archibald observed that sick soldiers who had been inoculated against typhoid showed a spike in agglutination for typhoid even though they were infected with paratyphoid.[33]

Often the body responds to a pathogenic infection by increasing the number of leukocytes (leukocytosis) but in the case of typhoid, leukocytosis is absent. Instead of increasing the number of leukocytes the blood serum clump, the bacteria and an agglutination test, *Widal reaction*, confirms the diagnosis of typhoid from the eighth day.[34] Similar clumping occurs when a person is infected with paratyphoid so a *...special technique...* was developed to differentiate the two diseases. Of a sample of *...350 cases investigated ... only 7 per cent were typhoid, 61 per cent paratyphoid "A", and 32 per cent type "B"...* which resulted in the development of a combined typhoid-paratyphoid vaccine. This vaccine was known as TAB (typhoid and paratyphoid A & B) and was available to all allied personnel.[35]

Searching for x(unknown)-rays

In 1879 the German-born physicist William Conrad Röntgen (1845-1923) proved that *...humid air can be heated more quickly than dry air, since water vapour actually absorbs radiation...* and published prolifically on all manner of problems relating to the physics. However, it was his single-minded interest in the conduction of cathode rays in 1895 which inadvertently led him to discover that *...new rays ... were illuminating the barium platinocyanide-coated screen at distances of more than a metre*. The usefulness of this discovery to medicine (especially orthopaedics) was blatantly obvious when he placed his wife's hand *...on a cassette loaded with a photographic plate, and on this he directed for fifteen minutes rays from his tube ... he saw the bones of his wife's hand depicted in light tones inside the darker shadows of the flesh surrounding them ... two rings she had on her fingers had almost completely stopped the rays, and were exactly silhouetted.*[36]

Fortunately, Röntgen was diligent in disseminating his findings to the broader scientific community so they could be replicated and improved upon. Allied armies greatly benefited from his discovery and during the First World War x-rays were commonplace. For example, Sister Tucker (AANS) enjoyed a moment of respite from transport duty during the Gallipoli Campaign when she and her colleagues visited Lemnos, where the tented First Stationary Hospital was situated, and found *...the theatre is a typical Australian shanty and at the other side of a division is the x-ray room.*[37] Acting Matron Alma Bennett (AANS) served in India where she was pleased to find that her hospital's *...operating theatre, x-ray room and path lab were annexes to ... the surgical ward.*[38] Staff Nurse A N Smith (AANS) was sent to 2 Australian CCS (ACCS) in France and her *...idea of CCS at that time was rather vague. So I was surprised to find that it consisted of a quite up-to-date hospital, in many ways, with excellent appliances and x-ray plant.*[39]

The enemy armies were well aware of the importance of x-rays because a month after the first x-ray was taken (January 1896) Röntgen was invited to the imperial court of Kaiser Wilhelm II to demonstrate his discovery; he was immediately awarded the Prussian Order of the Crown (Second Class). In 1901 he was awarded the first Nobel Prize for Physics.[40]

Wartime often prompted innovation and discovery. For example, during the First World War, analgesia was morphine-based and synthetic drugs such as aspirin had to be developed from scratch: The German-based Company, Bayer, was no longer inclined to trade with enemy countries. In response, George Nicholas, an Australian pharmacist, successfully manufactured acetylsalicylic acid in 1915 and two years later patented it under the *Aspro* brand name.[41]

Discovering radium and managing malignancies

There is little doubt that when Manya Sklodowska (1867-1934) was born in Warsaw during the Russian occupation, she endured many barriers to what was to become a habit of life-long learning. Her mind was sharp and her determination extraordinary. Eventually, she succeeded in following her sister to Paris in 1891, where she endured physical and financial deprivation to realise her goal, graduating in physics two years later.[42] This was the formal beginning of a career where her achievements in a male dominated area of science proved inspirational to women scientists who followed.[43]

Manya adopted the French spelling of her first name 'Marie'. In 1894 she met Pierre Curie (1859-1906) and the following year they married: Madame Marie Curie entered the pages of history. Despite the demands of motherhood and domestic duties she was determined to utilise her education and searched for a doctoral thesis question. Her scientific curiosity was ignited when Antoine Henri Becquerel (1852-1908) recorded that while researching uranium *...he had found that the salts of the metal gave off, spontaneously, rays similar to the x-rays that William Conrad Röntgen had discovered.* Marie and Pierre Curie collaborated with Becquerel and together they confirmed that radioactivity was a *...fundamental property of salts of uranium, thorium and other heavy metals.* In 1902 Marie and Pierre Curie painstakingly isolated the source of radiation, radium, and the following year Becquerel was awarded half, and Pierre and Marie Curie a quarter each of the Nobel Prize for Physics.

The discovery of the importance of radium to medicine was by accident. The three scientists suffered radium burns of various degrees but they universally healed and the idea that radium could be used to effectively destroy unwanted, diseased tissue was planted into the minds of scientists. In 1906 the Radium Hospital was founded in Paris, where research into the management and treatment of malignancies continues to assist people suffering from cancer today. Madame Marie Curie was awarded the Nobel Prize for Physics in 1911 for isolating pure radium.[44]

Anaesthesia and the joy of sleep

The amputation of a limb without recourse to an anaesthetic is difficult to imagine. One of the first men to experience the benefits of research into anaesthesia was Frederick Churchill, aged thirty-six, who had his leg amputated by Dr Robert Liston on 21 December 1846 at the Hospital of University College, London. The patient was rendered unconscious by the administration of an anaesthetic agent, ether, which was given by Dr Peter Squire.[45] Ether was a volatile liquid which, when inhaled, produced general anaesthesia and when applied topically was an antiseptic. It was a very useful product in the operating theatre but its volatility was a definite hazard.[46]

Pneumatic medicine, which involved experimenting with various *...specially adapted gases...* began in the 1790s. The gases were wafted, with bellows, over patients in a bid to reduce their pain. Eminent laymen such as James Watt and Josiah Wedgwood supported the research and subscribed to the establishment of a 'Pneumatic Institution' in Bristol by Dr Thomas Beddoes (a geologist) and a young student of medicine, Humphry Davy (1778-1829).

In 1799 Davy had discovered the intoxicating effect of nitrous oxide (laughing gas) which was used to create ...*a new pleasure for which language has no name*. Horace Wells (USA) was a dentist who observed that those under the influence of nitrous oxide did not appear to experience sensations of pain when injured. He allowed the gas to be administered to him while a colleague extracted one of his molar teeth – painlessly; this occurred in about 1844 and the analgesic benefits of nitrous oxide to dentistry continue today. The Pneumatic Institution closed in 1801 because of neighbourhood suspicion that the poisonous gases were being emitted into the surrounding air. However, Sir Humphry Davy went on to become one of the more influential chemists of his time.

Michael Faraday (1791-1867) assisted Davy and in 1815 he ...*noted that ether could be used to produce the same kind of intoxicating effect as nitrous oxide*. It was not his research into early anaesthesia for which Faraday, a self-taught scientist, gained world-wide acclaim but for the discovery of the laws of electrolysis (Faraday laws). Unfortunately, the value of ether and nitrous oxide for medicinal purposes was not immediately apparent. Instead ...*ether frolics*... and ...*laughing gas side-shows*... were more at home in the fairground than the operating theatres. It was serendipitous that Dr Crawford Williamson Long (USA) noticed, during one of these ether frolics, that one of the frolickers injured himself but appeared to feel no pain, Long used ether to deaden the pain of his patients during painful procedures but, unfortunately, he did not disseminate his work to the wider scientific community.

The extraordinary British doctor, John Snow, successfully demonstrated the practical application of ether for the purpose of operating on a patient at St George's Hospital, London.[47] By the time Frederick Churchill had his leg amputated in 1846, the place of ether within the discipline of anaesthesia was assured. In the nineteenth century, childbirth was a painful and often traumatic process. Once the beneficial results of Snow's ether practice became known, Dr James Young Simpson, Professor of

Midwifery at Edinburgh University, began to trial ether on women during childbirth. However, it became evident that ether was a cardiac stimulant and was dangerous to some patients.[48] Simpson sought a more portable anaesthetic agent and in 1847 he trialled chloroform (which had been discovered 50 years earlier) as a possible alternative.

Simpson and two of his colleagues, Drs Keith and Duncan, inhaled the drug, which *...rapidly took effect and the three men passed out simultaneously, almost as if they had been shot.*[49] The following week Simpson administered chloroform to a patient who had part of his arm amputated. However, it was Snow who conducted further experiments on the application of chloroform and it became the anaesthetic agent of choice for the next fifty years. Significantly, Snow administered *...that blessed chloroform...* to Queen Victoria during the birth of her fourth son and eighth child, Leopold in 1853. She found the *...effect was soothing, quietening and delightful beyond measure...*, which, no doubt, enhanced the popularity of the drug and the reputation of John Snow.[50]

Despite the colony's distance from England, it was reported that chloroform was used as an anaesthetic during the amputation of a man's limb at the Melbourne Hospital as early as 1848.[51] A decade later it was recorded that three operations, which required extreme delicacy and dexterity by the surgeon, were performed with the aid of chloroform in the rural district of Ballarat.[52]

The pioneering work of these scientists had a dramatic effect on the diagnosis of diseases, surgical outcomes in the operating theatre and the level of pain endured by patients. This was a period of scientific and medical curiosity which benefited soldiers so it was essential that nurse education developed at a similar pace. Hence, a priority for the women who were civilian nurse leaders at the end of the nineteenth century and military nurse leaders during the South African and First World Wars.

5 Colonial Army Nursing in the South African War 1899-1902

...ministrations to the wounded were invaluable and beyond all praise. They did a service during those distressful days which none but nurses could have rendered - *Sir Frederick Treves*

In 1857 Sidney Herbert - Nightingale's main political supporter - was invited to become chairman of the Royal Sanitary Commission, which had the optimistic objective of improving the appalling morbidity and mortality levels of British Army personnel stationed in India. Progress was slow because the baseline data from the many geographically and religiously disparate regions in India was not available; so the British military stations, which had materialised since British colonisation, did not have a reference point for improvement.

Nightingale the epidemiologist

Florence Nightingale, being a practical individual, obtained the necessary information from the military stations directly and created the *...second volume of the Indian Sanitary Commission's report, a folio of nearly 1000 pages in small type*. The epidemiological picture was graphic - the death rate for British soldiers in India was 69:1000. Nightingale was quick to point out that to deal with the sanitary conditions of the military stations without reference to the conditions of the nearby villages was a waste of time - sanitary reform was needed throughout India. She lobbied tirelessly to this end but to no avail. In 1864 she was approached by Sir John Lawrence, Governor of Bombay (present day Mumbai), to consider a scheme to deploy British trained nurses to India to work as part of the Indian Medical Service. Unfortunately, the Deputy Inspector-General in Madras visited Nightingale and tried to convince her that *...no matron was wanted. The Dr. ought to be matron...* which did not conform to the Nightingale model of nurse training.[1] It was obvious to

Nightingale that the Indian Medical Service was seeking a ready and reliable workforce instead of wanting to implement widespread public health reform through her nurses.[2]

However, in 1883 it was decreed that trained nurses would be appointed to every British military hospital with more than one hundred beds. This necessitated the establishment, in 1888, of the Indian Army Nursing Service (later known as Queen Alexandra's Imperial Military Nursing Service in India).[3] It was nearly a decade later that the Army Nursing Service Reserve (ANSR) was implemented by the third child of Queen Victoria, Helena, the Princess Christian of Schleswig-Holstein, in 1897; two years later there were 101 civilian nurses in reserve in the event of a *...pressing emergency*.[4]

Colonial army nursing and the Second Boer War (The South African War)

In 1885 Dr William Daniel Campbell Williams (1856-1919), the Honorary Surgeon at St Vincent's Hospital, Sydney, was appointed the Principal Medical Officer of the Army in NSW.[5] In February 1899, while Hester Maclean was gaining post-graduate experience in Australia, Nellie Gould was asked by (now) Colonel Williams (later Surgeon-General), *...to help form the Nursing Service in connection with his Army Medical Corps services. In May of the same year ... the little band of 26 nurses were sworn in*.[6] Gould, more than likely, was in the right place at the right time when approached by Williams, but her administrative experience as a civilian matron enabled her to foresee policy limitations in the slowly emerging discipline of military nursing.

The NSW Army Nursing Service Reserve (NSWANSR) was modelled on the British system of Princess Christian's Army Nursing Service Reserve. While the British reservists were unpaid in peacetime, the NSWANSR were provided with a uniform and paid a £2 allowance on joining and £1 thereafter each year.[7] Members were required to become 'efficient' by undergoing training each year and qualifying in first aid as well as receiving instruction on military organisation.[8] The Princess Christian reservists were required to have *...at least three years combined training and service in a civil General Hospital...* and when Gould led her nurses to the South

African War she was convinced of their capabilities as military nurses because ...*not one ... had had less than seven years experience*... nursing in Australia.[9] The belief that civilian nursing experience was sufficient to prepare a nurse for the carnage of a battlefield was undisputed at this time.

Not long after the approach by Williams the South African War was underway, and it was this conflict which brought the two different forms of nurse training and registration in Australia and New Zealand into close contrast. Unlike the expeditious formation of the NSWANSR, the New Zealand nurses had to assert their right to serve in the South African War. Nurses from the antipodes were first exposed to war nursing and army regulations during the South African War.

A Short History of the Conflict

In 1652 the first European settlers arrived in the Cape of Good Hope where the Dutch Cape Company established a base in South Africa. The Cape was governed by the Dutch East India Company until it was formally dissolved in 1799 at which point the Dutch Government took over the role. However, during the Napoleonic Wars the British occupied the Cape on three occasions and finally defeated the Dutch at the Battle of Blaauwberg in 1806 giving them permanent occupation. The area consisted of 26,000 colonists who were primarily Dutch but also had German and French descendants.

The Boers (meaning farmers) were a subgroup of itinerant farmers who resented the British administration, especially when they abolished slavery on 1 December 1834. During the Great Trek of 1836-52 more than 15,000 Boers moved towards Natal, but when the British annexed this area, they kept going further north. In 1852 the Boers established the South African Republic (SAR), which is also known as the Transvaal Republic. This was followed in 1854 by the creation of the Orange Free State; both were recognized as republics at this time by the British.

However, in 1866, the discovery of diamonds at Kimberley on the border of the Orange Free State changed the dynamics of the region. The great diamond rush attracted uitlanders (foreigners) from around the globe. In 1877 Britain attempted to annex the Transvaal and the First Boer War (1880-81) occurred. The Battle of Majuba

Hill was a defining defeat for the British and both republics were restored.
A few years later, in 1884, the discovery of gold at Witwatersrand in the Transvaal, making it the richest nation in South Africa, attracted the attention of Cecil Rhodes, a British expansionist. The Boers had insufficient manpower or infrastructure to manage these vast resources and so agreed to foreign, mainly British, support. These British foreigners were not allowed to vote until they had fourteen years' residence. This was considered unfair, so they took their grievances to Britain. The Boers were at risk of losing their political sovereignty as the Uitlanders outnumbered the native Transvaalers and the vote would give them control. Under the guidance of Cecil Rhodes, Dr Leander Starr Jameson, who was the Administrator of Southern Rhodesia, provoked an uprising of the Uitlanders but they refused to take up arms against the Transvaal Government so the Jameson Raid failed. Jameson was captured by the Boer Government within three days of his attempt and his incompetence reflected poorly on the British Empire.[10]

The South African War: 11 October 1899 to 31 May 1902

The South African War is also known as the Second Anglo-Boer War in South Africa. Following failed negotiations at the Bloemfontein Conference in June 1899 the British informed the Republics they were going to dispatch 10,000 troops. This gave the Boer irregulars and the militia time to attack British colonial settlements in the Natal colony. The Boers laid siege to Ladysmith, Kimberley and Mafeking and won victories at Colenso, Magersfontein and Stromberg. These victories were short-lived as the British troops, including colonials from Australia, retook them. Britain declared war on the Boer Republic on 5 October 1899 but the war was not won as decisively as expected. During the 'Black Week' of December 1899, for example, the English lost eleven guns during four battle defeats. The Boers had the benefit of local knowledge of the harsh landscape and they excelled in guerilla warfare.

Nursing in the South African War.

It has been estimated that 1,300-1,400 female British nurses served in the South African War; a relatively small number to nurse the casualties of a war in which it has been estimated that 450,000 British and colonial troops served.[11.] New Zealand sent approximately thirty nurses and it is estimated that 65 qualified nurses served from the various Australian colonies.[12] Nellie Gould, lady superintendent of nurses, led the first contingent of Australian nurses. She sailed with her superintendent, Julia Bligh Johnston and twelve other members of the NSWANSR aboard the *Moravian*, with the second contingent of soldiers (no nurses sailed with the first), on 17 January 1900.[13]

Mary Annie (Bessie) Pocock (1863-1946) sailed with Gould, for whom she developed an animosity. Pocock was an Anglican, born in Dalby, Queensland on Barunggam Country. Her young life was marred by disappointment when her fiancé died of tetanus three weeks before their wedding.[14] After his death she decided to become a nurse and commenced her training at SHSEH in 1890. She served at 2 British Stationary Hospital (2 BSH), East London, Cape Colony, in South Africa; 2 BSH later moved to Johannesburg in July 1900. The following month she joined 17 British Stationary Hospital (17 BSH), Middleburg, in the Transvaal, which was the closest unit to the front-line. Unfortunately, she contracted typhoid and was sent to England to convalesce. In 1902 she was still in London, where she received word she had been Mentioned in Despatches (MID) and was able to attend the coronation procession of King Edward VII in August of the same year.[15]

A third group of nurses sailed as part of 'The Bushmen's Contingent' from Victoria aboard the *Euryalus* which left Melbourne on 10 March 1900.[16] The Bushmen's Contingent was a tough group of men from the farming districts who had excellent horse and shooting skills. On arrival they had an arduous time at Elands River but managed to regroup at Mafeking before proceeding to ...*Kimberley, the Transvaal and Pretoria, fighting all the way*.[17]

Death, Disease and Awards

Frances (Fanny) Emma Hines, the fourth daughter of Patrick and Eleanor Hines who lived in the Inglewood district amidst the Victorian gold fields, travelled with her colleague, Janey Lempriere. Both women were educated at Faireleight Private Girls' School, East St Kilda and Lempriere was one of 16 South African War nurses who also saw overseas service in the First World War. Tragically, Fanny Hines died of pneumonia, complicated by malnutrition, just five months after leaving Melbourne.[18] During the last days of her life she was *...quite alone with as many as twenty-six patients at one time, no possibility of assistance or relief, and without sufficient nourishment...* at the Memorial Hospital at Bulawayo.[19] She died on 7 August 1900 and is remembered as the first nurse to die on active service from the colony of Victoria, not Australia: Australia was federated on 1 January 1901.

Fanny Hines was the only nurse known to have died.

Gertrude Greenway undertook 'private nursing' in Johannesburg from 1902 to 1906. She was ATNA qualified in 1900 and in 1907 also registered with the Transvaal Medical Council, before proceeding to Scotland and England for further nursing experience. She continued to travel the world and was 'on active service' during the First World War .[20] Nurses who undertook independent work during times of war are difficult to identify and it was a strain for families who waited for news from unofficial sources.

Awards

Like many precedents in military nursing, the presentation of awards to nurses was instituted soon after the Crimean War. Queen Victoria and the Prince Consort had been most impressed with the work of the nurses in the Crimea and became close personal friends with Florence Nightingale on her return. The Prince Consort designed a brooch of *...a St George's Cross in red enamel surmounted by a diamond crown; the cross bears the word "Crimea"' and is encircled with the words "blessed are the merciful"*. On the reverse is the inscription,... *"To Miss Florence Nightingale, as a mark of esteem and gratitude for her devotion towards the Queen's brave soldiers from Victoria R. 1855"*.[21] It was much later before other nurses who had accompanied Florence Nightingale were recognised. In commemoration of Queen Victoria's Diamond Jubilee in 1897, Sarah Anne Terrot, one of the last Sellonite sisters who served with Florence Nightingale at Scutari, was presented by Queen Victoria with the Royal Red Cross (RRC) at Balmoral Castle.[22]

The Royal Red Cross (1st Class) is a decoration (not a medal) for *...special devotion* *and competency in their nursing duties…* which was instituted by Queen Victoria on 27 April 1883 and was the first example of a British Military Order for females; Florence Nightingale was one of the first recipients. [23] Those who receive the highest honour of RRC (1st class) are members of the order and use the post-nominal RRC. The RRC (1st class) medal is a striking cross with red enamel and gold trim and includes the words 'faith, hope and charity' and the date 1883. The 2nd class award denotes associates of the order; those who receive this award are entitled to use the post-nominal ARRC. The medal is much the same as the first but has silver trim. The RRC was worn as a medal on a military uniform but after the war nurses, on occasion, wore it as badge on the civilian uniforms. In 1914 an emblem of bronze oak leaves, worn on the ribbon of the Victory Medal, denoted a nurse who had been Mentioned in Despatches (MID).[24]

See *Appendix 1* which shows that sixty-five nurses served and three (Rawson, Nixon and Bidmead) were highly decorated. In summary, seven nurses received at least one award; three were discharged (Armstrong, Brooks, Tchan), one left the unit (Lempriere), four were invalided out (Chatfield, Mansfield, Milne, Woodward), while one resigned (Naylor).

Matron Nellie Gould: The NSW Contingent

Wherever the NSW nurses moved during the South African War it was recognised that *…under the able leadership of Matron Ellen Gould…* they *…maintained standards and left their mark on generations of Australian nurses.*[25] Given that M. Rawson, who was the superintendent of nurses from Victoria, was awarded a RRC and a MID, it is somewhat surprising that Gould did not receive any awards in this conflict. One doctor who had a significant impact on Australian nurses in the First World War was Neville Howse, who received a Victoria Cross in the South African War. He was appointed the Director Medical Services (DMS) of the AIF and had over-arching responsibility for the AANS during the 1914-18 conflict.[26]

The British Army regrouped and by the end of the war in June 1902 they had managed to annex the Transvaal.[27] However, Britons were stunned by their Army's obvious deficiencies and the status and confidence of Britain was reduced by the end of the nineteenth century, even in the eyes of the new nation of Australia.[28] Not so, the status of military nurses.

When Gould's group of nurses left NSW, the New Zealand press correctly observed that *...some competent nurses from this colony...* could be of assistance in the war.[29] However, the New Zealand nurses faced similar problems to those experienced by nurses from the South Australia and WA colonies who were independently financed by the community. In the case of the WA nurses, the group was disbanded on reaching South Africa and while some were absorbed into the British Nursing Service others returned to WA.[30] However, unlike the New Zealand nurses who served, those sent from the Australian colonies were at least sanctioned by the War Office.[31] A number of New Zealand nurses paid their fares or were financially supported through community appeals because *...the New Zealand Government would not pay to send nurses to war.* Despite these obstacles a number of New Zealand nurses like Janet Williamson, who had the honour of being the first from her country to be awarded the RRC, served with distinction.[32]

Long before the Treaty of Vereeniging was signed on 31 May 1902, Queen Victoria had requested a Royal Commission into the 'Care and Treatment of the sick and wounded during the South African campaign' (24 July 1900).[33] Sir Frederick Treves was a surgeon of great renown who gave *...sensitive treatment...* to Joseph Merrick (known as 'The Elephant Man') who suffered from neurofibromatosis.[34] Treves was a member of the committee who considered the recommendations of the Royal Commission. He commended the service of the nurses, members of Princess Christian's Army Nursing Service Reserve, during the South African War; their *...ministrations to the wounded were invaluable and beyond all praise. They did a service during those distressful days which none but nurses could have rendered.*[35]

Queen Victoria died in 1901. King Edward VII succeeded her and his wife was previously Princess Alexandra of Denmark, reputedly one of the most beautiful women in Europe.[36] Queen Alexandra accepted the presidency of the reformed nursing service, an amalgamation of Princess Christian's ANSR and the Indian Nursing Service: in 1902 Queen Alexandra's Imperial Military Nursing Service (QAIMNS) was formed.

Queen Alexandra's Imperial Military Nursing Service (QAIMNS): 1902

A member of the QAIMNS is referred to as a 'QA' and in 1902 had to be civilian trained followed with three years' experience, between 25-35 years of age, of satisfactory 'social status' and have good reports from previous matrons. They were paid £37.10.00 in their first year with a £2 annual incremental increase until their salary reached £50 per annum; promotion was based on merit not seniority.[37] Uniforms consisted of grey dresses, muslin caps, grey outdoor bonnets and the important scarlet cape which Queen Victoria had bestowed on Florence Nightingale and her nurses when they returned from the Crimea.[38]

This was not a reserve but a service of elite, professional military nurses who served wherever the British Army was stationed. In 1902 the QAIMNS consisted of a matron-in-chief, two principal matrons (PMs), 27 matrons, 50 sisters and 150 nurses. They were needed in 27 hospitals throughout the Empire, including countries as far afield as Canada and Jamaica. The Royal Commission committee provided an *...extension of the powers of the Matron, of the Sisters and of the nurses in military hospitals.* The matron now had the authority to manage the hospital and also develop a syllabus of instruction for the Royal Army Medical Corps (RAMC) orderlies who were required to gain a nursing certificate.

In Britain two significant events occurred in 1907. The Territorial Army, accompanied by the Territorial Force Nursing Service, came into existence. The nursing service was later changed to Territorial Army Nursing Service and their members were referred to as 'TANS'. Eventually the QAIMNS Reserve (QAIMNSR) replaced the service which had provided personnel during the South African War.[39] In Australia, this prompted a review of Princess Christian's ANSR and by the time the First World War erupted there were numerous nursing and volunteer services which provided much needed nursing care on diverse war fronts.[40] An Australian nurse, Evelyn Vickers Foote (QAIMNSR and AANS) recalls working in Egypt during the First World War with a Territorial matron,...*Miss Newton (Territorial). She was a good sort. Discipline was strict. Doors locked at 9 p.m., but things were O.K., and we were well looked after.*[41] Indications are the calibre of the nurses in the various British and Australian nursing services was of a similar standard; civilian trained under the

Nightingale system.

The New Zealand Nursing Reforms

The contrast between the development of the NZANS and the AANS after the South African War was stark. The value of New Zealand nurses had been proved in the South African War but there was no foundation - no nursing reserve - from which to build an army nursing service. Janet Gillies (nee Speed) had served in the South African War and was outspoken about the need to create a nursing reserve in New Zealand. In 1908 the New Zealand Army Medical Corps Nursing Reserve was formed but recruitment was slow despite the best efforts of Gillies, a married woman, who was no longer practising as a nurse (which was a distinct disadvantage).[42]Unfortunately, the New Zealand Defence Bill, which was introduced into parliament on 2 December 1909, did not provide for the inclusion of the New Zealand Army Nursing Service (NZANS). The *...Bill was pushed through its three readings, its committee stages and signed into law...* in just under two weeks and only stipulated the need for four field ambulances in each military district (MD).[43]

Hester Maclean in New Zealand

Meanwhile, in November 1906, Hester Maclean was appointed the Assistant Inspector of Hospitals, New Zealand Department of Hospitals and Charitable Aid,) enabling her to further the reputation of New Zealand nurses. She claimed that New Zealand had *...the lowest infant mortality rate in the world...* because of the superior training of its midwives.[44] Unlike Gillies, Maclean did not have first-hand military nursing experience but she did have a position of some authority within the civilian profession. She never ceased to promote the importance of the qualified nurse and was the first president of the New Zealand Trained Nurses' Association. In 1908 Maclean became the founding editor of *Kai Tiaki* (The Guardian) and began to promote the need for a NZANS.[45] Just as Nightingale benefited from William Howard Russell's independent reporting of the Crimea Campaign, Maclean used nursing journals to encourage voluntary military service by civilian nurses during the South African War and First World War interregnum (1902-1914), thereby

creating a valuable reserve. From the time of her arrival in New Zealand with her friend Dr Agnes Bennett, Hester Maclean was decidedly a New Zealander.[46]
Viscount (later Earl) Herbert Horatio Kitchener, Commander-in-Chief of the British Forces in South Africa, visited New Zealand and Australia in 1910 to evaluate the state of the defences of both countries.[47] Maclean had, by this time, successfully manoeuvred herself into the consciousness of the higher echelons of the New Zealand military staff. When Kitchener recommended a defence scheme which included an *...army medical service and a nursing service...* this gave Maclean the impetus to push for a discrete military nursing service. Eventually, in September 1913, she was appointed the Matron-in-Chief of the New Zealand branch of the QAIMNS.[48] This result had two distinct aspects. The negative was that the NZANS was not yet a reality, which was in sharp contrast to the development of the AANS. On the positive side, a nurse had over-arching responsibility for the military nursing service in New Zealand.

6 Australian Army Nursing Service (AANS) 1902

... Often a Matron in Australia, found herself a Staff Nurse in the Army, under a Sister who had recently left her training school and perhaps only been a Sister for a year or less-
Nellie Gould

Eighteen months after federation, the separate nursing reserves in each of the colonies were officially combined to become the AANS on 1 July 1902. It was on this date that a general order circulated which changed colonial organisations to the Military Forces of Australia. The AANS replaced the army nursing reserves in the colonies but was still, in effect, a reserve and depended upon volunteers who were civilian trained and ATNA qualified nurses.

There were numerous personnel anomalies within the AANS which caused confusion, frustration and even anger during the First World War. Initially, the implementation of policy changes within the AANS was problem-free. However, the advent of war tested the theory of these changes. A serious barrier to the efficient operation of the AANS during the First World War was the failure of Surgeon-General Williams to appoint a nurse leader who had over-arching responsibilities for all MD. The AANS was divided into six MD which were aligned to the six Australian states: 1MD Queensland; 2 MD NSW; 3MD Victoria; 4MD South Australia; 5MD Western Australia; 6MD Tasmania. Unfortunately it took a period of administrative neglect during the first few years of war before it was decided to appoint an Australian Matron-in-Chief as the most senior nurse in the service in 1916.[1] Ironically, the much respected British Matron-in-Chief, (later Dame) Emma Maud McCarthy (1859-1949), was Australian born and while visiting Britain took up her training at London Hospital when she was 28 years old. Her record epitomises exceptional leadership in the South African War and the First World War.[2]

The structure of the AANS from 1903 included one PM and one matron for each MD plus a total of 96 sisters to be divided between the MD. Each State developed at different rates and in many ways was autonomous in the level of education and training provided to its reservists, but generally the level of personnel reflected the population base of the State.

The calibre of the nurses who were appointed to the senior AANS positions was justified during the First World War. While a number did not serve overseas because of their age, they provided important support services to their colleagues who did. For example, Hannah Elizabeth Glover, who trained at Winchester and Queen Charlotte Hospital, London, held a number of important positions in Victoria. She was also the Director of Residential Homes for Nurses and the Trained Nurses Club, and in 1902 she was appointed first joint secretary of VTNA. After training twenty-five AANS reservists she resigned as PM of 3MD in 1913, but three years later was a foundation member of the Edith Cavell Trust Fund which provided support for the First World War nurses on their return to Australia.[3]

Staff Nurses

Another serious personnel matter was the implementation of the 'staff nurse' (SN) position. The QAIMNS implemented this recommendation and Surgeon-General Williams followed the guidelines of the British without considering the variations in the civilian hospitals throughout Australia.[4] Although ATNA introduced recommendations for recognised training hospitals, there was no definitive, universal hierarchy of nurse rank. Some facilities had a 'staff nurse' position in place for recently qualified nurses, while other hospitals preferred the title of 'sister'. The title of 'sister' offered nurses kudos, and qualified ATNA nurses who had senior nursing positions within the civilian sphere found it demoralising to be referred to as a 'staff nurse' when they joined the AANS.[5] The AANS was a reserve for wartime emergencies, not a career path for military nurses like the QAs, who also provided nursing expertise to victims of peacetime catastrophes, such as earthquakes and tidal waves (Malta, 1908).[6] Gould recalled when the AANS changed in 1902 the ...*Lady Superintendent became a Principal Matron, otherwise no change*. However, she did concede the ... *idea of Staff Nurses was entirely new in Australia in the Army Nursing*

Service and it is due to the innate good breeding of the individual members of our service that we came through what was really an ordeal for so many equally qualified nurses ... Often a Matron in Australia, found herself a Staff Nurse in the Army, under a Sister who had recently left her training school and perhaps only been a Sister for a year or less.[7] Sister Haynes (AANS) concurred with this opinion. When writing to her mother she requested that she not ... *address the papers to Staff Nurse O. Haynes, but Sister. It is so galling to be addressed as a Staff Nurse when you are a Sister.*[8]

Orderlies

During the Crimean War a nurse claimed that orderlies were the ...*dregs of the army*... because they were ex-soldiers who preferred the safety of the hospital to the battlefield.[9] The reforms of the QAIMNS in 1902 included a policy under which it was ...*forbidden to accept presents of any kind from any patient.*[10] An incident in the Scutari hospital was particularly gruesome - a soldier patient went to his purse to pay an orderly for his assistance but when the orderly saw gold in the purse he attempted to take it. The patient resisted. The orderly struck him on the head and killed him with one blow. The orderly was tried and hanged for his crime, but it demonstrated the capricious nature of hospital life during the Crimean War.[11]

There was some improvement in the South African War but Sister Anderson from Victoria thought ...*the orderly system is not by any means to be commended. The men who take this work up are not as a rule of sufficient training or education to appreciate, as a trained nurse can, the gravity of the work.*[12] Reforms to the QAIMNS addressed the matter of education and training of orderlies but the AANS did not. However, during the First World War, Matron Kellett preferred the QAIMNS system of control over the orderlies and observed that a ... *Matron's position is co-equal with the C.Os. in an R.A.M.C. Hospital, and one thing which impressed me, and which I think we might cop in our Australian Hospitals, is that the Matron has control of the orderlies. To me it was a great ad-vantage being able to post the Nursing orderlies just to the wards I thought them most suited for.*[13] This change became the norm in Australian civilian hospitals after the war.

Voluntary Aid Detachment (VAD)

The Voluntary Aid Detachment (VAD) was a territorial association which acted through branches of the Red Cross and was ostensibly conceived in Britain by Surgeon General Sir Alfred Keogh. However, his notion that the VAD would be constituted by a group of ...*charwomen, maidservants, labourers*... was soon put to rest by the interest and determination of a cross-section of talented women and men. The VADs were launched in Britain in 1909 and by the time the war commenced 50,000 people had joined to serve as stretcher-bearers, cooks, drivers and nurse assistants.[15]
Initially, there was resentment towards VAD nurses by members of the AANS and the QAIMNS and this was further compounded if a VAD managed to circumvent the authority of the matron. This tended to occur when a woman of high social status became a VAD nurse and endeavoured to use her civilian influence within the war setting - often creating administrative complications for those trying to keep the activities of innovative women in check. However, the tireless work of VADs during the war became recognised and generally accepted by hospital staff and they were an important component of the staff establishment.

Vera Brittain left her studies at Oxford to reluctantly take up VAD nursing when her fiancé joined the Army. She quite openly acknowledged in a letter that ...*I shall hate it, but I will be all the more ready to do it on that account*. She told her diary he ... *has to face far worse things than any sight or act I could come across; he can bear it - so can I.* [16]
After the peace, the writings of Vera Brittain served to make the trials and contribution of a VAD nurse known to the wider community.

It was not unusual for an AANS nurse who married a soldier, and was subsequently discharged, to then join a voluntary community organisation and continue to nurse overseas. Controversy occurred when NZANS nurses, working in British hospitals, were obliged to resign on marriage and work as VADs who were not the responsibility of the military authorities. Nurses considered this a professional demotion which verged on an insult.[14]

Australian Red Cross Society

(Kathleen) Adele Brennan was the daughter of Mary Elizabeth and William Francis

Brennan, a prominent Sydney solicitor who had offices in Pendennis Chambers, George Street, during the war. Adele was sister to Florence Mary and William Keating Brennan; William enlisted in the 12th Australian Light Horse (ALH) Brigade in 1915 and was serving in Egypt when Adele left Australia in September 1916.[17] William may have been one of those soldiers who (when he innocently asked a qualified AANS nurse how his sister would go about joining) was treated to a stony response and pointedly informed that an AANS nurse had to complete ...*four years hard graff as a civilian hospital probationer and pass annual examinations.*[18]

Adele did what a number of unqualified women did during the war; she joined the Red Cross Society and became a VAD nurse.[19] Adele Brennan was one of thirty members of the Australian Red Cross Society who responded to an official request to provide staff for military hospitals in England.[20] She sailed from Sydney aboard the *Osterley* on 27 September 1916, Rania MacPhillamy who was determined to serve in Egypt to be near her fiancé, was also on board. Ronald Alexander (Ronnie) MacDonald hailed from a property (*Erudgere*) in the western districts of NSW and joined C Squadron, 1 ALH, with four of his mates from Mudgee early in the war. Ronnie was disappointed when he managed...*only the briefest glimpse...* of Rania on the wharf as he sailed away on the *Star of Victoria.*[623] Within a year he was worried ...*about how she would stand up to the heat, the filth and the dust of Egypt...* when she told him she had volunteered to work as a VAD at 2 Australian General Hospital (2 AGH), Ghezireh Palace.[21] Adele continued the voyage to England and was assigned for duty at 5 Northern Hospital, Leicester.

AANS Training

Apart from being ATNA qualified, the main difference between AANS personnel and VADs was the former also had basic military training. An AANS nurse in peacetime was required to ...*attend annually three out of the four lectures on Organization of Military Hospital, Hygiene, and Military Surgery...* and ...*qualify in first aid.* If the district principal medical officer (PMO) considered her competent, a certificate of efficiency was issued each year (1 July - 30 June).[22]

The level and type of instruction varied from State to State. For example, in 1903, nurses from Victoria (3 MD) attended lectures on topics such as AANS uniforms, pay rates and the delineation of roles in the Army. Examinations on subjects as varied as first aid, Army regulations, the role of Red Cross societies and the prevention of tropical diseases had to be passed. The Victorian AANS nurses were required to attend church and organise fund-raising events for soldiers. In contrast, AANS nurses from WA (5 MD) had a more intensive military experience when they spent one week in camp with troops during the winter months and attended lectures by military officers.[23] Principal Matrons of MDs were senior civilian nurses. They were able, albeit indirectly, to influence the education of AANS nurses in peacetime, which proved beneficial in wartime. For example, during the South African War, more soldiers died of disease than wounds.[24] This informed the ATNA curriculum.

Training in 'electricity and massage' proved to be of immense importance during the war and was a prelude to modern day physiotherapy. A working definition of massage in the 1950s claimed it was a *...scientific method of rubbing, kneading or stroking the superficial parts of the body...* and this in turn *...strengthens the muscles and stimulates the circulation of the blood.*[25] Ancillary massage treatments included the application of a heat lamp to decrease inflammation (thereby reducing pain) and 'electricity' which was used to stimulate muscles and nerves.[26] A number of ATNA nurses completed additional training in massage and held a massage certificate when they joined the AANS.[27]

Instruction in ophthalmic nursing was useful when soldiers suffering from the effects of mustard gas poured into the CCSs of France.[28] At first glance, lectures on paediatrics may appear to be of little value to a war nurse, although the youngest Australian soldier was only fourteen years old, but Australian nurses often found themselves in the midst of civilian tragedies.[29] Leela Brown (AANS) gave general and specialist care to the *...French civilians ranging in age from 3 months to that indescribable old age of the French peasant* ...who had become overnight refugees.[30]

Instruction in 'mental nursing' was part of the SHSEH training program from 1903 but was discontinued in 1911.[31] This was unfortunate for future military nurses who came face-to-face with tormented soldiers suffering from shell-shock. This term encapsulated a plethora of psychiatric conditions previously unknown to nurses.

7 Preparing for War

...approximately half of the 2,229 who served abroad were over thirty years of age
Rupert Goodman

When war was declared in August 1914, the only professional British nursing service, the QAIMNS, had 300 nurses in its ranks. The importance of the reserve, the QAIMNSR, was soon evident. Initially the QAIMNSR had 200 nurses who were deemed 'efficient' and another 600 who were available. By the end of the year, 2,223 civilian trained nurses had joined the QA Reserves, and when the war was finally over 10,404 nurses had passed through the ranks of the QAIMNSR.[1]
The situation was markedly different in Australia. In May 1914 there were forty AANS nurses who were considered to be 'efficients' who were part of the reserves and ready for active service in each MD. The first efficients were given the first chance of overseas service if and when a war was declared. One hundred ATNA qualified civilian nurses enlisted in the AANS and enlistments continued for the duration of the war.[2] The Official Medical Historian recorded the number of nurses who embarked for overseas service as members of the AANS were: 192 (1914); 549 (1915); 423 (1916); 791 (1917) and 176 (1918), bringing the total to 2,131 nurses.[3]. In 2011 an Army History Unit publication claimed at ... *least 2,286 – and possibly as many as 3,000 – AANS members served overseas.*[4] More recently others have asserted that about ... *5,000 Australian nurses are thought to have taken themselves to war...* but the truth lies somewhere in the middle.[5]

Statistics and Damned Lies

Over the past thirty years the author has cross-referenced the names of nurses with a service record (not all nurses who served have one) against the names of nurses mentioned by colleagues and patients in letters, diaries, photographs and newspaper articles. Obelisks in towns across Australia have been scanned for mention of a forgotten nurse, as have local museums. Official records are not a great source for identifying nurses who served. The author's final count is 2470 Australian nurses who served overseas during the First World War. The attached *Nominal Roll* differentiates between criteria for inclusion.

The names of nurses who served in India are included in the attached *Nominal Roll* because, despite India being an extremely debilitating theatre of war, it was considered to be 'home service' by the AIF. Therefore, the names of the nurses who served exclusively in India are not included in the Australian War Memorial Nominal Roll. Furthermore, ATNA qualified nurses like Jessie Dalgleish served as a VAD because she was unable to secure a position as a qualified nurse in any army service. John Edward Craig and Michael Frederick Hughes were two of seven ATNA qualified male nurses on the 1916 register. They were unable to join the AANS because of their gender and instead served with the AAMC.

Occasionally the names of nurses who are recorded on local obelisks and memorials throughout the towns and cities of Australia do not have an official record. Such a name may appear with an indication that she died during the war yet there is no record of her death on the commemorative or honour rolls of the Australian War Memorial; often they died outside the time guideline for inclusion on the Roll of Honour (4 August 1914 - 31 March 1921).[6] The primary sources of nurses have proved useful in identifying civilian colleagues whom they met up with on overseas active service but who are missing from all official sources. The 1916 ATNA register includes the names of nurses who were ...*on active service...* but were not on any official database. These nurses may have joined the British or allied Dominion nursing services or served in a voluntary capacity.

Enlistments

Australian nurses joined the AANS but were not considered to be part of the Army until they were called up for overseas service and signed their AIF attestation papers. A number of nurses were reluctant to wait for an opportunity to serve overseas with the AANS and elected to pay their own fares to England and join the

QA Reserves or even the Red Cross.[7] However, two nurses, May Dickson and Nora Kathleen Fletcher, who trained at the Coast Hospital, were in England when war was declared. Fletcher was invited to become matron of a *...northern English Hospital...* but declined the offer and eventually became the PM of the British Red Cross in France. Her service was remarkable and she was one of the most decorated Australian 1914-18 war nurses.[8]

The other Australian nurse, May Dickson, joined the QAIMNSR in England.[9] Born around 1880, she was thirty-seven when she finally returned to Australia after *...her health broke down...* due to the strain of the war. She did not reach her Sydney home because her condition deteriorated and she died *...of illness...* in Melbourne on 4 October 1917.[10] She has the distinction of being the first woman in Australia to be given a full military funeral but, sadly, was not the last. Sister Dickson was laid to rest at Coburg Cemetery, Victoria and although there is no record of her sacrifice with the QAIMNSR her name is recorded on the commemorative roll of the Australian War Memorial.[11] Irrespective of the uniform the sacrifice was the same.

In 1915 a newspaper appeal for Australian nurses to join the QAIMNSR resulted in 136 nurse's responses.[388] There is evidence that approximately 130 Australian nurses were either loaned to or recruited for service with the QAIMNSR. There are varying accounts from nurses about their experiences with the QAs but they were disappointed to find that their service was virtually unrecognised by Australian authorities. A number of Australian nurses who were living in England when war was declared joined the QAIMNSR or volunteer organisations such as the Red Cross and nine thousand trained or partially-trained nurses from the Empire served as VADs or orderlies in Britain.[12]

Australian nurses also joined USA Red Cross units and a number were members of the NZANS. The rationale for the decision of the Australian Government to come to a *...special arrangement...* with ten trained nurses from New Zealand who enlisted with the AANS is unclear.[13]There is some suggestion that a delay in the development of the NZANS prompted twelve New Zealand nurses to be sent to Sydney, where they were attached to the AANS in 1915.[14] They were included as *...additional to establishment...* to the staff of 1 and 2 AGH.[15]

Families of Nurses

To date, the author has identified seventy-five Australian families who had more than one daughter working as a military nurse during the First World War. The Lowrey family from NSW had four daughters involved in military nursing, while the Curtain family in Tasmania had four daughters in the AANS. It must be remembered that, apart from the large city-based hospitals, many Australian hospitals did not educate a high number of nurses. For example, the Western Suburbs Cottage Hospital had only eight graduands prior to 1913. Three of the eight served overseas with the AANS as well as another five who completed their training between 1914-17. The matron, Georgina Smith, was most likely prompted by her younger sister, Isobel Smith, to join the AANS. Unlike Isobel, Georgina was never called upon to serve overseas or in one of the many Australia based AGHs. It was fortunate that some competent and experienced nurses were not called upon to serve with the AANS, because they were needed in civilian hospitals.[16]

Identity and Uniforms

In many ways the design of the AANS uniform was as important to the nurses as the AIF uniform was to the Anzacs. Lieutenant A. T. White, an English clerk to General Birdwood, first used the acronym ANZAC when the Australian and New Zealand troops were still in Cairo, but the term did not gain common usage until after the landing at the Dardanelles.[17] Initially, the nurses of the AANS had two uniforms. The outdoor uniform was a long grey cape over a long grey dress and the head was covered with a small grey bonnet that had a chocolate bow and long silk tail. The ward uniform consisted of a long grey dress with starched collars and a stiff white apron plus a red or scarlet cape and a white veil. This was complemented with regulation footwear of laced walking shoes or boots and heavy black or grey stockings.[18]

The uniform design changed over the course of the four years but the scarlet cape remained. Australian nurses took great pride in their scarlet cape but it did cause occasional confusion for the British nurses who initially assumed every 'red cape' belonged to one of their elite QA Regulars.[19] British matrons had a *...great liking for Australian Sisters...* and had a sense of humour about the AANS uniforms, as one Australian nurse noted *...Miss Bleakley greeted us when we arrived jokingly by "here are the rival red capes"*.[20]

During wartime, uniforms were provided and an allowance was paid for their upkeep, being £16 per annum for maintenance or renewal, but the nurses often paid for the uniforms first and waited, sometimes in vain, for reimbursement.[21] When leaving for the front, AANS nurses were required to take *...one grey outdoor uniform, one grey outdoor cloak, two red capes, one outdoor bonnet, six linen collars, six cuffs, two pairs of ward shoes, one set of light underclothing, one set of heavy underclothing, one mackintosh, four white military caps, three grey indoor uniforms, four grey aprons, eight white aprons, one pair of wellington boots, one pair of galoshes, and one pair of lace up boots.*[22] The uniform was central to being identified as a 'military nurse' and it was important.

Elizabeth Rothery

One nurse who was keen to be identified as a military nurse was Elizabeth Rothery (AANS). Born in Hensingham, England, (circa 1882) her family migrated to Beechworth, but they later settled in nearby Myrtleford, Victoria (Ya-itma-thang tribe of Dhudoroa people) when she was about six years of age.[23] Elizabeth was one of a large family but three of her brothers died before reaching twelve months of age, creating an atmosphere of grief within the family. Norman, a younger brother born in Australia (1895), survived and, naturally, had a special place in the affection of his family.

Elizabeth attended a local primary school and later attended a private school at Beechworth. This was some distance from home so she boarded with a family friend, Miss Wilson. Initially she worked with her father in the general store until she decided to return to Beechworth and completed her training at the Ovens District Hospital, 1912. She later went to Melbourne where she successfully completed her midwifery certificate.

Elizabeth's father, Joseph, was a civic-minded man who approved of his children being part of the patriotic groundswell that overtook communities when war was declared. In November 1915, when Elizabeth was a private nurse at St Kilda, the family received the devastating news that Norman was KIA at Gallipoli. He was buried alive by shell fire, a cruel and all too common death. The local paper reported he was ...*buried with eight others. Poor, poor chap he rushed there for safety only to be trapped like a rat ... Poor little Rothery.*[24]

The death of a beloved brother did not deter Elizabeth from joining the war effort. . When she joined the AANS she was not immediately needed for overseas service so she continued to nurse in Australia. On 22 August 1916 she joined the AIF and saw service on troopships travelling between India, England and Australia.[25]

Salary and Conditions

During peacetime, AANS members did not receive a salary. The Standing Orders stipulated that ...*rates of pay and allowance for members of the Australian Army Nursing Service, when called up for duty, will be as laid down in Financial and Allowance Regulations*. There was provision for £1 per annum to be paid as a uniform allowance during peacetime.[26]

On 23 April 1915, Mary Stafford underwent a medical examination for admission to the AANS (4MD) and was found to be ...*in sound health, capable of doing hard work, and undergoing fatigue*. On acceptance into the AANS as a staff nurse she was offered payment of £60 per annum; a field allowance of 2/6 per day; free passage from and return to Australia; and a kit allowance of £15. The annual wage was on a par with the earning capacity of a civilian nurse at the time. For example ...*at Ballarat, from July 1915, all ward sisters earned £60 a year, instead of £52, after six months in their posts.*[27] The kit allowance meant the nurses had to purchase and provide their own uniforms, bed, bedding and mess furniture.[28]

The location of service had a bearing on whether the salary and allowances were adequate. For example, Staff Nurse Louisa Bicknell (AANS), who embarked on His Majesty's Hospital Ship (HMHS) *Kyarra* was paid 7/10 (7 shillings and 10 pence) per day en route to Egypt, which was sufficient funds to cover her expenses. Amy (Amelia Veda) O'Grady (AANS), a Catholic nurse from Melbourne, found the predominantly Hindu country of India was one of the most expensive placements for AANS nurses when she arrived in Bombay in 1916. Like many AANS nurses, she had assigned a small sum of her daily salary to be retained in Australia as savings but she soon realised that AANS nurses were financially disadvantaged in India at a number of levels. The caste system, which dominated Indian society, saw *...the performance of everyday tasks ...* as *... menial and simply lowers all white people in the eyes of the natives.* Therefore, Australian nurses were required to *...pay all manner of servants to do jobs they wished to do themselves.*[29] Given the nature of nursing, there were few 'menial' tasks that nurses could do without causing cultural offence. The AANS salary was paid and taxed by the Australian Government but initially was also taxed by the Indian Government.[30]

British nurses were able to take advantage of travel opportunities to Australia while stationed in India. For example, Sister TA (Muriel) Robertson (QAIMNSR) was given one month's leave in December 1918 to holiday in Australia following service in Calcutta. While on leave she resigned and the following month was given permission to remain in Australia. Unlike their QA colleagues, AANS personnel had to pay full transport costs, laundry charges and supply their own uniforms, as well as pay in excess of their mess allowance.[31]

Nearly five hundred AANS nurses served in India from 1916 to 1919 but many of this number also served in other campaigns.[32] The reason for this large and disproportionate number of Australian nurses in India and not in Mesopotamia, where the fighting was occurring, necessitated an investigation by the AIF into *...financial and other matters.* The inquiry found that *...in India the great part of the cost of nursing is borne by the Australian Government, which leaves the Indian Government only having to pay their own regulars and a very decreased number of Queen Alexandra Reserves in India.* After the war the Australian Government found it increasingly difficult to organise the timely return of AANS nurses to Australia which confirmed that *...the Indian Government depended on our nursing personnel for the effective persecution of the war in Afghanistan.*[33] This was a war in which Australia had no military involvement. Initially, Afghanistan was seen as a *...Muslim buffer state between British India and the Russian Empire...* and the control of the area was dependant on the authority of various Afghan tribesmen. Britain agreed to promote the post-war independence of Afghanistan in return for neutrality during the 1914-18 conflict. This pact was put at risk when the Ottomans joined the Central Powers because the religious affinity of Muslim Ottomans and Afghans was stronger than political alliances. Nonetheless, the Afghan leader, Amir Habibulla Khan *...maintained a generally peaceful balance of factional interests, and unrest on the Indian northwest frontier was restricted to minor local uprisings*. The British publicly affirmed Afghanistan's independence in early 1919 but Habibulla was assassinated in February and a decade of civil war followed.[34]

Officers and Gentlewomen

On 23 May 1916 orders were promulgated by the Director-General of Australian Army Medical Services, General Fetherston, stating AANS nurses were to wear badges of rank. A staff nurse, being the lowest rank, wore one star on each shoulder and was, in theory, equivalent to a second lieutenant but was paid as a private soldier. A sister wore two stars (lieutenant) and a PM or matron three stars (captain), while a Matron-in-Chief wore a crown - equivalent to a major - but was paid as a lieutenant.[35]

Matron Rose Creal in her SHSEH uniform and her AANS uniform provides a contrast between civilian and military attire. Her AANS uniform clearly shows three stars on the shoulder of her scarlet cape indicating that Creal held the rank of a captain. The system affording nurses the rank of officers was introduced in April 1916. Creal was a tall (169cm) woman who weighed 76 kg at the time of her enlistment in 1916. She has been described as a handsome woman and her dark complexion and her colouring (which was becoming grey by this stage) underscores her Irish background.[36.]

Age and Retirement Regulations

Rupert Goodman claims *...approximately half of the 2,229 who served abroad were over thirty years of age*.[37] This would be a safe approximation given that the early efficients were often senior nurses or matrons in civilian hospitals and were therefore older, more experienced and the first to serve overseas. For example, Rose Creal joined the

AANS in peacetime when the Standing Orders admitted nurses between the ages of twenty-one and forty years. Nurses could remain with the service until they retired at age forty-five, with a special provision for an extension not exceeding two years. These Standing Orders were modified during wartime by stating that AANS nurses had to be aged between twenty and forty-five years. Many senior nursing personnel were over forty-five when war was declared and they were already on overseas service when the standing orders were changed.[38] Even highly moral nurses like Rose Creal had to dance around the emerging policies. When she signed her AIF attestation papers on 14 August 1916 she claimed she was forty-nine, but when she was discharged in 1919 she was apparently only forty-five. In reality, Creal was born on 3 November 1865.[39]

The young entry age is also surprising because most hospitals preferred an entry age between nineteen and twenty-two for their trainees.[40] This varied considerably depending upon labour availability, and a number of later AANS recruits who trained from 1914 to 1918 were eager to serve as soon as they were ATNA qualified. Irene McPhail was one such eager recruit. She joined the staff of The Alfred, Melbourne, as a probationer and when she completed the three year course in 1917 she enlisted in the AIF on 8 November that year. Nonetheless, she was 24years old by that stage and it is difficult to imagine any AANS recruit, who had to be ATNA qualified, being eligible for the AANS by the age of twenty.[41]

Irene McPhail and the Impact of the Economic Downtown

The USA was developing into a nation built upon trade and banking, not heritage. Leaders of the American Civil War (1861-65) made use of technological advances such as breech-loading rifles, the telegraph, railroads and developments in ship design. The British considered the Americans to be indifferent to the upper classes and observed a lack of respect being afforded to the educated and wealthy.[42] In the USA, acquired wealth was deemed to be as socially legitimate as inherited wealth. The latter was still the mainstay of the British social hierarchy, but education and widespread literacy enabled other classes to question the wisdom of such a system.

The post-Civil War period witnessed a dramatic increase in the population base of the USA with fifty million people in 1880 increasing to seventy-five million by 1900. The exponential growth in consumer demand reaffirmed the capitalist base of the USA. However, the financial crisis of 1893 demonstrated that money alone does not assure the ambitious of power.[43] The gold-laden fields of Australia opened up new opportunities for prospectors from around the world.

In 1880 in the small rural town of Echuca, (Victoria, Yorta Yorta Country), an American butcher, James Junius McPhail, was initiated into the local Freemasons Lodge. He owned and operated his own butchery at Hare Street, Echuca, for twenty years but it is unclear why he resigned from the Freemasons in 1885. In 1887 James married Alice Maud Upton who was born in Sandhurst, Victoria (now known as Bendigo, Dja Dja Wurrung Country & Taungurung Country). Their firstborn daughter, Ida Maud (known as Maud), was born in Echuca in 1888 followed by another two daughters, Alice Mary in 1890 and Irene on 24 January 1893. The family was complete for a time.[44]

In the 1890s, Australia was in the grip of a severe drought, the world was enduring an economic depression and a number of Australians found themselves in dire circumstances.[45] James McPhail was one such person and in 1896 he sold the plant and rolling stock of his butchery.[46] A few months later, the family advertised for sale a number of elegant items, including *...splendid modern furniture, elegant Hapsburg piano, handsome drawing room suite...* along with more utilitarian items such as *...kitchen utensils and sundries.*[47] To compound an already difficult time, Alice McPhail became involved in a court case. The incident centred on the alleged theft of two gold bracelets (valued at £14) from Alice on 20 May 1896 when she boarded a train to Bendigo, where her husband was working as a butcher. At the time of the theft a labourer earned 15 shillings per week so the stolen gold bracelets represented the equivalent of five months' gross salary for an unskilled male.[48] The jewellery had never been advertised and Alice McPhail was taking her worldly possessions to Bendigo to join her husband. The alleged thief, a woman, was subsequently arrested and brought to trial.[49]

The family had fallen on hard times financially and endured a peripatetic existence. For example, in September 1898, James McPhail was working as a butcher at

Deniliquin, (NSW, Yorta Yorta Country), when he *...fell on a sharp hook, severely lacerating his arm from elbow to wrist.*[50] A few months earlier in February his eldest daughter, Maud, who was 10 years old at this stage, was living temporarily with Mr and Mrs Stickels of Shepparton, (Victoria, Yorta Yorta Country) and her parents were residing in the Elmore district (Yorta Yorta Country). One Saturday night in February, Maud, who was in the house in the company of a 16-year-old girl, *...was placing a kettle on the fire when her dress became ignited and she became enveloped in the flames almost instantly*. The poor child finally received medical attention from a local doctor at midnight but she died at 2am Sunday from the *...fearful injuries.*[51] The pain, shock and dehydration would have been sufficient to cause the little girl's death, which was no doubt more catastrophic owing to the absence of her parents. A year after her death, a son, Donald James, was born to Alice and James.[52]

Many Australians tramped vast distances to find work during the depression. Dependence on the generosity of family and friends, who often provided short-term care and accommodation for children, was not uncommon. Irene McPhail grew up during a period of familial and social instability which was reflective of Australia at the time. Irene's sister, Alice, opted for teaching, while Irene joined the staff of The Alfred, Melbourne, as a probationer. Irene now had a home.

Contrasting Wars

The South African War confirmed the worth of the civilian trained Australian nurse in a military hospital. Reforms to the QAIMNS and consequently its Reserve had a positive impact on the development of the AANS following Federation. Leaders of the British Army, Kitchener in particular, were aware of the value of a reserve of soldiers and a reserve of nurses to care for them. It was fortuitous that civilian nurses, influenced by matrons like Gould, who had seen service in the South African conflict, developed complementary policies with ATNA and the AANS.

However, the First World War was a different beast to the South African War. The ferocity of fighting causing horrific wounds and the involvement of so many countries over four years was unexpected. They had little idea of what lay ahead of them on troopships, in tropical outposts, desert hospitals or freezing CCS. In the beginning it was their family, their community, their colleagues, their country which motivated them to go. In the end it was their respect and love of the Australian soldiers plus camaraderie within the AANS which sustained so many for so long.

8 Feminism and AANS Leadership

... approached her parents about her pursuing a university education but her father did not want his daughter to become a "blue stocking" - J. Horsfield

The social histories of nurses who became leaders during the 1914-18 war provide a backdrop to cultural changes in Australia. The nurse leaders who emerged before and during the war had diverse backgrounds. To gain entry into an ATNA approved training program they had to be literate and numerate, but to complete the extensive schedule of work, training, examinations and social responsibilities which were expected of probationers they had to be extremely well disciplined. However, to follow this up with policy reforms in education, training and ultimately military nursing demonstrates that they are not only remarkable nurses, but remarkable women.

Jane Bell (1873-1959): Origins

Jane Bell was a remarkable woman and an extraordinary nurse leader. On the one hand she was a loyal advocate for nurses and on the other a strict, some may say unfeeling, disciplinarian. She was respected by some male medicos and loathed by others. It is not possible to discern what type of woman she was merely by reciting all of her achievements. Her young life was dramatically affected by tuberculosis (TB) despite never suffering from the disease herself. Tuberculosis is known by a number of names including TB, phthisis or consumption and will be henceforth referred to as TB. The tubercle bacilli (a rod-shaped bacterium) enters the lungs (via infected sputum, droplets in the air, contaminated eating utensils) or the digestive tract (via unpasteurised milk or other dairy products from infected cattle) but may spread to other areas of the body (miliary tuberculosis) via the blood.[1] A large family living in cramped conditions, whose diet most likely included unpasteurised milk, was particularly susceptible to the disease.

Jane Bell was born into such a family at Middlebie, Dumfriesshire, Scotland in 1873 and was one of William and Helen Bell's eight children. While she attended a small local school her father supported his large family by working the land. Catastrophe struck when, in quick succession, four of the children and Jane's parents died from tuberculosis. The parents and siblings of Jane Bell most likely succumbed to what was commonly called *...galloping consumption...*originating as *...a feverish cold ...terminates in a broncho-pneumonia ... which rapidly involves the lung tissue and shows no tendency to clear up...* and results in death.[2] Prior to research into and the development of antibiotics, the treatment for TB was very limited. After the Second World War, streptomycin, isoniazid and para-aminosalicylic acid (PAS) either singularly or in combination improved outcomes for TB patients.[3]

It was not unusual for the local community to take responsibility for children in this situation but *...normally the parish looked after orphans by boarding them out in the village*. For example, in 1806 a similar incident occurred near the village of Grasmere in the Lakes District of England where the poet (later Poet Laureate) William Wordsworth lived with his wife Mary and his sister Dorothy. An accident resulted in the death of a local couple who left behind six children aged fourteen years and under. The Wordsworth family organised a subscription fund to augment the parish resources which *...enabled the children to be well educated, placed in good positions and able to earn their own living when they grew up.*[4] Some 80 years later, in a village not too distant from Grasmere, Jane Bell and her siblings were offered the same chance by their community, but their placements were on the other side of the world.

In 1886, Jane, her brother and two sisters migrated to NSW with the assistance of the local Presbyterian parish.[5] The reason for sending Jane (who was just thirteen years of age) and her siblings to Sydney is unclear.[6] Sydney was a mass of social and political contradictions; a colony at a crossroads. The uneasy coexistence of diverse groups including those with convict ancestors, the 'new moneyed' from gold discoveries, the British ruling class, bushmen and city dwellers, farmers and factory workers created an atmosphere of tension. There is little doubt that a *...catastrophic* *contest between wealth and want, poverty and privilege...* was underway when young Jane arrived.[7] To compound the family's tragedy, Christine Bell, one of Jane's two remaining sisters, also died of TB on arrival in Australia; she is buried in the old Liverpool Cemetery near Sydney (Gandangara Country).[8]

Jane Bell's Early Career

Nursing was hard physical work but it offered women like Jane Bell and her sole remaining sister, Euphemia, an opportunity to be independent.[9] Jane Bell commenced her training at RPAH in 1894 when she was twenty-one and Euphemia undertook her training at SHSEH. Entry into a training course was cut-throat, with six hundred applicants for twenty to thirty nursing positions at SHSEH at the end of the nineteenth century.[10] A year after Jane Bell completed her three years of training on 7 February 1898, ATNA was founded, she successfully passed the ATNA examination and was registered on 8 September 1899.[10] She passed all her examinations with distinction, was awarded prizes in two successive years, and gained a reputation for administrative competence, becoming the first RPAH housekeeping sister.[11] Despite having excellent professional attributes, during the early stages of her nursing career Bell appears to have had difficulty acquiring positions. This is surprising because, in theory, she had a number of positive elements which would have impressed prospective employers.

Susan McGahey, her training matron, was a well-respected nurse leader and she provided Bell with a glowing reference. Bell was described as an excellent nurse, kind but firm in her management of the patients, painstaking and most persevering.[12] However, Bell did not have family connections in Sydney, which may have proved a disadvantage. However, between 1898 and 1902, Euphemia was matron of Bundaberg Hospital (Qld, Taribelang Bunda, Gooreng Gooreng, Gurang and Bailai Country). She vacated the position, as was the custom, when she married in April 1902. Nepotism apart, Jane took over from her sister and retained the position for two years. Her career was on the rise in September 1904, when she was appointed matron of the much larger and prestigious Brisbane General Hospital (Qld, Turrbal & Yuggera Country).[13] Present-day Royal Brisbane and Royal

Women's Hospital and henceforth referred to as RBWH. Jane Bell was matron of RBWH for a short period (1904-06). During her matronship Grace Wilson, a future military and civilian nurse leader of note, was in training (1905-07).[14] Bell had an excellent working relationship with the medical superintendent, Dr J. B. McLean, and was considered a competent, efficient and effective nurse leader. However, both nurses realized they needed additional qualifications. In the early years of the twentieth century, childbirth was considered a natural event and did not always require the attendance of a doctor or midwife. However, the discovery of gold in remote parts of the colonies resulted in women being isolated from medical care and there was a growing demand for nurses to become competent midwives.

Jane Bell's Further Education

The Australian nurse leaders who implemented the ATNA standards encouraged senior nurses to gain an additional nursing certificate, midwifery being the most common. Jane Bell was ambitious and she left Brisbane to become a student once more. She sailed to England where she completed four months of midwifery training at Queen Charlotte's Lying-in Hospital, London, on 4 February 1907.[14] Queen Charlotte (Sophia) was the wife of King George III. The Hospital was established in 1739 and continues to serve as a midwifery hospital, making it the oldest maternity hospital in England. After completing her midwifery training, Bell returned to her Scottish homeland and was employed as Senior Assistant Lady Superintendent (Deputy Matron) of Nurses at the Royal Infirmary of Edinburgh. During her three-year tenure at the Royal Infirmary she failed to secure a number of leadership positions in Ireland and London.[15]

The Board of the Melbourne Hospital sought overseas candidates for the most senior nursing position. The assumption that overseas qualified nurses were superior to Australian nurses was not uncommon at this stage. There was great respect for the Nightingale system but confidence in locally-trained nurses was not as high as for those who trained in Nightingale's country of origin. In many ways the First World War enabled the Australian-trained nurses to stand side-by-side with their overseas counterparts. During these four harsh years the worth and quality of the Australian nurse training system was confirmed.[16] Bell returned to Australia to take up the lady superintendent (matron) position of the Melbourne Hospital on 26 September 1910.

Grace Wilson (1879-1957)

Grace Wilson was born in the colony of Queensland on 25 June 1879 in South Brisbane and, like Jane Bell, she was of Scottish ancestry.[17] The religion of the Wilson family is not clear. However, Grace Wilson was buried at Christ Church, South Yarra which is today described as a *...progressive catholic Anglican parish which values Liturgy, Scripture, Reason, and inclusive Community...* and is part of the Anglican Church of Australia, Diocese of Melbourne.[18] Grace was the eldest of six children and her parents John and Fanny were sufficiently prosperous to enable her to attend Brisbane Girls Grammar School, although John's occupation as a 'clerk' indicates he would have worked hard for his success. Grace had two sisters and three brothers, Norman (1885), Roy (1887) and Graeme (1890).[19] She was known by her family as 'Gay' but always as 'Grace' within the nursing profession.

Little is known about what she did after she left school and before she commenced her training, aged twenty-six. During her training Wilson was consistently awarded excellent marks which culminated in her receiving the first gold medal for overall marks during the three-year course (December 1907).[20]

Grace Wilson left Australia to commence her midwifery training at Queen Charlotte's Hospital in the same year that Jane Bell graduated there as a midwife. Once qualified, Wilson acquired several years post-qualification experience in England at the National Hospital for the Paralysed and Epileptic (Albany Memorial) in London. One of the greatest achievements for a nurse was to be matron of her training hospital; Wilson returned to Queensland to take up the matronship of RBWH in July 1914 just one month before the First World War was declared.[21]

Eleanor Harvey in Western Australia

It was not until 1907 that a WA branch of ATNA was formed. Senior nursing positions in WA were filled by ATNA-qualified nurses who had trained in other States. Eleanor Harvey, the daughter of a doctor, was ATNA qualified in 1911 after training at the Perth Public Hospital.[22] Once she completed her training she became a theatre nurse but her interest and expertise lay elsewhere.[23] Harvey travelled to Dublin, Ireland and completed midwifery with honours at the Rotunda. The Rotunda is a world renowned centre for midwifery and a number of AANS nurses trained there, including one of Harvey's training colleagues, Kathleen McAleer.[24] On completion of her training Harvey gained valuable labour ward experience for about a year and then joined the staff of the Kent Fever Hospital. The importance of infection control by midwives was paramount due to the high mortality rate of mothers and babies from maternal infection (puerperal fever) and neonatal infections.

Harvey returned to Australia when her father was ill and her extensive education and experience resulted in her appointment *...by the government in April 1916 ... to the position of first Matron of the Fumitory or Industrial School in Barker Road Subiaco which was made available as a Maternity Hospital*. Eleanor Harvey was instrumental in transforming this makeshift maternity hospital in the Perth suburb of Subiaco into a specially designed facility for midwifery, the King Edward Memorial Hospital (KEMH). Opened on 16 July 1916, Harvey, an ATNA council member by this stage, ensured the KEMH met the standard for registration as an ATNA obstetric training school.[25]

ATNA and Obstetrics

The most distant colony from the east coast was the vast area of WA. Originally a small convict settlement the swathes of minerals, including gold, were soon uncovered bringing hordes of prospectors to the area. In reality, the women in rural and remote mining districts were attended by untrained midwives until ATNA introduced compulsory midwifery registration in 1913. The midwifery course included a six-month residence plus lectures for ATNA-qualified nurses. However, confusion reigned when untrained women were allowed to complete a twelve 12 month residence plus lectures. A training fee of ten guineas was charged to these pupil midwives and they did not receive any salary.[26] This 'privatisation' of nurse education caused a great deal of confusion and anger in the profession. In theory, the rules prohibited non-ATNA qualified nurses from attending to women during confinement except in an emergency. To become registered they had to successfully complete a course of midwifery at an approved ATNA midwifery training hospital. The private education of non-ATNA qualified midwives was compounded when the ATNA/RVTNA was established. For instance, despite her education and experience, Harvey had to successfully complete the ATNA midwifery examination before her name appears in the Obstetric Register on 14 June 1916 because she had only completed four months midwifery training, not six. Jane Bell resented being asked to sit the exam. She was prone to outrage, and resigned from the Council of the RVTNA in 1913 because the rules allowed nurses with *...a six months certificate from small Australian hospitals with a daily average of five occupied beds...*to be registered. However, nurses like her, who had successfully completed four months of midwifery in a world-renowned British hospital, were not.[27] While Harvey complied with the new rules by sitting the examination, Jane Bell would not.

Jane Bell and the Melbourne Hospital

Bell's initial leadership at the Melbourne Hospital was during a period of rapid change but she was not involved in the planning phase. This proved to be somewhat complicated for Bell, and no doubt, the builders. Bell relished involvement in the minutiae of decisions about things such as the size of sinks, shelving, floors, lighting, wards and the water supply; all of which are extremely important for the nurses. This was no small rebuild though. The ambitious project included a new hospital which was expected to occupy ten blocks in the centre of Melbourne. It was a state-of-the-art facility including all the mod cons such as electric automatic lifts, telephone systems, a new laundry and—something of an innovation for this time—an electric clock system to ensure uniform time throughout the hospital. The building project took from August 1913 until 1915 and it was not until 1916 that the Annual Report noted that it was completely finished and all building operations had come to an end.[28]

When Bell arrived at the Melbourne Hospital in 1910 the nurses' living quarters were described as 'Rat's Land.' Nurses worked tirelessly and then had to endure appalling living conditions when they did finally manage a few hours off duty. Bell insisted improvements in the nurses' home be incorporated in the new building. Bell was well aware of the benefits of the role of a Housekeeping Sister as this position had been introduced at RPAH when she was there. A qualified nurse had responsibility for the well-being of nurses when they were off duty.[29] Her reputation for demanding a disciplined nursing staff and her advocacy for the welfare of her staff were not incongruous. The nurses were not units of labour to her but the future standard-bearers of the profession, and (like those before them), they would in turn teach the next generation of Australian nurses. Nurses had to respect each other if the profession was to be assured of community respect.

Nursing Reforms at the Melbourne Hospital

It is difficult to know whether Bell's early life affected her future relationships. For example, on her arrival in Australia she was sponsored by the Presbyterian Church in Sydney and was *...put to service...* in doctors' homes.[30] Therefore, from the age of thirteen she was in a subservient role within a family home of medical practitioners. Despite her positive experience with the medical superintendent at Brisbane Hospital, Bell was plagued with resistance to her nursing reforms from the medical hierarchy. Coincidently, on 13 September 1910, two weeks before Bell's arrival, Dr William Moore, a long-standing and much respected surgeon resigned for unclear reasons. The board approached him to reconsider and withdraw his resignation, but he refused.

Within two years of Jane Bell becoming matron at the Melbourne Hospital, she persuaded the hospital committee to introduce female nurses to the operating theatre. She proposed a tutor sister be appointed in the theatre so the trainee nurses could gain supervised experience in their first year.[31] Bell received support from the hospital committee because they could see financial savings in the plan, which was introduced for a twelve month period. It was very successful and other training hospitals adopted it.[32] Surgical trainee nurses were instructed in operating theatre procedures and became proficient in assisting surgeons and anaesthetists.[33] This demonstrated a great deal of foresight on the part of Bell because these same operating theatre nurses were, in a few short years, assisting surgeons in CCSs and in makeshift theatres on hospital ships, repairing the damaged bodies of soldiers who had been wounded.

Suffrage

South Australia was the first colony to be settled by free settlers and the only colony where all women and men were given voting rights in 1894. After Federation on 1 January 1901, The Commonwealth Franchise Act 1902 gave Australian non-indigenous adult women the right to *...vote for and stand for the federal parliament in all states.*[34] All Australian States introduced women's suffrage, with Victoria being the last in 1905. During the First World War Australian-born women of *...British nationality who had married certain classes of aliens...*were not permitted to vote. Compulsory voting at Commonwealth General Elections was introduced in 1925.

The Labor Party moved to have the voting age of twenty-one years reduced to eighteen years in 1919 (given that soldiers who died were not old enough to vote on issues such as conscription) but it was not until 1943 that the Curtin (Labor) Government gave the vote to servicemen serving overseas during the war and for six months afterwards.[35]

It was not until 1962, following a successful referendum, that all indigenous men and women could exercise their right to vote. In this year the Menzies (Liberal) Government gave voluntary voting rights to Indigenous Australians. However, in 1984, the Hawke (Labor) Government made the Indigenous vote compulsory, in line with all Australian citizens.[36]

Rania MacPhillamy

Despite Australia being one of the first countries in the world to give women voting rights, many families were fearful of their daughters being too educated. For example, Rania MacPhillamy was the daughter of a wealthy property owner in western NSW and three of her brothers were sent to board at the prestigious Sydney Church of England Grammar School (known as Shore). She persuaded her father to send her to Ascham, but after two years (1905-07) and despite being a *...gifted student* *of literature and languages...* she was recalled home to attend to family responsibilities. Ascham was a progressive girls' school which offered matriculation classes *...but few parents wished to see their daughters extend their education to this level.* One of Rania's inspired teachers, Amy Molineaux, approached her parents about her pursuing a university education but her father did not want his daughter to *...become a* "blue stocking".[37] A reference to the literary salons hosted for intellectual women in the eighteenth century where fashionable silk stockings were shunned for more practical blue, knitted stockings.

Margaret Graham (1860-1942): Suffrage in South Australia

There is little known about the origins of Margaret Graham except that she was the daughter of a self-employed house painter, John Graham, and his wife Margaret (nee Farrer). She was born on 5 February 1860 in Carlisle, England and commenced as probationer at the Adelaide Hospital on 2 April 1891.[38] As previously noted, she was instrumental in the development of the RBNA, but early on in her career she had a significant impact on South Australian politics.[39] She was appointed charge nurse on 22 October 1894 and two months later, on 18 December 1894, legislation was enacted giving all men and women of South Australia, including indigenous men and women, the right to vote; making South Australia the second place in the world, NZ being the first, to give universal suffrage. However, Graham's name and the names of two other senior charge nurses are the only ones to appear on a petition in support of women's suffrage from the Adelaide Hospital. [40] Graham was dismissed from her position for insubordination on 15 February 1895 and she and another signatory were soon embroiled in a chain of events which escalated into a Royal Commission into the hospital's administration.

Nepotism at the Adelaide Hospital

There is little doubt that Margaret Graham was a 'blue stocking' and she exhibited no deference to men if she believed their behaviour to be unjust. When the sister of the colony's Chief Secretary Sir J H Gordon, was appointed to the position of night nurse superintendent, many charge nurses believed she was not the most qualified applicant. One charge nurse, Louise Hawkins, requested an independent inquiry by South Australia Premier C.C.Kingston into the promotion of Nurse Gordon. There were five other signatories to this request including Margaret Graham. Following a great deal of correspondence, Nurse Gordon's appointment was confirmed and the hospital board suspended Nurse Hawkins. The six charge nurses who were co-signatories to the Hawkins letter were asked to retract their statements; five did but Margaret Graham refused, resulting in her dismissal on 4 March 1895.

Graham proved to be a more dangerous individual outside the hospital environment than she was within it as she became an unrestrained critic. Eventually, due to her continued outspokenness on the matter, the hospital's medical superintendent offered her nursing positions with other hospitals; Margaret Graham publicly interpreted this as *...bribes for silence.* A Royal Commission into the incident recommended her reinstatement to the Adelaide Hospital in April 1896. Following Graham's reappointment as charge nurse, the matron, medical superintendent and the full complement of honorary medical staff, the colony's Chief Secretary and ultimately the entire hospital board resigned or were dismissed over the matter.[41]

Dr William Ramsay Smith accepted a position at the Adelaide Hospital during the industrial dispute, which prompted the British Medical Association (BMA) to question his professionalism and his honour.[42] He was one of two overseas doctors; *...Dr Ramsay Smith ... taking charge, with Dr Russell medical superintendent.*[43] As a coroner, Ramsay Smith was involved with research which resulted in the theft of 300 human remains belonging to the Ngarrindjeri people. His behaviour was considered to be unethical and he was suspended as the South Australian Coroner in 1903 for breaching the *Anatomy Act* (1884).[44] During the First World War he caused further controversy which resulted in the termination of the military career of one of Australia's more competent nurse leaders, none other than Jane Bell.

Margaret Graham was a serious political player and it was not long before she was appointed matron, a position she held with great distinction for more than twenty years (1898-1920). Graham was also committed to the AANS reserve during peacetime and was the serving PM (4 MD) when war was declared. When Graham left for overseas service she was replaced as PM by Ethelda R. Uren who held the post until she sailed for Salonika (the British name for Thessalonika) in 1917.[45]

Nellie Miles Walker: Tasmania

Jean Nellie Walker joined the AANS in 1906 and was appointed PM of 6 MD three years later. Another nurse from Tasmania also enlisted, Jean Roberto Walker.[46] PM Jean Nellie Walker added her father's middle name (Alfred Miles Walker) to her surname and used her middle name as a first name. Therefore, Jean Nellie Walker, born 16 November 1878 at River Forth (now known as Forth) near Port Sorrell in northern Tasmania (Palawa Country), daughter of Alfred Walker and his wife Louisa Walker, became known as Nellie Miles Walker (AANS). [47]

The family life of Nellie Miles Walker was not a typical. Within eleven years of their marriage Louisa and Alfred had nine children, including one set of twins, Alfred Miles and Nellie Ada, born in 1874. Alfred died at three years of age and a year later their last child, Jean Nellie, was born. Alfred Miles (Snr) died when Jean Nellie was just three years of age, leaving Louisa a widow with eight children aged between three and fourteen years.[48] There is no evidence that Nellie Ada also died but the use of her first name as Jean's middle name is suggestive.

Jean Nellie was privately educated until she enrolled at the Collegiate School in Hobart (1893). In 1906 she completed a three-year nurse training course at the Hobart General Hospital and joined the AANS the same year. She remained with her training hospital until 1908 when she began private nursing, a popular career choice at the time. In 1913 she completed six months' midwifery training at the Women's Hospital, Melbourne, and then served as matron of private hospitals at Tallangatta, Victoria and Darlinghurst, Sydney.[49]

The emergence of a nursing profession brought with it female leaders who not only saw an opportunity to improve working conditions for nurses but to also add their voice to women's rights more generally.

9 The not so Ordinary AANS Nurses

...great many of the prominent and successful men we hear about to-day would never have achieved such success had it not been for the excellent wives they had – H V Thorby

When war was declared in 1914 Australia was inhabited by men and women from a variety of geographic and social backgrounds. Some had successfully weathered the transition from colony to nation during an economic downturn. Many on the land were learning, the hard way, that the vast country was not only a source of mineral wealth and agricultural promise, it was also a land *...of drought and flooding rain...* and could not be tamed.[1] Nurses and soldiers who served in the First World War were an eclectic mix of personalities and characters. The quintessential Australian character stemmed from the collective social histories of those who served and those who stayed at home. Nurses and soldiers found a new home with their units, nursing or fighting.

Mary Stafford nursing in South Australia

Mary Florence Stafford was born in Nyngan (NSW, Wongaibon, Ngemba, Ngiyampaa & Weilwan Country) in 1891. Tragically, Mary and her sister were orphaned when she was just three years of age following the death of her parents, Charles and Lucy.[2] They were raised by their aunt, Miss Mackereth who remained unmarried, in Goodwood, a suburb of Adelaide.[3] Employment opportunities for a woman in Miss Mackereth's situation were already limited but taking on the care of two very young children who had no financial legacy was an act of extraordinary kindness and an indicator of personal strength. Correspondence suggests that Mary Mackereth loved her charges as if they were her own children.[4]

Mary Stafford made a sound financial and professional decision when she applied to start her training at the Adelaide Hospital. There can be little doubt that she had received a satisfactory education, possibly from her aunt, otherwise she would not have been accepted as a probationer in one of the more prestigious Australian training hospitals. Mary commenced her nurse training in 1911, completing four years at the Adelaide Hospital which was a registered ATNA training school since 1907. However, there was a slight variation in subjects because of Margaret Graham's preference for the RBNA, but *...the two syllabi included similar material.* Mary grew up in a female-dominated household and Margaret Graham had a significant influence on the women she trained.[5] During the course of the training Mary obtained first class certificates of efficiency in medical and surgical nursing. She was twenty-four years of age when she completed her three-year nursing course and once qualified, joined the RBNA.[6]

Doris Ridgway nursing in South Australia

The family life of Doris Ridgway was vastly different to that experienced by her Adelaide Hospital colleague, Mary Stafford. On 10 March 1887 the Reverend John Jones married Ada Mitton and Arthur John Samuel (known as John) Ridgway at the Hindmarsh Congregational Church, South Australia. Ada Mitton, the daughter of a grocer, grew up in Hindmarsh. Her parents were remembered as *...extremely nice gentlefolk...* by their grandson (aged 73 years old when interviewed) who recalled *...the wonderful aroma of grandfather's shop with its grocery bins and shelves laden with unadulterated spices, coffee and herbs, also smoked ham and bacon in quantity.* John Ridgway was from a farming family at *Tooriarra,* Salters Springs near Hamley Bridge (Ngadjuri Country) and during the first dozen or so years of their marriage Ada and John made a home for their fast-growing family in the Salters Springs district. They had ten children within the first thirteen years of their marriage - three daughters and seven sons.

Doris, who was known within the family as Dorrie, was the fourth, born on 13 November 1891. Sadly the ninth child, Arthur, was born and died in 1899. He lived just a few weeks and Ada *...right to her last days spoke wistfully of him and wished they could have saved him.* In 1900 when another son was born, Ada and John may have felt confident their family was complete, but in 1908 another daughter, Jean, was born. So they had ten living children, but the gap that Arthur's early death brought remained in the hearts of his parents.[7]

The selection of land by those who claimed to have farming experience was a matter of government policy. Nonetheless, the maximum amount of land allocated to any one settler was limited to 320 acres (*Land Act 1869*) so families often selected adjoining blocks to improve the economies of scale. This arrangement did not always work effectively at a practical level.[8] While Doris and the older children grew up at Salters Springs, there was a drastic change in the family's circumstances around 1900 due to a financial problem/misunderstanding with her father's family. The result was the loss of their property, which included their family home. John, Ada and their children moved to Hindmarsh and lived with Ada's parents for a short period while John re-established himself financially.

Eventually John and Ada managed to secure a dairy property in the Fulham district, where the family stayed for a number of years. Doris spent her very early teenage years doing the chores considered normal for a young woman during this era, such as helping her mother deal with washing, cooking, raising chickens, cleaning and the general education of the younger children. Unfortunately the dairy farm was not a success and the family moved again this time to the Grange area where the younger children enjoyed the close proximity of the sea.

Doris with her brothers and sisters attended school at the Grange before the family made another move to Woodville, where John worked for one of his brothers. Finally John and Ada's luck changed in 1906 when the government sub-divided a government land holding and they were allotted a block of scrub land at Brooks Plains, about eighty miles south-east of Adelaide. The land was cleared and a living was made from hay and wheat crops. In 1909-10 a permanent home was erected, it consisted of *...seven rooms and though no mansion, was very comfortable.* The industriousness of the family is apparent a few years later the farming enterprise continued to grow when two additional properties were purchased, taking the holding to about 4,000 acres.[9]

By this stage Doris was in her early 20s and she, along with older members of her family, begun to make her own way towards an independent life. The women of the family took up vocations that were acceptable for the times, such as marriage, nursing and teaching. Doris initially took up training as a teacher and then decided to commence her nurse training at the Adelaide Hospital. She commenced her training in early 1915 and completed her three-year course at the end of 1917. [10] Doris joined the AANS but did not get the opportunity to serve overseas.

Rural and Remote Nurses

There is no doubt that young girls who grew up in rural areas were well versed in the importance of women's work and the expertise required to perform it effectively. Women in the early 1900s did have a clear appreciation of their role within Australian society and felt valued for the contribution they made. A number of nurses went to war, quite specifically, to take care of their brothers.[11] This was a normal and expected role for a woman at this time. Career and vocational expectations for women were limited within mainstream Australia. Even four years after the war, when women had proved themselves in a variety of roles once considered the domain of men, the Minister for Agriculture, the Hon HV Thorby, gave the young female students this advice: ... *don't think of rushing into an office and tapping a typewriter all day. Far better is it to go into a home in the country, fit yourselves for your future lives as good country women.* He added a qualification by stating a ... *great many of the prominent and successful men we hear about to-day would never have achieved such success had it not been for the excellent wives they had.*[12]

Living in rural and remote areas was difficult for women wanting a nursing career. ATNA required a longer training period in a country hospital to compensate for the limited exposure probationers had to diverse conditions and disease states.[13] Fortunately the need for nurses to 'live-in', that is reside in the nurses' home, gave nurses from rural and remote areas a safe place to live while they completed their training. Consequently it was not unusual for young women to travel vast distances to train in city hospitals as the standard of training was considered to be more comprehensive.

Ada Thompson was one such woman who chose Royal North Shore Hospital

(RNSH) near Sydney (Guringai & Dharug Country).[14] She was born in 1885 at Dubbo, (NSW, Tubba-Gah Country) but by the time she enlisted with the AANS her mother, Marian, lived on a property *Wytonia* at Pallamallawa, a small town near Moree (NSW, Kamilaroi Country). On completion of her training Ada joined the AANS on 19 October 1917 and served at 4 AGH, Randwick (NSW, Gadigal and Bidjigal Country) before being accepted in the AIF. [15]

The Fremantle Six, WA - Irish and USA connections

In Western Australia the liberation of the 'Fremantle Six' exemplified how the strained Anglo-Irish relationship had made it to the new colonies. The Fenian Brotherhood had various origins but was strongest in ...*New York in 1858, for the express purpose of using Irish wealth in the United States against the English.*[16] Six Irishmen referred to as the 'Fremantle Six' were enduring hardships and deprivations in Fremantle Gaol, WA. One inmate, John Wilson, wrote a letter 'Beyond the tomb' to his Fenian Brothers in New York for assistance. The Brotherhood funded a most extraordinary rescue of the 'Fremantle Six' via the *Catalpa* in April 1876.

Rosa O'Kane and her Irish Connections

Irish migrants often held onto their history, fiercely and proudly and this made the family history of Rosa O'Kane extremely colourful. Her paternal grandfather, Timothy Joseph O'Kane, was born in County Kerry, Ireland, on 14 January 1820 and trained to become a priest at Maynooth seminary.[17] About forty years later another controversial student of Maynooth, Daniel Mannix, who completed eight years of study before his ordination in 1890, became the Archbishop of Melbourne. Mannix became the Catholic voice against conscription in Australia during the First World War.

The demography of Ireland changed dramatically when, from around 1848, the potato famine caused a ...*great wave of emigration ... to USA and Australia. The goldfields made Australia the magnet in the early 50s.*[18] In contrast to Archbishop Mannix, Timothy O'Kane led a more secular but no less radical life as a journalist, husband and father. He married Margaret Morris in 1852 in London and his only son, John Gregory, who was born in 1857 in Tralee, Ireland, had a rather exciting start to life when on the night of his birth the police raided the house looking for an agrarian terrorist group known as the 'Whiteboys'.[19] From about the 1790s this was the name adopted by rural rebels who were part of an organised campaign of terror to express peasant grievances. Although the protests started over the enclosure of common land, the injustices soon extended and there was widespread local support, making it difficult for authorities to repress the movement.

The marriage of Timothy and Margaret was steeped in controversy when Timothy sued his wife for divorce on the grounds of adultery with Lord Palmerston. Eventually, Timothy withdrew the action, changed his name to Thadeus John O'Kane and migrated to Queensland but not to a quieter life. He continued to work in journalism on a number of Queensland papers including as sub-editor of *The North Australian* in Ipswich (Tulmur Country), *Morning Bulletin* and *Northern Argus* (Rockhampton, Darumbal Country) before settling in the mining district of Charters Towers (Gudjal Country). Charters Towers continues to be a predominantly mining town and in 1874 he became the sole owner of a major newspaper, *The Northern Miner.* He continued to speak out against anything and anyone whom he perceived to be acting inappropriately. Consequently he was often sued for libel and had the extraordinary experience of being literally horsewhipped.[20]

In 1876 Thadeus' son John joined him at *The Northern Miner* as a reporter but soon became the business manager. The local schoolmistress Jeannie O'Kane who was no relation being the daughter of Dionysius and Rosetta O'Kane (nee Magee), married John in 1881. John and Jeannie had two sons, Frank (1882) and John (1884), and finally a daughter, Rosa who was born on 14 April 1890.[21] Rosa, being the only daughter and youngest child, had a special place in the affections of this prominent Charters Towers family.

Rosa was born the same year her controversial grandfather died, her father became the editor and, a year later, owner of *The Towers Herald.* Tragically her father died when she was just eight and he was forty-one years old. His wife Jeannie tried to retain ownership of the paper but it proved too difficult for the young widow with three children, so she eventually returned to teaching.[22] Nursing and teaching were respectable and acceptable professions for women at the time and Rosa O'Kane chose the former by training at the Townsville Hospital in north Queensland (Thul Garrie Waja Country & Gurrumbilbarra Country).[23] There can be little doubt that she brought to her career the idealism of her grandfather and the realism of her mother.

Hilda Williams and a Successful Migration to the West

A number of families travelled from the eastern colonies to WA when the railway was operational, and the motive was not always the pursuit of gold. William Williams Snr, a migrant from Holyhead, Wales, married Ann Sergeant from County Armagh, Ireland; they later settled in Victoria. Their son William Williams (Jnr) married Louisa Alice Walters of Box Hill (Wurundjeri Woi-wurrung Country). Louisa was the daughter of a mill sawyer, Ferdinand Walters, and his wife Kate (née Parlett). Staff families were once an entrenched and integral part of the British class system and Kate's family had been in service at Arundel Castle, Sussex, England. William and Louisa remained at Box Hill where their firstborn and only son, Arthur Stuart, was born (1887) but they ultimately had eight children.[24] Alice and Hilda, later to become nurses, were also born at Box Hill but it was decided to move the ever-growing family to the other side of the country to Claremont, WA. William Williams Jnr was a lay preacher in the Baptist Church and provided religious guidance to the good people of Claremont, Subiaco and Cottesloe (Whadjuk Nyoongar Country). He also built the Claremont Baptist Church. Hilda's parents raised a large family who were well educated and their lives had a sound religious basis.[25]

A Family at War

Alice Beatrice Williams, the second eldest child and eldest daughter, undertook her nurse training at Perth Children's Hospital, which she successfully completed in June 1912.[26] Alice wanted to join the AANS but many WA nurses believed priority was being given to nurses from the eastern states.[27] Alice grew tired of waiting for the 'call up', so she, like many others, paid her own fare to England, where she was accepted by the British Red Cross and *...worked at Ottershaw Park Hospital near Heathrow, a big private home which became a wartime hospital, owned by a German who lived in a small part of it during the war.*[28]

Alice's slightly younger sister, Hilda (b. 1893), followed her older sister's example and completed her nurse training in December 1913 at the Perth Children's Hospital.[29] She did not join the AANS but continued civilian nursing during the war. The exodus of qualified nurses volunteering for overseas service placed considerable strain on the human resources of the public and private hospitals in 1914-18.

Her parents may have been pleased to have Hilda at home because by the time Alice left for England their only son Arthur had already enlisted with the first AIF. He was a source of pride as his father was a well-respected builder in the Claremont-Nedlands area, so when Arthur became an architect his profession complemented that of his father.[30] Arthur joined in November 1914 and attained the rank of lieutenant with 3 Field Company of Engineers, but there were no safe jobs in the war and on 22 July 1916 while in *...France he was laying corduroy roads for the movement of tanks and he used his torch to look down a shaft – the light was noticed by a sniper who killed him.*[31] His family, especially his parents, never recovered.

10 War

... the weak were made to be devoured by the strong – Bismarck

On 28 June 1914 a Bosnian Serb, Gavrilo Princip, assassinated Archduke Franz Ferdinand, heir presumptive to the Austro-Hungarian throne, and his wife Sophie, in Sarajevo.[1] This event ignited a volatile set of reactions, culminating in a declaration of war by Austria-Hungary against Serbia. Austria-Hungary was assured of the full support of the powerful German military forces.[536] An Australian student of music, Ethel Cooper, was living in Germany at the time and she recorded in a letter (6 August 1914) to her sister in Adelaide that *...Germany mobilized – she has called out every man from 17 to 45*. Germany wasted no time in conscripting its civilian male population to the war effort.[2] Like a game of global monopoly, countries throughout the world staked their economic future on military alliances. The Russians aligned with the Serbs and consequently were at war with Germany and Austria-Hungary.

Given the outcome of the Franco-Prussian war (Germany still retained the two former French provinces of Alsace and Lorraine) France aligned with Serbia and Russia. Britain voted to support France once aware of Germany's intention to implement Alfred von Schlieffen's plan which included the invasion of Belgium, a neutral country.[3] British colonies, such as Australia, were automatically required to provide military support when war was announced in Australia at 12.30pm on 5 August 1914.[4] The Ottomans did not declare an alliance with Germany until November 1914 following serious diplomatic mistakes by Britain. No doubt many Australians had to resort to an atlas just to know where their allies and enemies were geographically located. Henceforth, Britain, Australia and allied countries will be referred to as 'allies'; Germany and her allies as the 'enemy'; fighting on the French and Belgian borders as the 'Western Front'; fighting on the Russian borders as the

'Eastern Front'; France, Britain and Russia as 'the Entente'.

Germany 1914-15

The Prussian Prime Minister, Bismarck, envisaged the benefits of a united Germany in 1868 when he claimed *...the weak were made to be devoured by the strong.*[5] Prussia was the strongest of the German states but when France declared war (15 July 1870) Napoleon III was convinced of the invincibility of his army. Significantly, both Germany and France had *...acceded to the 1864 Geneva Convention...* agreeing to comply with its articles and *...both had formed their own Red Cross national societies.* It was during this war that the term 'ambulance' was used to describe any source of support for the wounded.[6] The Franco-Prussian War (1870-71) saw the southern independent German states join Prussia to defeat France. In particular, the French keenly felt the loss of the provinces of Lorraine and Alsace and consequently fortified their exposed German border. However, the Germans had an alternative plan in the event that they had a need to invade France at a later date: The Schlieffen Plan. German troops would simply move through neutral Belgium to Paris.

At 6am on 4 August 1914, Herr von Below-Saleske, German Minister in Brussels, advised the Belgian Government that, to protect its own security, the German Army would enter Belgium. Belgium did not call upon France or Britain for assistance at this point. There was a chance that the threat of invasion may have been a tactical ruse by the Germans to cause France to redeploy troops away from the Franco-German border. Furthermore, the French Army may have been open to international criticism if it entered Belgium first. That evening, Kaiser Wilhelm II admitted to members of the Reichstag that our ... *invasion of Belgium is contrary to international law but the wrong – and I speak openly – that we are committing we will make good as soon as our military goal has been reached.*[7]

The Germans entered the fortified town of Liège on 5 August and within two weeks they entered Brussels; the Belgian Army made a strategic retreat to Antwerp.[602] The Schlieffen Plan failed, as the German troops did not envelop Paris from the left flank. On 25 August the German General Helmuth Moltke re-deployed four divisions to the Russian front because he believed a decisive victory over France had already been achieved – it had not.[603] A stalemate was reached by the end of 1914.[8] Trench lines were established; four years elapsed and a great deal of blood was spilled before the French and Belgian countryside was anything other than the 'Western Front'.[9]

Meanwhile, the music student from Adelaide, Ethel Cooper, was prevented from leaving Germany because she was suspected of keeping a diary and writing letters home to Australia. She did both, but evidence of neither was uncovered during the war.[10] The longer she stayed the enemy found it more dangerous to allow her leave so she remained in Germany for the entire war.

The Ottoman Empire

The Ottoman Empire began around 1300 CE, when Osman established a small principality in Anatolia. It expanded as other ethnic groups came under its umbrella and reached the peak of its power in the seventeenth century. The Turkish component was mainly from Anatolia (primarily present-day Republic of Türkiye) and became a minority to the other ethnic groups including Kurds, Greeks, Arabs, Bulgarians, Serbs, Croats, Albanians, Hungarians, Macedonians and Armenians. Many non-Muslims served the Sultan and these were known as 'devshirme' (meaning converted or recruited). Many were politically influential within the Empire.

The importance of the Dardanelle straits to the Islamic world was well established in 1914. By 1352 the Ottomans had crossed Europe via the straits of Gallipoli and began to annex the Balkans. Constantinople was the capital of the Ottoman Empire from 1453, it was renamed İstanbul in 1930. Over the next two centuries the Ottomans extended the influence of Islam from Vienna to Persia, present-day Iran, and from the Crimea to Yemen, virtually surrounding the Mediterranean Sea. The straits were well fortified with two castles on either side used for defence purposes.

Once the Empire stopped expanding, taxation levels increased, which in turn caused discontent and economic decline. Simultaneously, the Industrial Revolution gave England, France and Germany more prosperity and therefore more influence. Napoleon Bonaparte summed up the situation: *The major question is who shall have*

İstanbul, not whether the Ottomans survive.

In 1908 the answer came with Enver and the Young Turks. Following the French Revolution (1789) progressive ideas infiltrated diverse ethnic groups within the Ottoman Empire. There were a number of small uprisings which resulted in the emergence of small states. This put the Empire at risk, so France took Algeria and Tunisia; Britain occupied Egypt; Italy seized Tripoli.

The Young Turks emerged as a political force who wanted to unite diverse ethnic groups into an Empire of Turks. Enver, a distinguished battalion commander, led the Young Turks in the 1908 Revolution and secured İstanbul. By 1909 the Sultan was a merely a titular figurehead and a constitutional parliament was in place. The Young Turks were exceedingly popular with some groups. During the 1912-13 Balkan Wars the Ottoman armies offered six weeks of resistance against Bulgarian, Greek and Serbian forces. In 1913 a coup d'état saw Enver and the Young Turks displace parliament and depose the Sultan, who was kept under house arrest until he died in 1918. The terms 'Turk' and 'Turkey' were adopted as nationalistic symbols by the Young Turks and became official in 1923 with the formation of the Republic of Turkey. Therefore, Australians fought the Ottomans at Gallipoli, although the geographic area is part of present-day Turkey.

Enver assumed the title Paşa, which translates as General, and ruthlessly oppressed opposing minority groups including the Armenians. Germany had an interest in the oil reserves of Mesopotamia (present day Iraq) so to secure access she cultivated a diplomatic relationship with Enver Paşa. Nonetheless, there was an element of mistrust toward Germany. When the Triple Entente and Central Powers were lining up against each other, the Ottomans approached Britain to join the alliance of the Central Powers. They approached Britain three times and were rejected three times so, in May 1914, they went to Russia for a pact but were also rejected.

Despite no formal alliances with Britain or Germany, the Ottomans continued to do business with both countries. For example, in December 1913 German General Otto Liman von Sanders arrived in İstanbul to reorganise the Ottoman Army and the Ottomans commissioned the British to build two new warships, funded by public donations.[11] Britain misjudged the mood of the Ottomans when on the eve of war it requisitioned the ships for its own navy which, in effect, left the Ottomans unaligned and with limited defences.

On 2 August 1914, Enver Paşa entered a secret alliance with Germany but Mustafa Kemal, an influential Young Turk, opposed the alliance. He reasoned that if the Entente lost the war, the Ottoman Empire would cease to exist and if it was victorious the Empire would merely be a satellite for Germany. However, the alliance was assured when on 9 August Enver Paşa allowed two German warships (*Breslau* and *Goeben*), stranded in the Mediterranean, to escape through the Dardanelles. When they reached Constantinople the Germans sold them to the Ottomans and a German admiral was made Commander-in-Chief of the Ottoman Navy.[12] This decision had long-term consequences in the Mediterranean. For example, in 1917 an Australian nurse, Gladys Walter, was invalided home via Egypt but the four-day journey from Salonika took fourteen days because the *Goeben* and *Breslau* were a continuing threat. When she finally arrived in Alexandria she saw the wrecks of the allied ships ...Osmanieh *and the* Aragon *and the bodies of some of the victims floating about*.[13]

The First AIF Contingent

The plain khaki army uniform was not the first military uniform donned by the men of the First AIF. On 29 September 1908 the Minister for Defence, Thomas Ewing, introduced compulsory military training under the auspices of the Deakin Government. The Australian Labor Party (ALP) was in opposition at the time and supported the introduction of compulsory military training (the correct spelling at this time was *Labour Party* but for ease of historical narrative *Labor Party* will be henceforth used). A number of leading politicians were of the view that *...war should not be thought of as a curse, but rather a fate that periodically overtook nations just as disease overtook individuals*.[14] When the Labor caucus elected George Pearce as the Minister for Defence in November 1908 there was no change of policy because the 'Citizen Army' had been part of the ALP policy platform since its inception as a federal parliamentary party in 1901.[15]

Young men from farming districts throughout Australia rushed to enlist in the prestigious ALH regiments.[16] In 1914 the average weekly income for Australian men was £2 9s 3d with soldiers getting £2 2 0 or six bob (shillings) a day. Given this was a time of drought and many early recruits hailed from the country this was decent money for 'Australian Cockies'; men scratching a living from the land. [17] In contrast a British recruit only earned one shilling per day when the average weekly wage was £2 5s.5d).[18]

Hostilities between the allies and the Ottomans formally started on 31 October 1914 and the first contingent soldiers, who left Australia in November, were en route to England for training when they heard the news via semaphore.[19]

11 Australian Nurses in German New Guinea

...he was shot in the spine early in the day and later died on the Berrima *– Stuart Braga*

Soon after the declaration of war, Britain requested the capture of the German administrative centre of Rabaul because it was considered to have strategic importance for the enemy.[1] Since the 1880s the territories of New Guinea had been ruled by the British, Dutch and Germans, but the declaration of war necessitated prompt action to change this situation. German radio outposts posed a threat to the security of British operations so an Australian naval and military expeditionary force, including the AAMC led by the South African War hero Dr Neville Howse, was dispatched in September 1914. Howse sailed on the troopship *Berrima* with doctors Pockley, Maquire and Donaldson and no nurses. On 11 September the force landed at Kabakaul, near Rabaul, and Howse appointed Pockley in charge of the small AAMC detachment with the landing party. Tragically *...he was shot in the spine early in the day and later died on the* Berrima.[2]

Both Pockley and Able Seaman WGV Williams, the man Pockley had stopped to attend, *...died during the afternoon.* It is not clear which of them was the first casualty of the First World War but there is no doubt that Brian Colden Antill Pockley was the first member of the AAMC to die while protecting another man's life.[3] Sister Rose Kirkcaldie worked with him at RPAH and was saddened by his death because he *...was a fine personality and of great professional promise, and it was typical of the man that he should give his Red Cross brassard to one of his men and go into action himself unprotected.*[4] Many AANS nurses were bereft because they not only trained with him but received lectures from his father, an Honorary Ophthalmic Surgeon at RPAH.[5]

The parent who was left to mourn the loss of his son was not anonymous because Australian nurses were diligent in their duty to keep the next-of-kin informed of how their soldier husband, father, son or brother died. Nurses were painfully aware that they were often the last to see them alive and information about how the soldiers felt or spoke immediately prior to their death mattered to those at home. Many were unlikely to visit the grave, if the soldier was fortunate enough to have one, in a distant part of the world.[6]

Transport Nursing

At the outbreak of the war the Royal Australian Navy was in its infancy but a number of sailors, soldiers, medical officers and nurses who served on transports and naval ships were members of the AIF, which incorporated the AANS.[7] Each had a different uniform but the overarching identity was one of being an Australian. AANS nurses crossed the world's waterways a number of times during four years of war. As previously explained the collation of statistics during the war was not a fine art. Nurses who were assigned to an AGH were often needed on transport duty. That is, soldiers who were sufficiently recovered were transported back to their unit unaccompanied by nurses on troopships. Alternatively, those who required further treatment or convalescence in England required nursing staff on the voyage on hospital ships. Australians who were not likely to be fighting fit again were sent home on hospital ships.

Problems arose when nurses were needed to work on troopships as there were insufficient numbers to warrant a hospital ship or they were unavailable. Hospital ships were ostensibly protected from attack but nurses who served on troopships were not. When a ship was torpedoed or struck a mine the identification of those on board and those who perished was not infallible. This was especially true for transport nurses. Furthermore, Australian nurses who married, changed their name, left the AANS while overseas and later joined other nursing or volunteer organisations no longer existed - officially. The oceans of the world were dangerous as the war was fought along the trade routes as much as national boundaries.

Nurses on the Australian mercantile fleet auxiliary *Grantala*

It was decided to send reinforcements, including nurses, to New Guinea but fortunately the only fighting had already occurred at Kabakaul with six dead and four wounded.[8] Rose Kirkcaldie was not an AANS reservist but when war was declared she was in the right place at the right time. Sister Kirkcaldie was working at her training hospital (RPAH) in 1914 when she received a telephone call from a friend telling her that a hospital ship was being *...fitted up at Garden Island in Sydney Harbour*. She made an impromptu trip to the *...well known interstate steamer, the Grantala...* where she, by chance, met *...Dr Horsfall – an ex-naval officer – who was to be the PMO of the ship*. Within a few days she mentioned the situation to a number of other friends from RPAH who also went directly down to visit the ship and made themselves known to Dr Horsfall.

Kirkcaldie did attempt to join the AANS and found *...a large throng of women filled the office and over-flowed into the corridors*. It was soon obvious that the general population of women did not realise that it required training and education to become a qualified nurse. Finally, Kirkcaldie was received by a harassed matron who had spent much of her day *...listening to applications by women unqualified as nurses*. The ATNA standards proved to be invaluable because they provided a clear standard of nursing which was a prerequisite for entry into the AANS. It also brought to public consciousness the level of training required to be a 'sister' or qualified nurse.

However, Horsfall was either unaware of the processes in place for AANS entry or chose to ignore them, as he contacted Kirkcaldie and her colleagues directly with a telegram which read *...Services accepted. Prepare to sail shortly*. Needless to say the matron of RPAH was dismayed when seven of her qualified nurses left at short notice for service on the *Grantala*. The AANS leaders were not impressed and did not recognise the service of the nurses who sailed with the *Grantala*. The PMs of each MD were also keenly aware of the need to ensure a high standard of care for those at home as well as for the soldiers overseas.

The local *...shop worked overtime to provide uniforms...* and the RPAH staff purchased a deck chair and rug for each of their colleagues; the war nurses then embarked on the *Grantala*, now in the *...prescribed hospital ship colours of white and green...* at midday, 30 September 1914.[9] The seven nurses who served on the *Grantala* included Matron Neale, Sisters Kirkcaldie, Collis, Bertinshaw, McMillan, Clouston and De Mestre. Their first port of call was Townsville, where they were met by Miss

McGrath who was also an ex-RPAH colleague. Kirkcaldie clearly states that Matron Neale was in charge, which is at odds with claims that Sarah de Mestre was matron.[10] The narrative of Sarah de Mestre was *...taken down in longhand by Medical Collator AIF...* whose handwriting verges on the illegible but it does state that *...I was off to matron "troopship" Grantala.*[11] Irrespective of who was, or who thought they were in-charge the staff had all worked at RPAH and they *...formed a happy little family.*

The nurses enjoyed the Queensland hospitality of Miss McGrath and then boarded the *Grantala* which made its way through a number of islands. The nurses had no idea their eventual destination was Rabaul, capital of Germany's New Guinea territory and the chief objective was to destroy *...the powerful wireless station.* The nurses received their first casualties, mainly gunshot wounds, but remained on the ship in the harbour. They were joined by the French cruiser *Montcalm* and relations between the two ships *...grew very friendly...* as the Australians nursed a number of their sick sailors. The nurses remained on board for a fortnight but an invitation to have Sunday tea with the land force officers enabled them to finally visit the town. Tea was served in the old German Club which was now the officers' mess and a lovely afternoon was spent visiting 'China Town' and the botanical gardens. The ship encountered the trade winds en route to Fiji, where Kirkcaldie and her colleagues spent *...several happy weeks...*at Suva before returning to Sydney just before Christmas.[12]

Nurses in New Guinea

In December 1914 May Gibbon (RRC), who graduated from RBWH in 1910, was one of four nurses who sailed to Rabaul but her status remains unclear as she is occasionally referred to as 'matron'. Her sister Beatrice Louise Gibbon (ARRC), who also trained at Brisbane (1913), sailed with Jane Bell on the *Kyarra.*[13] May Gibbon was most likely accompanied by Sisters Marian Adelaide MacLean (1 MD), Agnes Bissett Nelson (2 MD) and Catherine Elizabeth Letherbridge (1 MD), who served the community and patients at Namanula Hospital, Rabaul with Matron Flora Robertson (2 MD).[14] Hester Maclean also sent seven New Zealand nurses to Samoa to replace German nursing staff.[15]

Malaria

When the monsoon season (January 1915) arrived on the islands *...more than half of the garrison was ill with malaria...* and the mosquito was known to be the culprit.[16] Symptoms include frequent attacks of chills followed within a few hours by fever. Depending on the parasitic species (*Plasmodium falciparum* being the species that usually results in death) the attacks recur at various intervals. For example, tertian malaria causes attacks every other day while quartan malaria is said to exist when the attacks recur at three-day intervals. Apart from the fever and profuse perspiring, which often results in absolute exhaustion, other symptoms include headache, nausea and body pains.

There was no effective inoculation against malaria. The method of transfer is by a protozoan parasite which is carried in the bloodstream of a mosquito and finally to the salivary glands in the mouth. The transfer of the protozoa to the human bloodstream is via the bite of the mosquito.[17] The complex life cycle of a parasite and the many types of mosquitoes continue to make the development of a vaccine extremely difficult. It was more than a century later, in 2021, that the World Health Organization recommended the widespread use of a vaccine for specific countries and limited demographics; a second vaccine was released two years later.

Howse implemented precautions against the debilitating disease including hammocks with mosquito netting, daily quinine and the need to boil all water. He returned to Australia because it was evident there would be no further fighting and therefore no need for his special skills; he did persuade the authorities to send *...medical men with knowledge of tropical diseases...* to New Guinea.[18] Drs CL Strangman and (later Sir) Raphael Cilento dedicated their working lives to eradicating the disease. Dr Strangman worked with May Gibbon and her nurses in a bid to reduce the immense suffering caused by the disease. Matron Gibbon was awarded the RRC but her service left a more enduring legacy as she also acquired sub-tertian malaria.[19] Nurses who were returned to Australia in 1915 discovered that during their absence they had lost any chance of placement with AANS units on the first two ships, which sailed in November 1914 and January 1915. This did not deter Rose Kirkcaldie who later travelled to England where she joined the QAs with her RPAH friend, Elsie Welman.[20] Despite being stationed in New Guinea as members of the Tropical Force Detail, these remarkable nurses did not have their contribution recognized on their return to Australia.[21] This has since been rectified.

Prisoners-of-War

Surprisingly, Gibbon found five German doctors and three nurses still working when she arrived. It would appear that they were not treated as POWs but were repatriated in January 1915. During the First World War no Australian nurses became POWs but this tragically changed in the Second World War. The mistreatment of Australian nurses by the Japanese in POW camps and the Banka Island massacre, where 22 AANS nurses were machine-gunned to death (Vivian Bullwinkle survived) is lamented by Australian nurses to this day.[22] Nurses were often the first women to be seen by emancipated POWs and when John Wheat, a submariner on *AE2*, was released during a prisoner exchange in 1918 he *...saw the Australian hospital ship Kanowna sail into the harbour. It did us such a lot of good to see the bright smiling faces of the nursing sisters on board ... after three and a half years.*[23] The treatment of the 3,647 Australian soldiers who were captured during the war varied depending on the humanity of their custodians.[24]

12 The First AANS Contingent to Egypt 1914-15

Germany mobilized – she has called out every man from 17 to 45, and ten million are in camp this week –Ethel Cooper

Australian nurses continued their training, hoping to join the AANS as soon as they were qualified. Those already ATNA-registered rushed to enlist, hoping for an overseas placement. Initially, the British authorities requested that twenty-five senior army nurses be sent to England for service wherever the British felt it necessary. The nurses expected to sail to England aboard the *Omah* but instead sailed on seven different ships with the first contingent of the AIF.[1]

Nellie Miles Walker: HMAT *Euripides*

When war was declared, Nellie Miles Walker was provided with a reference from Dr Sheldon (Molong Private Hospital, Forbes Street, Darlinghurst) stating that she was *...quite competent in all branches of nursing (being in charge of above hospital).*[2] Her mother Louisa was distraught at her daughter's imminent departure for overseas service and owing to her mother's ill health, Nellie's brother, Albert Edward, was her designated next-of-kin.[3] PM Nellie Gould recorded that *...On 29th September, 1914, Principal Matron Gould, EJ, Matron Johnston, J Bligh, Sisters Frater, P., Kellett, AM, Twynam, and the Matron of the Tasmanian AANS who happened to be working on Reserve in Sydney, ... Miss Walker, J., were detailed for duty on Transport "Euripides"...* which indicates Miles Walker had not moved to NSW permanently. Although she was a PM during peacetime she left Australia as a sister from 2 MD.[4] It was not uncommon for the records to incorrectly state the MD of origin and instead list the MD from which the nurses departed.[5]

When Nellie Gould sailed she was PM of 2 MD, a senior civilian nurse and an experienced military nurse leader, but she was not 'in charge' of the other nurses. In addition to the lack of a clear policy on leadership, Gould was not universally liked. She was accompanied on the *Euripides* by Sister Julia Bligh Johnston, a life-long friend and colleague. Born in Windsor (NSW, Dharug Country) Julia Bligh Johnston was the granddaughter of an architect who established a Protestant church and supported the infamous Governor Bligh (hence the inclusion of Bligh in the family name). Her father, James, was a magistrate and coroner. Following a private education at Ashfield Ladies College, Julia worked as a teacher and companion for a short period. She commenced her nurse training at Launceston Hospital, Tasmania, but later moved to Sydney and completed her training requirements at SHSEH, where she most likely met Nellie Gould.[6] They became firm friends and served together in both the South African War and the First World War.

Maud Kellett: HMAT *Euripides*

The indomitable (Adelaide) Maud Kellett (AANS) also sailed on the *Euripides* and was kept busy because *...we brought an epidemic of Influenza on board with us ... We lost two bonnie boys on the trip across from Pneumonia follow-ing Influenza. The Sick Parades, morning and evening, were always very largely attended. Many cases of Boils, Eye infection, Ear trouble, Septic-fingers, and the minor ill of the flesh, especially colds, much Mist-Tussi being used on the voyage.* Kellett was a competent theatre sister from SHSEH, a position she held on the voyage. Her ability to quickly adapt is evident because *...the second day out, we had a case of appendicitis ... Fortunately I had sterilised many dressings, sheets, etc. while waiting at Albany* (Menang Country), *so by the time the basins, etc. were boiled ... Next day we had another case of appendicitis, this one being gangrenous which naturally did not do as well as the first.* Sadly, there were two deaths on the *Euripides* and Kellett witnessed her first sea burial which *...seems much more impressive than a burial on land.*[7]

In summary, *Appendix* 2 shows the leaders of the nursing establishment were among the twenty-five chosen to sail with the first contingent and twenty were awarded, at the minimum, a MID. Eleven became members of the Royal Red Cross (RRC) and six were made Associates of the Royal Red Cross (ARRC). Ten received more than one award and two were given honours in recognition of their service from the country in which they had served with distinction. See *Appendix 2* for a summary of the first contingent nurses' achievements.[8]

Like the soldiers, the nurses of the first contingent expected to arrive in England for service in France. This was a fluid situation and the nurse leaders were quick to accept change at a moment's notice.[9] Unfortunately, the DGMS failed to see the importance of appointing a nurse leader with ultimate responsibility for the AANS.[10]

Hilda Knox: Second Contingent Sails: 1 AGH, Egypt

Hilda Knox, an experienced charge-nurse at the Homeopathic Hospital in Melbourne, accepted a SN position with 1 AGH on 21 November 1914. The demotion was tolerated by most nurses who wanted to serve overseas under any circumstances.[15] The Homeopathic Hospital originally operated from 153 Collins Street as a dispensary for outpatients to assist the poor of Melbourne, but was later enlarged to accommodate inpatients in 1877, when the hospital was relocated to Spring Street.[16] Hilda Knox was born (1884) in 'Kelly country' (north eastern Victoria) four years after the notorious bushranger's death.[17] Her father, James Knox, was a civic minded man who was the Shire Secretary of Benalla (Yorta Yorta Nation) for a number of years. Hilda was one of the 161 nurses who sailed with the Jane Bell contingent which left in December 1914 and arrived in Egypt about seven weeks later. Minnie Kate Porter and another AANS nurse, Valerie Woinarski, were aboard and Valerie claimed that *...of the voyage of the* Kyarra *the less said by any of us the better.*[18]

Jane Bell: *Australian Hospital Ship (AHS) Kyarra*: 1914

On 24 November 1914, Jane Bell was notified that she would board a ship the following Saturday. She left the Melbourne Hospital in capable hands: Miss Pace was appointed acting lady superintendent and Sister Fleming was the acting assistant lady superintendent.[11] The first contingent had sailed and Bell was placed in charge of the *Kyarra* which departed the following month. Initially, the hospital ship had sufficient equipment and supplies for 1 AGH and 2 AGH (520 beds each), two stationary hospitals and one CCS.[12]

Interstate Rivalry

Despite the success of ATNA/RVTNA, there was an unhealthy rivalry between the states and even between hospitals within the same state. This was not helped by the lack of a clear leadership position in the AANS. Surgeon General Williams was deemed to be subjective about the appointment of AANS nurses to senior positions at the two main hospitals in Egypt. Jane Bell had a short history in the AANS but was appointed PM of 1 AGH. Mary Knowles graduated from the Adelaide Hospital in 1892 and was a member of the South Australia Branch of the RBNA.[13] She had been matron of 4 MD since its inception and had a longer AANS history than Bell, but was appointed to the position of 'Sister' at 1 AGH.[14] This situation did little to alleviate interstate animosity.

William Ramsay Smith

Initially, doctors were given military rank and nurses were not. Lieutenant Colonel (Dr) William Ramsay Smith was the commanding officer at 1 AGH and, for reasons which are unclear, Ramsay Smith and Bell did not like each other. They were both from Edinburgh but Ramsay Smith arrived in Australia in July 1896 during the 'hospital trouble' at the Adelaide Hospital so he was well known to Margaret Graham who was also nursing at 1 AGH. He believed that Mary Knowles, matron of the same military district as he, had seniority over Bell and was entitled to be matron of 1 AGH. When Bell arrived in Egypt she was informed by Ramsay Smith that she was to be a house matron; a serious demotion and an insult to someone with the experience and reputation of Bell. Bell, as a Nightingale nurse, correctly believed all nursing-related matters were her domain and Ramsay Smith believed that all aspects of the hospital, including the nursing staff, came under his authority. Bell requested clarification from the DGMS and she retained her position. Tensions simmered.

Jane Bell and Controversy at 1 AGH, Heliopolis: 1915

Failure of the AIF to appreciate the history of civilian nursing and the development of the AANS underpinned the subsequent furore.[19] Bell's immediate task was to convert Heliopolis Palace into a functioning hospital with the capacity to nurse the casualties of the proposed Dardanelles Campaign. Gould was appointed Matron of 2AGH and was commissioned to alter Mena House, a hunting lodge near the pyramids, into a functioning military hospital. The Heliopolis Palace was previously a four-storey hotel plus basement. The building included a large restaurant, dining room and billiard recesses as well as the great hall and rotundas. Many of the hotel rooms could only accommodate three to six beds, so were allocated to the staff. Ablution facilities, apart from the standard hotel bathrooms, were far from satisfactory for the extremely ill and dependent patients who were soon filling the vast foyer of the large hospital.[20] A train line directly to 1 AGH enabled ease of access for casualties who were transported by rail from the port town of Alexandria to Cairo. Bell and her nurses coped with war casualties which ranged in number from 520 to 2,500.[21]

A Crisis of Confidence

Bell and Ramsay Smith were never in accord and this had an impact on all aspects of the hospital's management, especially when the wounded soldiers started to arrive in April 1915. Ramsay Smith enjoyed the support of his registrar, James Barrett (1862-1945), a Melbourne doctor, but other medical officers from Melbourne and Sydney requested transfers because they objected to Ramsay Smith. The nursing fraternity also took sides. Nurses who had trained at the Adelaide Hospital found 1AGH to be …*a beastly place, the heads don't agree and we are not wanted.*[22] Emma Cuthbert (AANS) from Victoria sailed with Bell and enjoyed the voyage. On arrival at 1 AGH she found that …*there were no patients and nothing ready for the hospital work*… but matron quickly organised the appropriate allocation of staff as well as the living quarters for the nurses.[23] When Leila Smith arrived at 1 AGH in May 1915 the tension was at its height. She reported directly to Knowles and the next day Bell saw about 36 of the nurses. Despite the problems Smith found the conditions at 1 AGH …*pretty good*… as she undertook relieving shifts for the staff.[24] However, by this time, the discontent of the doctors attracted the attention of authorities in Australia; complaints about 1AGH were being discussed in the Commonwealth Parliament and an investigation was instigated.[25]

The situation at 1AGH deteriorated to such an extent that both Bell and Ramsay Smith were recalled to Australia. When Bell reached Fremantle she read that a court of inquiry had been instigated in Egypt during her absence. She was more shocked to read that the newspaper claimed that she had been recalled because of the findings of the inquiry.[26] Knowles gave evidence at the inquiry that she had seniority and therefore was entitled to be matron of 1 AGH. Gould claimed there was conflict between senior nursing staff because the number of AANS efficients was disproportionate to the number of available senior positions.

Witnesses, mainly doctors, claimed that Bell *...was a capable Matron but she had a temper which did not go with the position.*[27] The doctors found it quite impossible to understand why Bell objected to their allocating nursing staff; they did not understand the role and responsibilities of a civilian matron. Civilian doctors were not employed by the hospital, unless in training, and the role of the medical superintendent was vastly different to that of the matron. Matrons were also nurse educators, whereas doctors gained their education from a university. Furthermore, matrons were, in effect, responsible for the morality, health and social safety of their nursing staff. Bell, like most competent matrons, felt this responsibility keenly. She attempted to ensure her nurses felt confident and safe in an environment which was professionally, geographically, culturally and socially foreign - she could not afford to have her authority undermined.

Jane Bell RTA

Bell tried, without success, to get the opportunity to put her side of the story on the record. Her position with the AANS was terminated and she returned to the matronship of the Melbourne Hospital. The incident created friction even within the civilian nursing establishment and a number of nurses resigned when she was reappointed matron. Ramsay Smith's position with the AAMC was also terminated. Dr James Barrett was sent to England as an invalid and he later co-authored a history of this period without reference to Bell.[28] The Official History notes that Bell was an experienced and competent nurse and that circumstances, not her individual failings, caused the crisis at 1 AGH.[29]

The Bell and Ramsay Smith inquiry had some positive results, as the AIF realised that a review of how the AANS functioned in a war situation was needed. The other finding was that despite the chaos and uncertainty at 1 AGH, when the sick or wounded soldiers arrived, Australian nurses did not rest until their needs were met. Gallipoli was a defining moment for Australia and a watershed for Australian nursing.

Casualties arrive in Egypt

In the intervening months casualties were transferred via hospital ships to the port of Alexandria and then entrained over rough country to reach 1AGH and 2AGH hours away. To reduce the strain on the soldiers many were triaged at Alexandria. It was not uncommon for AANS nurses to be assigned to British hospitals during the war. Grace Burns, who sailed on the *Kyarra* in November 1914, recorded that *...in the middle of April 1915 a number of the Nursing Sisters of No. 2 General, were detailed to go to British hospitals in Alexandria. I was among four to go to No. 17 General Hospital at Victoria, not far from Alexandria. I stayed at this hospital until the following August, and I must say, those few months abroad will always stand out as the most trying that I have experienced abroad.*[30] Burns and her colleagues met the casualties directly from the hospital transports prior to their transfer by train to Cairo. Burns remained with the AANS but not all nurses who were loaned to other services were able to return to their Australian units.

***Kyarra* (April 1915) Reinforcements**

Reinforcements continued to arrive to enable the continued running of 1AGH. Norma Mowbray and Louisa Bicknell nursed together at 1 AGH but it is unlikely these women met in civilian times. The war brought nurses from different parts of Australia together for the first time. Louisa Bicknell and her colleagues, Special Reinforcement of 1 AGH, sailed on the *Kyarra* on 3 April 1915 from Sydney. Kate Porter and Theresa Tyson embarked in the eastern states, and Minnie Lightbody boarded in Fremantle.[31]

Bicknell worked at Mooroopna Hospital, Victoria (Yorta Yorta Country), for three years before moving to Melbourne and commencing her formal nurse training at the Women's Hospital. By the time war was declared, she was a qualified RVTNA nurse with many years' experience, including district nursing. She owned and operated a private hospital in Bairnsdale (Tatungalung Country) but readily accepted a SN position with the AANS when the opportunity arose.[32]

Norma Mowbray was a Queenslander, born in St George (Mandandanji, Kooma & Bigambul Country) in 1883; she enlisted with the AANS as a SN on 11 November 1914. She was 31 years old and a mole on her right check was her only distinguishing mark when she enlisted. Her personal belongings indicate she was a serious cigarette smoker as every travel box included an ashtray.[33] Nurses were not allowed to drink in public places unless it was wine with meals but they were allowed to smoke cigarettes in private. During her war service she could be forgiven for indulging in both, whenever and wherever possible. Such behaviour would have resulted in her immediate return to Australia, as it was considered a blight on the professionalism of the AANS.

Nellie Gould 2AGH Egypt

Once the landing was underway Nellie Gould was given 24 hours' notice to prepare her hospital and staff for the influx of casualties who began to arrive five days later. Olive Haynes, from South Australia, was shocked by the casualties who began to flood into the hospital. She also thought of those who had died, finding it…*terrible to think of all who haven't come back – the 9th and 11th have just about been wiped out … All the South Australia men were in the 3rd Brigade. They say there are only about 200 left that are not wounded or killed.*[34]

Initially, 2 AGH was located at Mena House, …*a large tourist hotel adapted for a hospital…* situated at the base of the pyramids.[35] Nellie Gould took over as matron when her complement of 96 Australian nurses arrived in Egypt on 20 January 1915, but it had to be closed as an acute hospital on 12 June of the same year owing to the heat.[36] She had to move the entire plant and staff of the hospital to Ghezireh. When the Suez Canal was opened in 1869, Ismail Pasha (1830-95) received the inauguration guests at this recently built hotel, which was situated on a small island on the Nile.[37]

Ghezireh, like many of the luxury buildings which were requisitioned as hospitals during the war, proved to be difficult to modify into functional hospital wards but war often brought out the skills of innovative individuals.

The AANS nurses adapted to the appalling wartime conditions by falling back on their inherent professionalism but ...*those of the wounded who knew them previously were shocked at the change which the strain had produced in them.*[38] Gould had to contend with the administration of Mena House as a hospital but more importantly, she had to deal with the collective and individual grief of her nurses. It was not unusual for a nurse to hear of the death of a beloved brother or fiancé while tending to the wounded.[39] Gould managed 2 AGH in two different and difficult locations in 1915, during which time more than 10,000 patients were admitted.[40]

In the main the nurses focused on their nursing but some found the military regulations irksome. Sister Haynes preferred to work at 2 AGH than at any other hospital but she found the rules and regulation of the Army ...*quite mad*... especially during the Egyptian summer when the ...*matron has a fit when she sees us without our capes.* It wasn't long before the Australian nurses ...*wore their scarlet capes with the same pride as the Australian soldiers wore their slouch hats.*[41]

Grace Wilson: 3 AGH to England: May 1915

News of the casualties from Gallipoli created a groundswell of enlistments in the AIF and the AANS. Grace Wilson, who was commissioned to lead 3 AGH, set sail on RMS *Mooltan* (15 May 1915) destined for England with an expectation of future service in France.[42] The 3 AGH consisted of sufficient plant and equipment for 1,040 acute hospital beds. News travelled very slowly and the journey from Australia to Egypt took seven weeks. By the time 3 AGH reached England it was obvious to authorities that its staff were needed to treat the Gallipoli casualties. So, on arrival in England, Wilson and her nurses were immediately recalled to Egypt, where they awaited further orders. The delay was costly to the soldiers of Anzac who were enduring great hardships due to a lack of medical and nursing care. [43]

13 A Sexual Revolution and the Impact on Military Nursing

… March 1918 a woman with venereal disease could be arrested for having sex with her husband if he were a serviceman, even if he had first infected her-Britain's Defence of the Realm Act, 1914

Ronnie MacDonald survived Gallipoli and was fortunate to have his fiancée, Rania MacPhillamy, waiting for him in Egypt. The war gave her the opportunity to leave her family responsibilities on the property because her parents could hardly object to her travelling overseas to nurse because it would be unpatriotic. Sadly, their reunion was marred by Ronnie's confession of a long past sexual encounter and their relationship faltered.[1] He was not alone in sending letters of confession during and immediately after the war.[2]

One of the more contentious policy issues during the South African War related to the appropriateness of sending female nurses, as opposed to male orderlies, to a war zone. Many military men did not consider the front-line an appropriate place for women and preferred male orderlies to provide acute care before transferring the soldier to a military hospital.[3] The critics were assuaged, to some extent, by the resilience and effectiveness of the South African War nurses.[4]

Until this time, male assistants had been in charge of the management of operating procedures. Male surgeons, like most of the general population, believed the male anatomy should remain a mystery to unmarried female nurses and found their participation in the activities of the operating theatre unorthodox, even alarming. Women who became nursing volunteers during the First World War were *…overwhelmed with nervousness and embarrassment … thanks to the Victorian tradition which up to 1914 dictated that a young woman should know nothing of men but their faces and their clothes until marriage pitchforked her into an incompletely visualised and highly disconcerting intimacy.*[5] Due to the insight of a number of Australian nurse leaders prior to the war AANS personnel had been allowed to join the surgical staff during procedures on males.

Venereal Disease

One of the recommendations arising from Queen Victoria's Royal Commission (1900) is unambiguous: *Venereal cases clearly ought to be treated only by orderlies.*[6] A precedent in civilian hospitals was established whereby female nurses were not permitted to work amongst such men; where infected women were treated is unclear.[7] During the early stages of the First World War special hospitals were erected to deal with cases of venereal disease (VD). The problem was acute when the soldiers first arrived in Egypt. By the end of the war Australia had one of the highest rates of infection, with a conservative estimate being not less than 100 cases for every 1,000 soldiers (10%).[8] Diseases like syphilis were painful and the long-term effects, such as dementia, cruel.[9]

Nurse training for males proved difficult in the early 1900s because they were not permitted to attend women and children but they were able to care for men, including those suffering from venereal diseases. In 1913 John Edward Craig successfully completed his course of nurse training at the Coast Hospital and passed the ATNA examination. During his training he worked in the 'locked' venereal disease ward and was respected for his expertise in the area. The Coast Hospital trained four male nurses prior to 1917 but they were responsible to the medical superintendent not the matron. In total, the ATNA Register included the names of seven male nurses in 1916, but it was not until the 1970s that it became more acceptable for male nurses to undertake general training and enter the mainstream of the profession.[10]

Wardsmen (orderlies/attendants) were paid more than female nurses so there was little incentive to undertake four years' hard training for males. Unlike his female training colleagues Sarah Furnifull and May Dickson, John Craig was not able to join a nursing service during the First World War but instead served in the Australian Army Medical Corps (AAMC) as a private.[11] Edith Blake, who also trained at the Coast Hospital, joined the QAIMNSR and served at the 17 British General Hospital (17 BGH), Sidi Gaba, near Alexandria, Egypt in 1916. This hospital and 16 BGH were in Egypt during the Dardanelles Campaign and were staffed almost entirely by men before being replaced by AANS.[12]

A Sexual Watershed

There was a sexual watershed during the First World War. Soldiers were tempted by offers of sex and many realized they may die without making love. Many endured the pain of leaving the love of their life at home with a promise of marriage on return. The women left behind often endured a long life of spinsterhood, along with the social contempt that status engendered. Alternatively, a quick marriage prior to enlistment often left many young women widowed with small children, along with the financial distress that situation caused, especially during the depression years. It is easy to forget that women had little control over their reproductive lives until the middle of the twentieth century when the contraceptive pill was made available - marriage equated to pregnancy. Widows were permitted to join the AANS because there was, theoretically, no risk of pregnancy.

Nurses were placed in a precarious social position during the war: they were single women who were drastically outnumbered by men — young men who were likely to die or be maimed in the near future. It has been claimed that only two or three AANS nurses married while on active duty because they were pregnant, but how many had sexual relationships outside the confines of marriage is impossible to estimate.[13] The records of nurses who were posted overseas are incomplete but those that are available indicate that 108 of some 1,805 nurses gave marriage as their reason for resignation.[14]

One such nurse was Nellie Irene Honeywill who on 17 January 1915 at Mena Camp married *...a popular South Australia footballer, Private Phillip de Quetteville Robin ... in the officers' mess tent. Nurses at the time, although not commissioned officers, were granted the privileges of the officers' mess. With the officers' mess being the most suitable venue in the camp approval was given to them to be married there.*[15] The next record of Nellie de Quetteville Robin (nee Honeywill) is that she died in November 1915 in England having already lost her husband Phillip, who was KIA on 28 April 1915. A short and tragic marriage.[16]

If Australian nurses endured rape in the First World War the crime remains unrecorded: sex was not discussed, so such an atrocity would most likely have been borne in silent shame by the victim. After the war, civilian nurses were considered to be *...knowledgeable about sex which caused them to be targets for considerable sexual aggression...* but how they gained this knowledge about sex is not apparent in the nursing syllabus. For example, Matron McNevin was described as *...courageous...* when she gave a one hour lecture on sex each year to her senior nurses at the then Prince Henry Hospital. The year was 1943.

In reality, Australians could not return home for leave and were isolated from their families for up to four years. During leave in Britain many Australian soldiers were infected. For the first time in their lives, they were confronted by women soliciting sex in a *...open and unashamed...* manner.[18] The official Australian medical historian claimed that, prior to the war, venereal disease was almost exclusively the domain of the prostitute class. The belief that sexual *...continence...* (abstinence) was an *...essential attribute of manliness...* and *...incontinence...* (activity) was *...somehow harmful...* was condemned in the military literature. Furthermore, the authorities warned soldiers that women who granted sexual favours to men could not be regarded as safe because *...the amateur, no matter how clean looking, is just as dangerous as the regular prostitute.*[18]

Initially, the Army had a policy of returning all soldiers suffering from a venereal disease home to Australia. The strategy was designed to humiliate them but it became unsupportable owing to the large number of soldiers who frequented, initially, the Haret el Wasser (brothel) district in Egypt and later the prostitute districts of France, especially Amiens.[19] For example, Dr Neville Howse (Director Medical Services, AIF) sought permission for an Australian soldier to marry a nurse (who was four months pregnant) because it was preferable to the soldier marrying one of *...the whores of Amiens.*[20] The central paradigm was women were responsible for the sexual transmission of venereal diseases implying that women who had pre-marital sex were *...amateur prostitutes.*[21]

Soldiers were considered blameless because they were tempted by women and this social belief was enacted in Britain with the introduction of the Defence of the Realm

Act (passed 8 August 1914). [22] There is no doubt this law infringed civilian rights, especially for women, because after … *March 1918 a woman with venereal disease could be arrested for having sex with her husband if he were a serviceman, even if he had first infected her.*[23] The reality was that young men, many likely to be killed, and young women, many likely never to experience the long-held dream of happy matrimony, elected to risk disease and pregnancy outside the confines of marriage.

A possible consequence of this sexual revolution is cited in a pathology text book published in 1920 which makes the extraordinary claim that …*syphilis constitutes one-third of human pathology.*[24] The truth of the claim is impossible to verify but what is apparent is that the problem was a major public health issue during and, of course, after the war when the soldiers went home to their wives and sweethearts.

Contraception

Earlier civilisations tried all manner of contraception. Ancient Egyptians used crocodile dung, in pessary form as the acidity acted as a spermicide, but this form of contraception did not catch on over the centuries.[25] In some countries Roman Catholics are not permitted, theoretically, to use contraception on religious grounds to this day. Abstinence has been a long-held form of contraception, although very unreliable due to poor compliance rates. Governments also attempted to influence the reproductive lives of women by introducing despicable policies. For example, in 1912 the NSW Government attempted to increase the population, except for …*Asiatics, aboriginal natives of Australia, Papua, or the islands of the Pacific…* by offering women who delivered a viable baby (one which survived for at least twelve hours) a one-off payment of £5 in a bid to rectify the declining birth-rate of white Australians. Abstinence was considered to be the best protection against pregnancy and this was reinforced by a community ethos of keeping unmarried women (including nurses) as ignorant as possible about sexuality.[26] No action, at a policy level, was taken when the level of maternal deaths from backyard abortions rose dramatically after the war. Dr Millard worked at the Coast Hospital and was concerned when the number of abortions rose from 54 (1919) to 497 (1925); he claimed …*the practice of abortion must be increasing enormously in the metropolis* [Sydney], *as the patients who are seeking admission are probably only a small proportion of those on whom this criminal operation is performed.*[27]

Infection and pregnancy were two major deterrents to intercourse during the war. The early identification of signs and symptoms of venereal diseases was a problem. No soldier wanted to be sent home in disgrace. The Army did, later in the war, reconsider its policies. For instance, there was a review of financial disincentives. Initially, soldiers reporting for treatment who were then hospitalized had their pay docked for the duration of the treatment. There were 'blue light depots' along unit lines and at AIF headquarters in London where soldiers could access treatment anonymously. Preventative measures were rudimentary. For instance, 'French letters' were issued to soldiers and the content of the envelopes were condoms which became synonymous with the term.[28] Condoms had to be purchased by Australian soldiers on leave in Britain. Given that condoms were made of sheepskin, the protective qualities were not assured and educational programs on the immorality of premarital intercourse, was in the main, ineffective.

Nonetheless, VD was rife throughout the troops in all locations of the war. The diagnosis of venereal disease was via microscope, but treatment was not evidence-based and was painful. Gonorrhoea was treated by three methods; sealing up, massage and plugging. Silver salt and a glycerine of B. Naphthol were *...used as anterior injections, whilst Pot. Permang.* [Potassium permanganate] *is used as a posterior irrigation.* The process for the evaluation of the treatment was ad hoc and required the doctor to judge each case *...according to the degree of tenderness present and the irritation produced.*[29] Syphilis was treated by the application of saline dressings to any lesion. While the treatment was, no doubt, ineffective, the causative organism, *Treponema pallidum,* had been identified in 1905 by Schaudinn and Hoffmann.[30] At least, the use of a microscope enabled a differential diagnosis of the various venereal diseases.

Needless to say, the impact on any nurse infected with VD or becoming pregnant was socially and professionally catastrophic. Matrons of the AANS were responsible for the moral and physical health of their nurses and it would have been devastating, at a personal and professional level, if an Australian nurse was infected. When

Matron Grace Wilson arrived in Egypt she was considered to be particularly intolerant of any of her nurses not respecting curfews or social and military rules of association with soldiers.[31] It is somewhat surprising that Vera Brittain, an English VAD, was instructed to 'special' (provide one-to-one care) a soldier suffering from syphilitic cancer at Queen Alexandra's Hospital (Millbank) just prior to the armistice. A visiting medical officer was appalled and claimed that *...it wasn't a job for a girl...* and *...one of the older nurses ought to have taken it on.*[32] By war's end the roles and responsibilities of nurses and women were much altered.

Marriage and Pregnancy

Despite clear guidelines in the AANS standing orders stating *...a candidate for enrolment as a Sister must be ... single, or a widow...* adherence to said guidelines was variable. Matrons in the AANS and the QAIMNSR used their discretion throughout the war.[33] A number of matrons, like Jane Bell, found nurses who married were an embarrassment to the AANS and had no tolerance for nurses who relinquished their careers for marriage.[34] Others, like Rose Creal, were more understanding but were obliged to conform to the regulations.[35] However, there is evidence that the British marriage regulations were not strictly adhered to, because Maud McCarthy (British Matron-in-Chief) recorded in 1915 that five married nurses were given special permission to remain in the QAIMNSR while another fifteen resigned so they could be married.[36]When the NZANS became a reality in 1915, Hester Maclean campaigned for the right of married nurses to join and be retained in the NZANS. Initially, a ruling that...*NZANS members would not be allowed to marry on active service and those who did so would have to resign...* was made. Maclean repeated her protest and in February 1917 the policy was amended *...NZANS sisters on active service abroad must not marry without special permission and ... they may be retired from the Service or placed on the Reserve.* A month later it was reversed to the original order. Confusion ensued, especially for the New Zealand nurses who served in British or Australian hospitals. Given that only fourteen New Zealand nurses, from a pool of five hundred, married during the war the constant revision of the policy was regrettable.[37]

14 Gallipoli and the Reality of War

...plague of blow-flies from dead bodies in August was phenomenal (at Lone Pine maggots were swept up from the trenches in bucketsful) – AG Butler.

The decision by Kaiser Wilhelm II to ignore Bismarck's advice and open the war on two fronts - France via Belgium to the west and Russia to the east - proved to be strategically disastrous. Similarly, the allies' decision to divert troops to Kut-al-Amara, the Dardanelles and Salonika demonstrated a lack of appreciation of the logistics involved in finishing an advance, especially if it was somewhat distant from the original objective.[1] However, there were a number of strategic imperatives associated with these decisions. For example, the British recognised that to maintain control of resources in India and Persia, victory in Mesopotamia (present-day Iraq) was essential. The importance of Palestine was evident when the third Battle of Gaza (Battle of Beersheba) in October 1917 was supported by *...the war's heaviest artillery attack outside Europe, with as many heavy guns per yard of front as in the battle of the Somme. Furthermore, aerial supremacy meant that their fire was better directed and coordinated.*[2]

The Dardanelles

The Austro-Hungarian and German armies advance on the Eastern Front prompted Russia's leader, Tsar Nicholas II, to request the allies to create a diversion. The Dardanelles Strait was chosen as it served a twofold purpose. It would relieve pressure on the Russian Army and open up the strait to the allies thereby facilitating the easy movement of troops and supplies via the Black Sea. The naval operation in March and the invasion in April 1915 was a strategic failure, but the campaign was a cultural turning point for the Australian and New Zealand soldiers who landed at

Gaba Tepe.[3] The initiative and bloody-mindedness of these troops in the face of overwhelming odds gave rise to an enduring, reverential respect for the term 'Anzac' (which entered the lexicon after the landing).[4]

Tragically, soldiers died even before the battle had commenced by such ordinary things as insect bites. Such was the case for the English poet Rupert Brooke (1887-1915), a member of the Royal Naval Division, who died of septicaemia (blood poisoning) on the island of Skyros in the Aegean Sea the day before the landing. He was considered to be part of the *...gifted and golden youth...* of his generation. [5] It may have been just as well because Gallipoli in April 1915 was not a place for poets; not a place for anyone.

Sea Assault

When the Ottoman Empire entered the war at the end of October 1914 it consisted of twenty million people, half of whom were Turkish. History had taught them that the Dardanelles would be of strategic importance and within three days of their alliance with Germany the allies began shelling the Dardanelles fort. In response the Ottomans began immediate improvements to existing forts and also laid 350 mines in geometric patterns along the straits. The British naval attacks commenced on 19 February but were delayed until weather conditions improved. Six days later the attack began in earnest and a number of fortifications received direct hits, which caused extreme anxiety to those in İstanbul. Despite bombardments at Gaba Tepe by *HMS Queen Elizabeth*, one of the largest battleships in the world, one third of the allied fleet was sunk by mines without reaching the Narrows. The Turks commemorate 18 March as the day in which they succeeded in repelling the enemy against all odds. The sea currents, geography of the coastline and tenacity of the Ottomans had foiled the allied attempt at invasion by sea.

The British Commander-in-Chief, General Sir Ian Hamilton and Lord Kitchener decided on a land invasion. Enver Paşa ordered the German General Otto Liman von Sanders to command the Dardanelle forces. Instead of a European and Asian defence, Liman von Sanders decided on a north and south protection of the Dardanelles and set up command at Gallipoli.He was in an unenviable position militarily because his Ottoman soldiers had no historical or social connection with Germans and the language was a barrier, even for the execution of simple orders. The religious and cultural beliefs of the Ottomans had no universal correlation with the Germans. Despite these differences there *...was a loyalty between German and Ottoman soldiers – not to be underestimated even today.*[6]

The proposed invasion was expected by the enemy but the exact time and location was not known. Mustafa Kemal was now a Lieutenant-Colonel leading a roving division with a view to identifying areas that required reinforcements. He was later known as Kemal Atatürk ('Father Turk') due in no small measure to his extraordinary leadership at Gallipoli. Liman von Sanders had correctly assumed Gaba Tepe was the most likely landing place and had reinforced the area with barbed wire defences and extra soldiers. It was inadequately defended though.

The Landing

At 8am on 25 April 1915, 8,000 allied soldiers were put ashore at Ari Burnu which was being defended by only 500 Ottomans. The Australian soldiers were mistakenly put ashore about a mile north of their intended landing place at Gaba Tepe, on the western side of the Gallipoli peninsula. They faced high ridges and rugged terrain instead of the expected open plain and gently sloping hills. The small number of Ottomans at Ari Burnu meant that the allies penetrated inland quickly. It became clear to Lieutenant-Colonel Mustafa Kemal that if the enemy reached the peak (260m) of Chunuk Bair, which dominates the entire region, the Ottoman positions would be totally exposed. He saved the situation by rushing his 57th Regiment and mountain gun artillery (not just the one battalion of the 19th Division which he had been ordered to do) to Ari Burnu. The Ottomans were seriously outnumbered but Mustafa Kemal told his men they must face the enemy and they did; the regiment was made famous because all were killed.[7] Mustafa Kemal was ordered by Liman von Sanders to drive the infidels into the sea and the Anzacs were ordered by Hamilton to *...dig, dig, dig, until you are safe.*[8]

Bravery of Doctors

Officers from both sides gave universal orders at the close of day...*send the doctors to carry off my wounded.*[9] On the peninsula Howse was one of a number of doctors as well as orderlies working in CCS. Medical officers tried to classify the wounded as a 'light casualty' by applying a white tab to the soldier's uniform or a red tab to indicate he was a more 'serious' case. The chaos of the landing meant ...*the theoretical scheme of evacuation ... was quite impossible.* This confusion had an impact on the casualties who were transported to the two main hospital ships waiting off the coast. The AANS personnel on the *Gascon* expected the seriously wounded to arrive while those on the *Clan MacGillivray* were prepared for less serious cases. Instead they were confronted with men suffering from horrific wounds. Once the medical officers had triaged the soldiers as best they could, the soldiers were transported by a small launch, an open ferry 'lighter', from a makeshift pier at the beach. These exhausted, dehydrated, wounded men had to then endure the agony of being transferred to the larger hospital ships. The work of the AAMC was relentless at Gallipoli, and during 1915 nine members of the corps died as a result of their devotion to duty.[10]

Gascon

Six Australian nurses served under a British matron on the *Gascon* on the day of the Anzac landing: Ella Tucker, Clem Marshall, Minne Kate Porter, Sophie Durham, Clarice Dickson and Daisy Richmond.[11] Ella Tucker recorded what she saw and how she felt on the day of the landing which was a ...*Red letter day. Shells bursting all round, we are off Gaba Tepe. The soldiers have commenced to land, there are Men of War, & Transport Boats, in every direction round us, an occasional shell bursts quite near us. The wounded commence to come on board about 9.a.m. – four die in the first boat that comes over – the patients just pour into the wards from the barges and boats ... I start straight away at dressing; I'm responsible for about 76 patients in the Ward, & about 40 which I have on mattresses on the fore-deck, with the assistance of a medical student, we get through all the dressings by about 2.a.m. Have quite a lot of compound fractures which I put up temporarily ... I press on with many anxious looks at the paler faces down the long line of bunks – infer that haemorrhage might pass un-noticed – several times I go back along the lines of dressings*

& find a dressing saturated, & have to apply more dressing & pressure. The boys are bricks – they smoke on & patiently wait their turn ... all this time we can hardly hear ourselves speak with the banging which is going on outside. The ship just shivers with the extra heavy reports but we are much too busy to think of what is going on – even forget that we haven't had a meal till the steward says there is a cup of tea in the pantry sisters – about 6 o'clock. The last dressing is finished about 2.30 a.m. & the men are nearly all sleeping. Matron comes into the Ward, and absolutely bundles me off to bed. At 5.30 a.m. up and in the ward again – the Orderlies look after the feeding of the patients – we can't attempt to wash them, or make their beds. I commence straight away at dressings & and go on solidly until 10-30 p.m. There are 557 patients on board & only 7 nurses, so we can't attempt to do anything else for the men, except their dressings. It nearly breaks your heart to see them lying – looking hot and dirty – & not able to sponge them & make them comfortable.[12]

At a practical level Tucker refers to a number of nursing emergencies on the first day. The risk to life from haemorrhage was acute. As mentioned earlier, Robertson did not develop the practice of adding sodium citrate to blood for another two years and 'on-the-hoof' transfusion option was not feasible. The continual application of pressure to the wound and the reapplication of bandages to promote clotting was the only option available to the nurses.

The Australian nurses on the *Gascon* adapted to military nursing. Awards are not the only measure of competence and many excellent nurses did not receive any. Nonetheless, Richmond, Marshall, Minnie Kate Porter and Clarice Dickson were recognized for their war service.

Daisy Richmond

Daisy Richmond proved to be an excellent military nurse but her earlier life and training did not prepare her for what she had to face. She was born 3 March 1883 in Maitland, South Australia, the daughter of the Reverend F. Richmond. The family later moved to Boorowa, NSW, where her father was the Anglican Minister. Daisy Richmond worked as a teacher before commencing her nurse training at SHSEH, completing the course in 1911. After nursing in Sydney and Melbourne she joined the Bush Nursing Association in 1913 and developed expertise in nursing women and children in remote areas. Like many in the AANS she learnt fast.

Vera Brittain's cousin was shot while landing at Suvla Bay. He did not die from the bullet but from being left unattended for a week at Mudros, during which time sepsis took hold. She, like many around the world, was shocked to realise *...that lives were being thrown away through the inadequacy of the medical services in the Mediterranean.*[13] Mudros harbor on the Greek Island of Lemnos was the staging post for casualties who were later transported to Egypt. It would take until August before 3AGH was eventually established at Lemnos.

AANS and QAIMNSR on the *Assaye: Bessie Pocock*

The reputation of Bessie Pocock as a leader and disciplinarian was mixed. For example, during the Gallipoli Campaign she served on the *Assaye* with Australian nurses who had sailed on RMS *Mooltan* and were subsequently loaned to the QAs. The nurses included Staff Nurses Vickers Foote, Gilliland and Day. The latter two refused to work with Matron Pocock, who claimed a medical officer had requested the removal of Staff Nurse Gilliland from his ward because she was *...useless.*[14] The accuracy or otherwise of this claim is impossible to discern but the acute staff shortages on the hospital ships at the time make it difficult to comprehend. Furthermore, it was the norm for a nurse leader to defend her staff against any such accusations until they were verified by another nurse. Nurses assessed the competence of other nurses.

Kathleen (Kitty) Power

Evelyn Vickers Foote recalled *...we were all Australian sisters, except one Irish girl, trained in Dublin, Sisters Day, Howman* [Hoyman], *Gillebrand* [Gilliland], *and O'Cooke.'*[15] The Irish girl, Kitty Power, born in 1888, was only young when she commenced her training at St. Stevens Hospital in Dublin. She completed four-and-a-half years and then a further two-and-a-half years as a sister and superintendent. She was a member of the QAIMNSR for more than four years, commencing around 1912.[16] This would account for her immediate inclusion in the Dardanelles campaign because she would have gained military training during her time in the reserve.

The procedure for joining the AANS from the QAIMNSR was easier for Kitty Power than it was for Australian nurses CL Despard, Beatrice Mawson and Vickers Foote. Despite being loaned to the QAIMNSR when they enlisted in Australia, they had to return to Australia and enlist in the AANS. The three seasoned military nurses boarded the ill-fated *Mongolia* at Port Said on 13 June 1917 and the journey was so terrifying that only one, Vickers Foote, eventually re-enlisted with the AANS.[17] The administrative protocols of the AIF were not always logical or consistent.

Conversely, it was relatively easy for Kitty Power, who signed her attestation papers on 9 March 1916 while stationed in Egypt, to join the AANS. On the date of signing she recorded, in her own hand, that she had been a member of the AANS since 24 August 1915 and prior to this date had been a member of the QAIMNSR.[18] There are numerous instances of Australian nurses travelling to England to join the QAIMNSR but the reverse happening was rare.[19] However, it was not unheard of for English men, living in Australia, who wanted to get home to England, but could not afford the fare, to join the AIF. A well-known example is John Kirkpatrick who, along with his dutiful off-sider, was immortalised in Australia as 'Simpson and his donkey'.[20]

AANS Service in Egypt

Although it is safe to assume Kitty Power served on the *Assaye* she becomes historically visible as an AANS nurse once she signed the attestation papers. Although she signed her attestation papers at 4AAH (Egypt) in March 1916 she left Melbourne on the *Morea* on 24 August 1915 and joined the AANS on 11 August 1915. This suggests she most likely found herself in Australia after accompanying casualties back to Australia from Egypt.

10 AGH to Egypt via England

Once in Australia, Kitty Power needed to get back to the war so she responded to the call for special reinforcements to staff a new unit, 10AGH. This unit was expected to take over the functions of 1AAH, Harefield, London. Owing to administrative confusion the staff of the proposed 10AGH was dispersed to various convalescent hospitals throughout England. Eventually the nurses were sent to units in Egypt.

Kitty disembarked at Suez where she was taken on strength with 1AGH (Heliopolis) on 21 September 1915. On 22 March 1916 Kitty Power was temporarily transferred to 3AGH, where she most likely worked with Anne Donnell and May Tilton.

4 AAH, Abbassia: Infection Control Nursing, 1916

Following service at 3AGH, Kitty Power worked at 4AAH, which was a 420 bed infectious disease hospital in Abbassia.[21] In 1916 Pauline E Pierre Humbert AANS), who also worked at 4AAH in 1916, was *...vaccinated four times without any result...* on her voyage on the RMS *Mooltan* from Australia which indicates a certain lack of robustness in the inoculation process. Although Power clearly showed vaccination marks on her left arm there is no way of knowing if she received the cholera vaccination while in Egypt. Sister Pierre Humbert found *...the staff had very comfortable quarters and a fairly good mess...*, and although they were required to wear caps and gowns for infection control purposes *...they had them laundered at their own expense.* [22] Given that in June 1916 4AAH admitted 150 typhoid cases in one day, the laundering costs were likely to be prohibitive on an AANS wage. In August 1916, 4AAH was transformed into a Turkish POW hospital where seriously ill patients were nursed and those requiring less intensive care were transferred to a Red Crescent hospital. To the Ottomans the 'red cross' emblem was a negative symbol associated with the crusaders. Instead they adopted the 'red crescent' which had the same humanitarian connotations as the 'red cross' had to allied armies.[23] Kitty Power and Letitia Moreton, who also served at 4AAH prior to her departure from Egypt, may have become immune-compromised while caring for the soldiers who had a vast array of infectious diseases at 4AAH.[24]

***Mooltan* (May 1915) reinforcements: Charlotte Berrie, Agnes Corfield and Mary Stafford**

Two Australian nurses who sailed with Matron Grace Wilson were Charlotte (Chassie) Berrie and Agnes Corfield, who embarked on RMS *Mooltan* on 15 May 1915 from NSW (2 MD).[25] A select number of Australian nurses on the *Mooltan* were assigned or loaned to British nursing units and effectively ceased to exist as

Australian nurses from an administrative and historical perspective.[26]

Chassie Berrie was born in Brisbane on 14 April 1885, the daughter of a mining engineer, Peter McGregor Berrie, and his wife Agnes (née O'Lachlan). Her family, including two sisters, moved to Cairns (Gimuy Walubara Yidinji Country) in northern Queensland in 1903 where Peter worked as an engineer and Agnes worked as a domestic at the Shamrock Hotel.[27] In 1912 Charlotte completed her training at RBWH and the following year she undertook 'home duties' as she cared for her father in Bamford (a suburb of Brisbane).[28]

Details of Agnes Corfield's life are scant but she was born in 1892 in Maryborough, Queensland (Gubbi Gubbi Country) and also completed her training at RBWH in 1914, just in time to enlist for war service.[29] Berrie and Corfield spent the war in Egypt and Palestine.

When the *Mooltan* reached Adelaide, Mary Stafford's service record claims she was a brunette with a fresh complexion and of medium build when she embarked. She had undertaken private nursing and had gained experience in the wards when she left Adelaide on 20 May 1915. Unlike Berrie and Corfield, who were henceforth known as QAs, Stafford was fortunate to be a member of the AANS throughout the war.[30]

3 AGH Egypt: August 1915

A photograph of Grace Wilson at the time of her service shows an attractive woman of 36 years, medium build (167cm, 64kg) with an olive complexion and dark brown hair and eyes. Her youngest brother of six children, Graeme, an engineer in the 2nd Light Horse Brigade, left Queensland on 24 September 1914 with the first AIF contingent. He was just 24 years old when he left whereas Grace was much more mature and had travelled widely. At the time of leaving, Wilson was still PM of 1 MD and Matron of the Brisbane Hospital. She, and her family, anticipated Grace meeting up with Graeme but on arrival in Egypt she was greeted with the news that Graeme was 'Killed in Action' (KIA) on 19 May 1915 at Monash Gully.[31] Reportedly he died instantly from a sniper's bullet.[32] One of Grace's other brothers, Norman, served from 1915 to 1919 while still another, Roy, was rejected by the AIF as medically unfit due to an injured knee.[33] Nonetheless, the death of one child was too much to bear. Not unusually, but nonetheless heart-breakingly, after the war Graeme's mother made her way to London, seeking advice from the War Office about where she might find the remains of her dead son.[34] Locating an identifiable grave amongst the many in Monash Gully was near impossible.

The Battle of Lone Pine: August 1915

Grace Wilson had to put her grief aside as she was given the herculean task of establishing 3AGH on Lemnos. Wilson and her nurses arrived at Lemnos in August, four months after the initial landing, but they were confronted with a high number of casualties. Ian Hamilton made the ill-fated decision to break the stalemate at Gallipoli and finally push through to the Dardanelles. Like the landing, the results in terms of meeting strategic military objectives and containing the burgeoning casualty numbers were poor. In particular, the Battle of Lone Pine, which was part of the feint designed to divert the Ottomans as allied reinforcements attempted to counterattack the strait, was a bloodbath. Within four days 80 Australian officers plus 2,197 allied soldiers and approximately 5,000 Ottomans were killed.[35] Lessons from the landing, regarding the transfer and triage of casualties, had not been learnt.

Matron Grace Wilson, 3 AGH, Lemnos: August 1915

The unnecessary diversion to England and a delay of a few days in the harbour of Mudros on Lemnos caused Wilson to despair of ever getting down to work. She recorded on her arrival ...*Things are just too awful for words ... about 40 miles from the firing line. We are the first women to come so far, except for the Sisters on the hospital ships ... imagine a bare piece of ground, covered with stones, from the size of pebbles to boulders – the men in their clothes lying on it – waiting – and we Sisters imprisoned on a ship opposite, also waiting and doing nothing – and you have 3AGH after touring for eleven or twelve weeks.*[36] Eventually, they were transferred onto the island where they were ...*met at the pier of West Mudros by a staff sergeant with bagpipes playing us into camp!*[37] She must have thought she was in a pantomime.

It was now that the calibre of Grace Wilson's leadership manifested. She soon restored order despite the plant and equipment for 3 AGH not arriving for another six weeks. Wilson, through leadership, reinforced the nursing ideal of the best possible care with the available resources. This was not always easy as Sister Howitt (AANS) found …*when the patients came in, we had nothing for them and had to tear up sheets and towels etc., to wash and bandage them with. We had to use sanitary utensils to wash them in and this chaos continued for three weeks, until the equipment arrived.*[38] Each tent or makeshift ward contained …*many very sick men; many were suffering from Dysentery, various … Fevers, Rheumatics, Gastritis and Pneumonia…* as well as other patients with wounds from the August offensive.[39]

Matron Wilson herself was critical of Australian nurses for not taking the time to appreciate the importance of completing requisition forms and tallying statistics because they were under the impression …*these things are stuff and nonsense.*[40] After Lemnos, she realised the value of good relations with the quartermaster and tried to instil in her nurses the need to be competent in all areas of military nursing: Not just at the bedside but in administration too.

The lack of clean water was one of the biggest issues for the nurses. Sister Charlotte Donnelly (AANS) noted that…*The water was very bad, and we had no way of sterilising it. We had many dysentery patients from the Peninsula, and the water made them ill … The theatre was going day and night, and in about six weeks time, we were fully fitted up.*[41] Given the range of surgical cases and seriousness of wounds, removing the dried and thickly encrusted dressings from blood-soaked soldiers was a difficult task. Sister Florence Maud Howitt (AANS) …*was transferred to the theatre. There was not very much here, and we had to make shift with anything we had. The cases were of all kinds – Laminectomy and amputations.*[42]

Grace Wilson had concerns about the welfare of her nurses because their living conditions were primitive due to a combination of extremes in weather and inappropriate accommodation. Her nurses were at risk of strain from over-work, disease, dehydration, starvation and exposure to the elements. For instance, one nurse checked her bed each night for …*snakes, moles, scorpions and centipedes…* and generally managed to …*catch something.*[43]

Outcome of the August Offensive

It became clear to the military authorities by the end of August that the second attempt at taking the Dardanelles was a failure. In one four-day period the British and allied forces sacrificed 12,000 men whose corpses, along with those of the enemy, became part of the Turkish landscape.[44] Soldiers who were not killed outright were transferred to hospitals in Egypt, including 2 AGH.

On 17 August 1915 the Commander-in-Chief of the British Expeditionary Force, General Sir Ian Hamilton, sent a report to Lord Kitchener detailing the outcome of the August offensive at Gallipoli. He used the opportunity to claim *...how nearly this operation was a success complete beyond all anticipation...* and rather poetically explained that *...unfortunately, the 54th Division broke in my hand, leaving me like a fencer with a broken rapier.*[45] The health consequences of the ill-fated August offensive at Gallipoli are best summarised by the Official Australian Medical Historian who recorded in less lyrical terms that the *...plague of blow-flies from dead bodies in August was phenomenal (at Lone Pine maggots were swept up from the trenches in bucketsful).*[46]

***Orsova* reinforcements: 2AGH, Egypt: August - December 1915**

Reinforcements were sent on the *Orsova* in August including three competent nurses from Victoria. Letitia Moreton, aged 23, said goodbye to her family, who returned a few weeks later to farewell her cousin, George Victor Moreton.[47] Letitia sailed with two other Staff Nurses, Blodwyn Williams and Edith Moorhouse, who both hailed from Ballarat.

They arrived at 2 AGH in August 1915 and the next day Williams *...went on duty in a medical ward with 100 beds. That night I had my first experience of convoys of sick and wounded which I shall never forget, it was simply dreadful to see the poor boys, absolute wrecks, nothing but skin and bone, and the heat and flies were a great trial at times, still the boys were always bright and cheerful in the midst of it all how little we have had to grumble about, compared with what the boys have had.*[48] Pressure on the three new recruits was acute as they dealt with the influx of casualties. Edith Moorhouse was now working with Letitia Moreton who found *...Military nursing is quite different to other nursing and it takes quite a while to get used to it.*[49]

Edith Moorhouse: Biography

Edith had already dealt with a great deal in her life and she soon became a competent military nurse. Born in the small country town of Kyabram (Victoria, Bangarang & Yort Yorta Country) in 1886, she was the fourth child of Frederick and Deborah Moorhouse (née McCleary) who were married in 1879. She had two older sisters, Mary and Jane, an older brother Mathew and a younger sister, Sarah. Any chance of an emotionally secure childhood was destroyed when she was just five years old when her mother died. Her father died the following year.[50]

Her father's sister, Helen, had married William Ponsford, a prominent businessman in Echuca. Her paternal uncle, Henry Moorhouse, was a surveyor who also lived in the town.[51] It appears that the young orphaned family settled in Echuca and Edith was most likely cared for by her uncle Henry and his wife Louise. The local community of Echuca, which was a short distance from Kyabram, embraced her as one of their own.[52] Henry and Louise's son, Leslie Victor Moorhouse, was two years younger than Edith and as they grew up together they were more like brother and sister than cousins.

By the time war was declared Edith had demonstrated that she was a competent young woman, completing three years of general nurse training at Mooroopna Hospital and registering with the RVTNA. The hospital was near where she had grown up and Edith had five years' experience as a qualified civilian nurse, including infectious nursing experience. She was a 'Sister-in-Charge' when she enlisted with the AANS in 1915. It is more than likely she met Louisa Bicknel who also worked at Mooroopna Hospital prior to enlisting. Edith's cousin, Leslie also enlisted with the AIF and attained the rank of Captain.[53] Henry Moorhouse had retired to Hawthorn, Melbourne, and was Edith's, and his son's, next-of-kin.[54]

Three weeks after her arrival in Egypt, Moreton wrote that she liked being part of 2AGH because *...they are very good to the patients here. Since we came we have admitted over 800.* By the time the *Orsova* reinforcements arrived in Egypt, the staff of 2 AGH had been dispersed to different physical locations because of the climate. Mena House was re-opened as a convalescent hospital and later Moreton was sent to the Ghezireh Palace Hotel where she found Nellie Miles Walker was a...*wonderful* *matron, such a splendid manager.*[55] This view of Miles Walker never faltered throughout the war. She was competent and kind, an essential combination for any nurse.

Edith Moorhouse's service was not linear. She served at 2 AGH (Mena House) from August until October 1915 with Letitia and Blodwyn and was then sent to 2 Convalescent Depot at Ras el-Tin, located on the outskirts of Alexandria and considered quite 'unsatisfactory' as a convalescent hospital.[56] After a month Moorhouse returned to Australia on 18 November 1915 on transport duty aboard the *Nestor,* which left Egypt with the soldiers who had been evacuated from the Gallipoli Peninsula following the August offensive. Her return was not permanent as she was part of 2AGH by this time and she wanted to return to her unit, to her soldiers.

Hospital changes in Egypt

A summary of the change in the status and roles of the hospitals during August 1915 included:

1: Mena House was reopened to accommodate 400 men. PM Nellie Gould.

2: Abbassia Army Barracks, Cairo was taken over by 1AGH and became 4AAH, which was staffed by 6 Australian Field Ambulance. 4AAH was expected to cater for a few hundred patients. In 1916 PM Rose Creal was in-charge when it became 14AGH.

3: A fine civilian hospital at Choubra was taken over by 3AAH. The staff and cases were transferred to Choubra Hospital, which became an infectious hospital.

4: 3AAH was reopened on 10 August and 850 light cases were nursed in this pavilion (sporting club) hospital.[57]

5: 3AGH was established on Lemnos. Matron Grace Wilson.

Gallipoli began to freeze and the soldier's suffering intensified. A request was made to Lord Kitchener for another 100,000 soldiers and he reconsidered the invasion strategy resulting in the entire allied force being evacuated by the end of December.[58] Meanwhile, AANS nurses continued to enlist and when they arrived at locations around the world they carried on the earlier work of their colleagues.

Matron Grace Wilson, RRC

After the successful evacuation of soldiers from Gallipoli the nurses of 3 AGH remained on Lemnos until 13 January 1916 and were then transferred to the Abbassia Army Barracks near Cairo, where they awaited new orders. One of Wilson's nurses, Anne Donnell, recorded in her diary *...We hear Matron has been awarded the Royal Red Cross and aren't we pleased!* Less than two weeks later, at the end of May, the nurses organised a special dinner to honour their matron. Officers who had also served on Lemnos were invited and in response to a toast by Colonel Stawell who noted *...how Matron's bright personality and influence had helped us all on to bigger efforts...* Matron Wilson *...said the honour of the Royal Red Cross was for us all, not for herself alone, that it could only be given to one, and that she could not have done what was done without the united help of us all.*[59] The RRC was the first military award bestowed on Grace Wilson but it was not the last. Before the First World War was over she was MID four times.[60] The diary entry by Donnell on 31 May 1916 is particularly moving as she describes the speeches given and the table design/menu. Australian civilian trained nurses made the transition to competent military nurses under confronting circumstances in 1915. Like soldiers, they had no idea what to expect but they faced the war wounds and the diseases with courage and stoicism, always considering the soldier's suffering and suppressing their own. These ATNA trained women were now military nurses.

15 War Wounds and Disease

......the deadly bitter seriousness of war ... purifies and deepens the entire human being – David Oppenheimer

During the Renaissance, the church reinforced the long-held doctrine that the mind and soul belonged to the metaphysical world. Abnormalities of the mind were the result of moral deviations and those afflicted were *ipso facto* evil. While this view was recognised as being scientifically invalid during the early twentieth century, uncertainty about how to differentiate delinquent behaviour from neurotic or psychotic conditions persisted.[1]

Morality or Madness

The impact of the war on individuals was diverse. Henry Maudsley (1835-1918) and Mercier (1852-1919) had developed their thesis on ...*moral insanity.* At the same time, the theories of Freud and other psychoanalysts were gaining momentum.[2] The Nancy School (1880-90) in France had inspired Freud, Jung and Adler and, as a consequence, the psychoanalytic school of thought. The original research of Janet (1907) on mental dissociation and Charcot who identified the condition of 'hysteria' helped establish psychoanalytic terms in the medical language.[3]

A number of Australian trained nurses, who were now leaders in the AANS and New Zealand, including Nellie Gould and Hester Maclean, were ATNA registered mental nurses.[4] Gould gained experience at the Hospital for the Insane, Rydalmere (NSW, Dharug Country) while Maclean worked at the Bay View Asylum, Sydney.[5]

When the psychoanalyst and protégé of Sigmund Freud, Carl Gustav Jung, had visions of world destruction in early 1914, the declaration of war in August confirmed in his mind that his visions were prescient and not due to neurosis.

Therefore, he believed he had an ...*obligation to probe the depths of my own psyche.* He did this throughout the war in neutral Switzerland and claimed the neurosis of his patients, during these years, was due to the...*spirit of the age.*[6] Conversely, David Oppenheimer, a classics scholar and member of Adler's Society for Free Psychoanalytic Research, became a German officer during the First World War and found ...*the deadly bitter seriousness of war ... purifies and deepens the entire human being.*[7] Both conclusions did little to assist the vast number of soldiers, and some nurses, who endured the physical and psychological terror of shell-shock.

Shell-shock

The term 'shell-shock' was used by the Duke of Wellington and had therefore entered the military lexicon long before the First World War.[8] Nonetheless, the ...*study of the "mind" was, in 1914, philosophic and introspective rather than scientific...* and only the more complex syndromes, like dementia praecox (premature dementia) and paranoia, attracted the attention of physicians and researchers.[9] It was anticipated by the military and medical authorities that any soldiers exhibiting signs of mental illness would not survive the process of ...*weeding out...* during initial training.[10] This idea failed to take into account that a psychologically healthy individual, once exposed to the trauma of war, would be adversely affected by the experience. Consequently, doctors and nurses were ill-prepared for the diverse and severe mental health issues within the ranks.[11] Conscripts were thought to be more cowardly than volunteers so they were thought to be more likely to succumb to shell-shock. This notion was put to rest when Australian soldiers, none of whom were conscripts, developed the condition, often after a number of years of serving bravely.

The official medical historian, AG Butler, claimed the Gallipoli campaign offered treating medical officers a rare opportunity to review wartime conditions of a unique, self-contained cohort. That is, it was of a specific duration, was limited to one area of land and comprised a complete experience.[12] Initially it was believed that shell-shock occurred after a physical shock to the brain, usually the frontal lobe, resulting in lesions of varying sizes. This hypothesis was soon replaced with another: The unconscious need to escape into disease, like hysteria but without the weaker, feminine connotations.

Disordered Action of the Heart (DAH)

In September 1915, a medical officer, Colonel Purves-Stewart, examined the apparently healthy soldiers in the trenches at Gallipoli. He found 77 per cent were anaemic and 50 per cent had tachycardia (rapid pulse) which was ...*not due to sudden exertion or emotion* ...while 74 per cent suffered from shortness of breath. If the link between anaemia and the cardio-pulmonary symptoms was understood at the time, it was not explicitly reported. This condition, labelled Disordered Action of the Heart (DAH), was considered to be psychosomatic in nature but offered ...*hope of an understanding of the interaction of mind and body in disease.*[13] Eventually it was recognised that ...*simple terror*... is not pathological but is a normal response to ...*a threat to life.*[14] This research did little to help understand the cause of shell-shock.

Management of shell-shock at 2AGH

Matron Gould and Dr Springthorpe, a senior physician, served together at 2 AGH. They researched the signs and symptoms of shell-shock and developed a treatment plan which had some benefits.[15]

It was in the early stages of the war that ...*nervous functional disorders were classified into:*

a) neuroses involving the motor apparatus and common sensibility, the special senses, and speech;

b) neurasthenia (including "trench spine");

c) psychoses (minor psychoses, mental stupor, insanity).[16]

Gould also worked with Dr AW Campbell, who introduced rudimentary treatment. The soldier was given a few days to 'settle down' and then encouraged to whisper so normal speech would return, but it was noted that progress was compromised if the soldier experienced another shock during his recovery.[17] The introduction of ...*Corps Rest Stations*... gave the front-line soldier a chance to recover from the bombardment of battle and reduce the likelihood of symptoms becoming chronic. Occasionally morphia was given and the soldier was rested for an hour and then sent back to the front, but the outcome of such treatment was not scientifically evaluated.[18] There is little doubt the AAMC and AANS was better prepared for the physical, as opposed to the psychological, impact of war.

Operating theatres

The makeshift operating theatres were in constant use and nurses were confronted with horrific wounds. The operating theatres of the auxiliary hospitals were tailored from all manner of buildings. For example, 1 AAH had been an amusement centre known as Luna Park. The 'mysterious cavern' acted as a dressing room while the operating theatre had once been the ticket office.[19] Fortunately, the pre-operative protocol was sound and required each theatre sister to be responsible for her own patient. Esther King recalled she took her patient from the ward and *...prepared the theatre, took her own dressings, sterilized instruments, and lotions.* The equipment in the theatre *...consisted of a Primus stove ... with two stools ... a few anaesthetics on a box. Linen ... from the Q.M. for each case and used it unsterilized...*but fortunately...*this all improved in time.*

Sterile techniques often failed due to lack of antiseptics.[20] Instruments were boiled in soda water for ten minutes, except scissors and knives which were either placed in carbolic acid or methylated spirits *...for a few minutes.* Sutures and catgut were in high demand and sterilised in various ways. Silk sutures were by far the easiest to prepare, no more than two layers were wound onto glass rods and boiled for 30 minutes, then placed in a glass jar of carbolic acid with a tightly fitted lid.[21] Needless to say, it was not unknown for patients to acquire infections during surgery or, for that matter, for nurses to become infected while attending to post-operative dressings.

Death from Sepsis: Louisa Bicknell, 1AGH, 1915

All too soon into the war it was recorded that on *...June 25th 1915 ... the first Sister from 1 AGH. Sister Bicknell ... died ... after a short illness.*[22] Louisa Bicknell (1879-1915) died of sepsis within three months of joining the AANS. She was the first Australian nurse to die during military service. The term sepsis covered a multitude of infections from the relatively minor, which a strong immune system could deal with, to death. However, most cases during wartime resulted in a quick death.

Back in Australia on 3 July 1915 a small column appeared in the death notices of a Victorian newspaper. It read... *BICKNELL. On the 25th June, at Heliopolis, Egypt, Louisa Annie Bicknell, dearly loved sister of Mrs. A.A. Connell and J.G. Bicknell, Campaspe, aged 36.* A week later the same newspaper announced that Staff Nurse Louisa Annie Bicknell had been ...*Called Home*! A reference, no doubt, to her spiritual home because by this time she had been buried at the Cairo War Memorial Cemetery, Egypt.[23]

Louisa was afforded a full military and Christian burial, which was in keeping with her status as an AANS nurse and her Anglican faith. Her nursing colleagues became mourners and they include Sisters Grewar, Kate Porter, Tyson, Mowbray and Woniaski; four of these five women were themselves dead by 1921.[24] When John Bicknell and Eliza Brooks married in 1869 they did not envisage their youngest child, a daughter, being a casualty of a world war.[25]

Like many relatives of the 60,000 Australian servicemen and women who died, Louisa Bicknell's family mourned her from afar. Elmore in rural Victoria was a world away from Cairo. Her ageing parents had to also deal with the additional trauma of recently receiving word from Louisa that she was in ...*splendid health*. The slow transport of mail via ships resulted in letters being received out of order. Grieving parents, who had already received the dreaded telegram, often found cheery letters from deceased sons and daughters in their letterbox, sometimes months later: Creating a new and all too poignant hell.

Florence MacKenzie: A slow death from sepsis.

Sepsis could be a slow death. Despite precautions, bacteria from the trenches would find their way into the hospitals via the soldiers' footwear and clothes. Conditions in the trenches were appalling and it was near impossible to prevent cross-infection. Florence MacKenzie, aged 35, was dressing a septic case when she accidentally stuck a safety pin into the middle finger of her right hand. She had already had two years military experience on Hospital Transports nursing the sick and wounded from Egypt, London and Australia. Florence was nominally attached to 1 AGH but nursed in AAHs in England and Egypt awaiting another full load of casualties.

After her injury she was invalided to Australia in July 1917 where a month later, 31 August 1917, she was admitted to 8 AGH (Fremantle). Her finger was obviously infected and despite incisions into the finger and her palm the infection would not heal. The following month her middle finger was amputated but unfortunately, arthritis, stiffness and limitation in the movement of other fingers occurred post-operatively and she became debilitated, losing more than a stone in weight.[26] Despite her medical notes making reference to her tiring easily during her convalescence, she had to make a living.

There were no pensions or government support for nurses who had served. As was often the case with ex-soldiers and nurses, once Florence MacKenzie was discharged from the AIF on 16 November 1917, she ceased to exist. Her immediate whereabouts remain unclear but in 1919 she did secure a position as matron of Cue Hospital in outback WA, 660 kms north of Perth (Wajarri, Badimia, Wutha and Tjupan Country). Cue was once a thriving town of 10,000 in the 1890s when it became the centre of the Murchison goldfields. Matron MacKenzie was only in the position for a number of weeks when she became ill with dysentery and died suddenly. She was buried in March 1919 about ten kilometers away at the Day Dawn cemetery.[27]

Diphtheria

The diphtheria bacillus is highly contagious and is rapidly spread by droplets escaping from the mouth, nose or throat of an infected person. Without recourse to antibiotics, the primary management was isolation nursing. One of the more alarming aspects of the disease is that the diphtheria bacillus can produce a toxin which spreads throughout the body and can affect the nervous system and heart permanently.[28] Although an anti-toxin was given to counteract the risk, those who were infected often had such mild symptoms they were unaware they were infected until the condition was sufficiently advanced to be fatal.[29]

Enteric Conditions: Typhoid, Paratyphoid, Dysentery, Cholera

The August Offensive led to an alarming rise in the prevalence of various diseases often described under the umbrella term 'enteric'. This is a generic term used to describe conditions affecting the intestine including cholera, diarrhoea, dysentery, typhoid and paratyphoid. When outbreaks of cholera occurred during the Gallipoli Campaign, AIF soldiers were strongly urged, although not compelled, to accept the risk which accompanied inoculation. However, when a confirmed outbreak of the disease occurred amongst the ALH the AIF decided ...*compulsion was to be exercised.*[30] Three soldiers elected the disgrace of court-martial rather than risk inoculation.[31]

Normally, diarrhoea is considered a symptom of a disease but, due to the difficulty of confirming the diagnosis,specific enteric diseases such as typhoid, paratyphoid, cholera and dysentery were often given a provisional diagnosis of 'diarrhoea' until further confirmation.[32] Accurate diagnosis was complex because the signs and symptoms were similar. The appalling level of vermin running from trench to trench, corpse to corpse, added to the burden on doctors who had to work under horrific and unsanitary conditions while trying to accurately diagnose diseases they had rarely come across in peacetime.[33]

Dysentery and Cholera

The mode of onset and symptoms were similar for all enteric conditions.[34] Dysentery and cholera are similar in onset because they are lower intestinal infections. The patient presents with fever, stomach cramps and the sudden onset of diarrhea which is often streaked with blood and pus.[35] Asiatic cholera is the most common form of the disease and is caused by *Vibrio cholera,* a spiral bacterium. In 1914-18 vaccination did not assure complete immunity. Today the oral cholera vaccine (OCV) can help prevent and control the disease. Factors including the quality of the local water supply, community sanitation, herd immunity and the integrity of the individual's immune system have a direct impact on infection rates within the ranks.[36]

Once infected with cholera, it takes between one and five days for the intestine to become inflamed to such an extent that a sloughing necrosis of the lining of the gut occurs. This results in the intestinal tract distending with a thin watery fluid which painlessly and continuously seeps from the bowel. Death from the effects of persistent vomiting and diarrhoea, which ultimately causes dehydration and an electrolyte imbalance due to the loss of alkaline substances, is quick. There is some evidence that the importance of electrolyte replacement was not known at this time, as there is no mention of cholera patients receiving intravenous infusions of sodium bicarbonate which would have negated life-threatening acidosis.[37]

Nursing strategies for cholera

Evelyn Vickers Foote was a remarkable nurse who was loaned to the QAIMNSR and later returned to Australia so she could join the AANS and once again serve. She found cholera to be ...*the most terrible disease I have seen. Cases would die on the stretcher 12 hours after they were taken ill. We dressed in rubber costumes with masks, overalls, and rubber boots. The vomiting was so terrible we had to have masks, Jacanet* [type of gauze] *across nose and mouth, with a wad of wool soaked with a strong smelling antiseptic. We were isolated ... The cases usually died or got better within 24 hours. The cases practically lived on Pot.Permang., two pints per day to drink, as well as solid tablets. There was a transfusion of saline (hypertonic) into a vein.*[38]

Potassium permanganate is a drug which owes its antiseptic properties to the liberation of oxygen in the presence of organic matter. Hence these dark purple crystals (permanganates form the basis of Condy's fluid) most likely diluted in a solution of 0.1 per cent, were used to clean the intestine of cholera patients as well as hydrate them.[39] Surprisingly the management of cholera today is relatively unchanged, although more attention is paid to the importance of replacing specific electrolytes at the correct ratio and the use of antibiotics. Nevertheless, the same principles of prompt diagnosis, isolation, positive electrolyte balance and re-hydration still apply.[40]

Typhoid, Paratyphoid: 3AGH, Lemnos, 1915

The research of Georges Dreyer, a medical officer serving in France, was furthered by another medico at Lemnos (3AGH), Captain Archibald.[41] The symptoms of typhoid and paratyphoid are very similar, although the latter is usually milder and has a shorter incubation period, and the onset of symptoms is often more immediate.[42] However, during a particularly severe epidemic at Gallipoli toward the end of 1915 medicos were able to isolate specific differences.[43] Finding a correct diagnosis ensured appropriate treatment and a better outcomes for the sufferer.

Typhoid fever is a bacterial infection (*Salmonella typhi*) which enters the body through the intestinal tract from contaminated food and water. Once inside, the typhoid bacillus is picked up in the bloodstream where it multiplies. The early symptoms are headache and perhaps a sore throat – both of which are not terribly alarming during wartime. Fever and increasingly severe diarrhoea was a sound clinical indicator of typhoid. Once ulcers developed along the lining of the intestine, perforation and subsequent haemorrhage were the biggest risks to life. Nurses were alert to clinical signs such as rising temperature and the development of either constipation or yellowish, greenish, watery diarrhoea. These changes often gave rise to periods of chills and sweating accompanied by no appetite.

Nursing Management of Typhoid

The nursing management of typhoid was basic and the main aim was to reduce the fever. Under ideal conditions, patients were nursed in isolation and ice packs and sponge baths were used to reduce the patient's temperature (see previous discussion of the Hare typhoid bath). Dehydration was minimized by ensuring the patient's fluid input remained greater than fluid output, thereby keeping him in a positive balance.[774] Nurses closely observed patients for any signs of intestinal bleeding including a rapid, thready pulse and quick, shallow respirations. Such changes were suggestive of a life-threatening perforation at which time the patient may have experienced *...intense abdominal pain and tenderness, frequent vomiting, a rapid pulse, and a sunken and anxious face.*[44]

Choubra Infectious Diseases Hospital: Maud Kellett: Egypt 1916

In 1916 the Choubra Infectious Diseases Hospital was a designated specialist typhoid hospital. Maud Kellett was appointed matron but she was not initially pleased with the appointment because *...the word Choubra seemed to strike terror to my* *heart, thought it was away in the desert somewhere, and only Natives near...* but she was pleasantly surprised to find it was located not too distant from Cairo and it was a *...fine civil hospital...* which accommodated 400 infectious patients.[45]

Amy O'Grady and Kitty Power in Egypt

Amy O'Grady and Kathleen (Kitty) Power had a great deal in common once they enlisted with the AANS. However, there is no evidence they were acquainted before their wartime service when they left Melbourne. Amy's brother, Reverend James Henry O'Grady, most likely spent the war years knocking on the doors of homes with the unwelcome news of a beloved relative who was wounded, dead or missing-in-action.[46]

Amy was transferred to Choubra hospital in March 1916 and the working conditions were strenuous. She worked a long day (7 am-8 pm) followed by a short shift (7 am-1 pm) every alternate day, and was usually allowed one day off each week.[47] The Egyptian summer was extremely tiring for nurses who wore a heavy ward uniform underneath an array of infection control paraphernalia. This was necessary to act as protection from the many serious infectious cases with which they were in constant contact.[48] Even Kellett, who was tireless, recognised the *...work was so continuous and strenuous, nurses only did three months here, six changing every fortnight.*[49]

James Martin: *Glenart Castle*, 1915.

Not all soldiers found their way to a specialised hospital. The youngest member of the AIF, Private James Martin, who claimed he was eighteen but was only fourteen years old, died of typhoid on the *Glenart Castle.* It is difficult to contemplate the distress the symptoms of typhoid caused this child soldier: A young boy dying without family on a ship off the coast of Gallipoli on 25 October 1915.[50]

Gangrene

History is often limited by the mere description of events. However, it is the bombardment of the senses which stays with participants of a war. For example, the symptoms of gangrene depend on the site of infection but *...may include fever, pain,* *darkening of the skin and an unpleasant odour.*[51] On 24 May 1915 a ceasefire was called between the Ottomans and Anzacs. Between the hours of 7.30 am and 4.30 pm 4,000 bodies, at varies stages of decay, were buried. If the ghastliness of the situation is put to one side the question remains: what did such a day in history smell like? An Australian soldier who *...felt eternally grateful to the Ottoman medico who gave him pieces of scented wool to block his nostrils...*knew the answer.[52]

While Doris Ridgway remained in Australia completing her training at the Adelaide Hospital, two of her younger brothers, Hugh and Eric, volunteered for overseas service with the first AIF. Eric joined the 9th Light Horse Regiment and while both brothers were away the family was, understandably *...filled with apprehension.* Eric remained in Egypt after the evacuation of Gallipoli, but a few months before Doris completed her nurse training he was accidentally shot and later died from gangrene on 1 July 1917. The only treatment being amputation and that was only possible if it was confined to an extremity. Naturally *...this cast a gloom over the household, and the same thing was happening throughout the district.* While Ada and John were dealing with this latest tragedy, it was indicative of the patriotic times that Eric's slightly younger brother, Victor, should feel that *...it was my duty to take my brother Eric's place, so enlisted and in due course was sent overseas.*[53] This was a time of familial and community sacrifice.

16 Nursing in Egypt 1915-16

I never dreamed a little animal would lie there like that…You should have seen them laughing and running for me to see the fun, so I did not let on that I had left it there – Letitia Moreton

The evacuation of Gallipoli was an outstanding success due to allied forces' ability to keep the plan secret. The enemy could literally see the allied trenches so a progressive retreat would have alerted them. Instead Australian General White held the frontline positions while the back lines withdrew. When considering the logistics of the evacuation it was not unrealistic for the officers to expect 2,000 casualties but instead the figure was nil. Fred Tomlins (1 ALH) noted that in the end only 1,500 soldiers were maintaining the enormous network of trenches with only one man for every seven to eight yards along the Anzac-Suvla line. The men boarded the ships and were taken to Mudros Harbor on Lemnos where they encamped for the night, were given basic rations and transported to Egypt the next day.[1]

The first site of an Australian military battle retained the corpses of 7600 Australian soldiers and 2,500 New Zealanders. Those who managed to leave with wounds numbered 19,000 Australians and 5000 New Zealanders. Australian and New Zealand nurses who were waiting on the ships, at 3AGH on Lemnos, in the AGHS and AAHs in Egypt had also died while trying to save those who had survived Gallipoli.

Letitia Moreton: Egypt: Christmas 1915

Christmas 1915 was a time of mixed blessings for the soldiers who had survived Gallipoli. Survival was often accompanied by guilt and grief as many absent friends were remembered. Nurses went beyond the call to ensure Christmas was memorable. Letitia Moreton and her colleagues spent their first wartime Christmas providing their patients at Maadi Rest Camp with a feast of ham, turkey, chicken and plenty of plum pudding accompanied with alcoholic beverages. How she spent her Christmas is unclear but within two days of returning to 2AGH on 7 January, 1916 she was herself recuperating from influenza at the Nurses' Red Cross Rest Home at Zizinia, Bacos Remlah via Alexandria.[2] Considering the 2 AGH nurses had cared for 988 recorded cases of influenza during 1915 it is hardly surprising that Letitia succumbed to the condition herself but fortunately she recovered.[3]

Norma Mowbray: Egypt: 21 January 1916

The New Year did not start well for the AANS nurses in Egypt. On 10 January 1916 Norma Mowbray was admitted to hospital with bronchitis but was discharged a few days later on the fourteenth. A week later on 21 January 1916 she died of pneumonia at 10.40am but there is no record of her being re-admitted to hospital prior to her death. While her service record claims she was buried the day she died, one of her colleagues made a detailed account of her funeral the day after her death. Sister Agnes Katherine Isambert (AANS) recorded on 21 January 1916 that *...Poor Mowbray died. Scott and I went into town and ordered wreaths. Her mother will be broken-hearted.* The next day Agnes found the funeral a very *...trying experience...a miserable day ...every one depressed.* The body of Norma Mowbray was taken to the cemetery and six of her AANS colleagues acted as mourners and walked beside the pallbearers. They *...followed the coffin covered with the Union Jack to the motor hearse...* and they *...walked beside the coffin, the Sisters and Officers following, while the band played the Dead March. The two Chaplains walked in front of the hearse to the graveside. After the brief service, the firing party fired three volleys, the Last Post was sounded and it was all over.*[4] Norma Violet Mowbray, aged 32 years, died as a SN of the AANS and was given an Anglican burial with military honours. Her grave is not too distant from her colleague Louisa Bicknell.

Norma's mother, Elizabeth, received her daughter's Victory Medal, a memorial scroll and King's message in 1922. The following year another relative, Mona Mowbray, took possession of her memorial plaque.[5] Norma's name is etched in bronze on the Roll of Honour at the AWM but history did not record if this was sufficient to comfort her heartbroken mother.

Agnes Corfield: QAIMNSR: Egypt February 1916

Agnes Corfield, Chassie Berrie and Norma Mowbray trained at Brisbane Hospital. Sister Agnes Isambert recorded nearly two weeks after Norma Mowbray died that *...Sister AB Corfield, a Queensland nurse with the Imperials died yesterday from influenza.* Agnes Corfield (QAIMNSR) died on 2 February 1916 but unlike Louisa Bicknell and Norma Mowbray who were respectfully acknowledged as Australian nurses, she was not.[6] Corfield's slightly older and more senior training colleague, Chassie Berrie, was still serving with the QAs in Egypt but it is not known if she attended her funeral. It is known that Agnes wrote to her best friend, Lizzie Ryland, while on active service so she was mourned.[7]

A newspaper in Maryborough, Queensland, *The Chronicle* reported Corfield's death and claimed she was a nurse from Bundaberg, aged just 24 years, while the community of Beaudesert records her as one of their own.[8] The headstone of her grave in Chatby Military Cemetery, Egypt, clearly indicates she was a Queenslander as well as an Australian; there is a record of her sacrifice by the British nursing services.[9] In 1923 a subscription to raise a monument for French and allied nurses was opened by Madame Juliette Adam. The monument is located on the Esplanade Ceres in Reims and includes the name of the Australian nurse Agnes Corfield.[10]

Communication from home: Royal Mail Steamers (RMS) like the *Morea*

One Australian Light Horseman was lamenting his forgetfulness about not bringing sufficient writing material with him to the peninsula claiming *...mail day is always looked forward to here and causes as much excitement as a charge.*[11] It was one of the few, and for many, the only link to home. Unfortunately, letters from home did not always contain welcome news. Family and friends died and romances were terminated while nurses and soldiers were living a life unimaginable back home. A number of nurses and soldiers, impatient for letters, often found their beloved parents had not answered because they themselves had died: A situation more common at the end of the war during the influenza pandemic.[12]

The war was conducted at a great distance from the shores of Australia so the Australian soldiers, nurses and public at home were in a perpetual state of waiting for news. Royal Mail Steamers (RMS) like the *Morea* performed the invaluable task of transporting the news, concerns and gossip between the military personnel and those on the home front. Occasionally RMS transported a small number of passengers and even troops, but this practice was unwise because the enemy also knew the psychological importance mail had on the morale of troops, so mail ships made excellent U-boat targets.[13] Fortunately, Amy O'Grady, Kitty Power and Elsie Grant were safely transported to Egypt on the *Morea*, leaving Australia in August, 1915. On arrival Kitty Power briefly met up with Anne Donnell at 3AGH.[14]

Elsie Grant: AANS: 1AGH: August 1915: *Morea*

Elsie Grant, aged 25, already had a credible nursing record when she enlisted on 19 August 1915. On completion of her training at Mackay District Hospital (Queensland, Yuwi Country) she was appointed Sister and gained six months' further experience. Her clinical specialty was the operating theatre but she must have had exceptional administrative skills. Unusually, for someone of her age, she obtained the position of matron, Emerald Hospital, where she worked for eighteen months before joining the AANS.[15] Elsie's mother, Ellen, lived at Manly (Queensland, Quandamooka Country) from where she bade farewell to her son, Allan, as well as her daughter. Elsie travelled overland to Sydney where she embarked on the *Morea,* departing 21 August 1915. Unlike a number of her colleagues Elsie did not elect to defer any of her pay while overseas.[16] A wise move in hindsight when she saw service during the winter months on the Somme, in the CCS operating theatres, and had to often buy rations.[17]

On arrival in Egypt she proceeded to 1 AGH where she became close friends with May Tilton. May wrote a thorough account of her war service and often mentions Elsie.[18] SN Grant had a mild attack of bronchitis on 9 January 1916 and was readmitted ten days later with influenza, from which she made a recovery.[19] Ellen Grant received word that her daughter was ill but the message had been sent to her at the wrong address causing a few days' delay. The controlled panic of a mother can be discerned as she writes *...I sincerely hope I will not hear that worse symptoms have set in...* before reiterating the correct address.[20]

Marquette tragedy: Mediterranean Sea: 23 October 1915

Nellie Gould and Hester Maclean were in Egypt in 1915 when the troopship *Marquette* was sunk off the coast of Salonika on 23 October. The *Marquette* left Egypt with 741 people on board, including 36 nurses who were to form the staff of 1 New Zealand Stationary Hospital (1 NZSH) in Salonika.[21] A torpedo struck the starboard side of the ship causing the enormous vessel to sink within 10 to 15 minutes resulting in 167 deaths, including ten nurses.

The soldiers and nurses survived the day-long ordeal by clutching onto pieces of flotsam and jetsam in the freezing Mediterranean Sea. Edith Popplewell and her colleague Lorna Rattray clung onto a piece of wreckage all day until Lorna told Edith *...that she mustn't hold her any longer.*[22] Popplewell, born in Ballarat and trained at the local base hospital, 1904-07, returned to New Zealand after the war, where the shocking memory of releasing her colleague to the sea remained with her.[23]

A rescue mission including the *Grantully Castle,* staffed by Australian nurses, and the *Canada,* staffed by French nurses, arrived in the late afternoon. An Australian, Marie Cameron, was the matron of the ill-fated 1 NZSH. She suffered a cerebral haemorrhage (stroke) while in the water awaiting rescue and endured life-long hemiplegia as a consequence. A great deal of care and attention was given to the nurses including Marie and *...medical staff on the* Canada *probably saved her life.* Cameron's sister (AANS) was stationed in Alexandria and nursed Marie until her transfer home, still *...nursing a teddy bear from which she would not be parted.*[24] On her return to Sydney she lived the remainder of her long life as a semi-invalid, dying more than thirty years later.[25]

Acting Matron Miles Walker, 1 ASH

Nellie Miles Walker had a varied tour of duty in Egypt. Along with other nurses from the first contingent, she eagerly awaited the arrival of the *Kyarra* once it was decided they would stay together and staff Australian hospitals. The hazards of transport duty during the Gallipoli Campaign were well known to her and the staffing levels and available resources on these ships were notoriously poor. They were the subject of an official inquiry after the peninsula was evacuated.[26]

The competence of Miles Walker was apparent and from February to August 1916 she was given the position of Acting Matron of 1 Australian Stationary Hospital (1ASH), Ismailia. The hospital was a former French convent located north of the Suez Canal between Suez and Kantara.[27] While 1 ASH was not particularly busy until the Battle of Romani in early August 1916, the location of the hospital and the extreme climate were enervating for the nurses and many suffered from general debility. Fortunately, the staff and patients were served well by Miles Walker, who was universally considered to be one of the kindest nurse leaders to serve with the AANS.[28] Kindness was important but the changing nature of the war meant that the civilian-trained nurses had to also develop a high level of competence in areas of military nursing.

Beatrice Watson: ***HMAT Orsova:*** **November 1915**

It usually took about four to five weeks, depending on the frequency of ports of call, for a ship to sail from Melbourne to Egypt.[29] The sea voyage was not a cruise but constituted a considerable workload for nurses who inoculated soldiers and nursed the sick. There is a great deal of evidence they were not well rested when they arrived in Egypt, where they were thrown into the reality of military nursing.

HMAT *Orsova* had been built in 1909 for the Orient Steamship Navigation Co Ltd, London, so nurses like Beatrice Watson would have enjoyed a pleasant voyage in such a ship under peacetime conditions. During the war many commercial ships were requisitioned for troop transport by the government of the day. The ship was substantial as it weighed 12,036 tons and could reach a speed of 18 knots. Nurses often sailed on troopships, so they were not afforded the relative safety that a clearly-marked white cross on the side of a hospital ship offered. HMAT *Orsova* had a blessed life as it survived the war and was finally broken up in 1936.[30]

Beatrice Middleton Watson was born in Caulfield (Victoria, Wurundjeri Woi Wurrung & Bunurong Country) in 1882.[31] She trained at the Children's Hospital,

Melbourne, and successfully completed a certificate in infectious nursing before enlisting with the AANS in October 1915. A month later she was accepted for AIF service. At this time her father, William Galley Watson, worked for the agricultural business Dalgetys and lived with her mother, Jane Ada of Middleton, in Kooyong Road, Elsternwick (Boon Wurrung Country).[32]

Beatrice is described as brunette with light brown eyes and dark complexion. Her height, 157 cm, and weight, just under 64 kg, suggest she was of slender build.[33] So it was that Staff Nurse Watson left Melbourne on the *Orsova* on 12 November 1915 and reported for duty at 1 AGH in February 1916. Her infectious nursing certificate may have come to the notice of Kellett or Miles Walker so she was detailed for service at 2 Auxiliary Command Depot, Ismailia.[34] Within a month of her arrival Beatrice was admitted to 1 ASH on 28 February 1916 for influenza. As was the custom, all nurses who are ill receive the special attention of matron.[35] At the same time, Mary Stafford had succumbed to influenza and was admitted to her own unit at 1 AGH but then spent a few weeks recovering in a convalescent hospital.[36] Fortunately the severity of influenza varied considerably and they both made a good recovery.

However, Beatrice was readmitted on 1 June and died the next day of 'cerebral'. Her medical record initially stated she ...*died of disease (abscess of brain)*... but the additional diagnosis of ...*cerebral haemorrhage*... was added later.[37] The abruptness of her death and the absence of any clinical information about her symptoms suggest she may have had cerebrospinal meningitis, which is also known as 'spotted fever'.[38] There are a variety of forms but during the war the most likely cause was meningococcal meningitis. Meningitis refers to the inflammation of the meninges – the membranes that surround the brain and spinal cord. Beatrice's symptoms most likely included vomiting and a severe headache which does not respond to analgesia.[39]

The bacterium is present in the throat as well as the spinal fluid, which may explain the accepted use of a nasal spray treatment. Sister Gertrude Agnes Grewar (AANS) recalled, during an outbreak on transport duty, that when ...*Cerebro Spinal Meningitis broke out all contacts had to be isolated, and every man on board had nasal spray treatment at certain intervals. At the time the ship did not have a spray house, and this treatment was carried out individually and given by the AMC officers and men.*[40] During the war one of the main management strategies for cerebrospinal fever was isolation and an increase in the distance between beds which proved effective.[41] However, another more invasive treatment, with an uncertain prognosis, was the injection of *...10-40 cc of an anti-meningococcic serum after the withdrawal of a similar quantity of cerebro-spinal fluid ... about 30 per cent die if serum is used; about twice as many if it is not.*[42] The use of such a serum was not recorded on Beatrice's medical record.[43]

At the time of her death Nellie Miles Walker was her matron and she would have felt the loss of one of her young nurses keenly. The cruel duty of writing a letter to Beatrice's parents would have weighed heavily on this dedicated matron. Miles Walker herself, often wrote to her own mother at such times, seeking solace from someone she herself loved dearly. Beatrice's funeral was attended by her AANS colleagues and her soldier patients. The grave of Beatrice Middleton Watson in the Ismailia War Cemetery in Egypt is dominated by a large cross, but gives very little away about the woman who rests there, except that she belonged to the Church of England and was an army nurse.[44] Of course, she was much more.

Australian Comforts Fund (ACF)

In June 1915 it was proposed by the Minister for Defence that the Australian Branch of the British Red Cross Society should take over welfare responsibility for invalided soldiers. Voluntary organisations like the Young Men's Christian Association (YMCA), Belgian Relief Fund and War Patriotic Funds proliferated and eventually amalgamated into the Australian Comforts Fund (ACF) in 1916.[45] Rania MacPhillamy remained in Egypt and did excellent work with the ACF, which brought entertainment and comforts to soldiers in Egyptian hospitals.[46]

The Red Cross Wounded and Missing Enquiry Bureau

In October 1915, Vera Deakin (daughter of Prime Minister Alfred Deakin), arrived in Cairo with her friend, Winifred Johnson. They had joined the Australian branch of the British Red Cross Society in Melbourne and found their niche as competent managers by creating the 'Australian Wounded and Missing Inquiry Bureau', winning her public respect and gratitude. Matrons and nurses were often the last people to see a soldier or a colleague when they were sick, transferred or died. The Bureau became a central point of contact for matrons regarding the deaths and the status of casualties. Vera, aged 25 years, was appointed OBE in 1917 for her remarkable work.[47]

Snapshots-from-Home League of Australia

Another excellent initiative was the YMCA Snapshots-from-Home League which started in Britain in 1915 and was adopted in Australia a year later. The cost of a camera and the development of photographs were prohibitive to many Australian families and soldiers. The League distributed application forms to soldiers and their families. Once completed the League sought amateur photographers to volunteer to go into the soldier's homes and photograph the family. The League distributed the photographs to the soldiers free of charge. By the end of the war many soldiers had not seen their parents for four years and some had not seen images of their new siblings. Married soldiers had not seen their children grow up; babies were now toddlers; children had grown into teenagers. Families at home were also relieved to receive a photograph of their son, father or husband as the soldiers also applied. In Australia during the First World War 6,000 amateur photographers volunteered from 800 local League areas and sent 150,000 photographs to serving men. The YMCA Snapshots-from-Home League scheme continued throughout the Second World War.[48]

Changes to the AIF and AANS 1916

Following the evacuation of Gallipoli at the end of 1915 the AIF was reorganised into 1 Anzac Corps, which went to France in March 1916, and II Anzac Corps, which remained in Egypt.[49] The reformed ALH, now known as the Anzac Mounted Division, became part of the II Anzac Corps in Egypt.[50] The 14 AGH, led by Rose Creal, was established in the middle of August 1916 as the main AGH for II Anzac Corps.[51] On her arrival, 20 September 1916, Grace Wilson was eager to leave Cairo and lead her 3 AGH nurses to England and ultimately France. A number of

Australian nurses, including Letitia Moreton, remained in Egypt with British units until the transfer orders to Europe for 2 AGH were confirmed.

Anzac Day 1916

Once she had recovered from the effects of influenza in 1916, Staff Nurse Letitia Moreton remained in Egypt and was lent to 4 British Auxiliary Hospital. A number of Australian soldiers, many Anzacs, spent the first anniversary of the Gallipoli landing in a saddened state. Acting Prime Minister Pearce officially named 25 April 'Anzac Day' in 1916 but it wasn't until 1923 that it was accepted as an Australian public holiday.[52] It is difficult to explain to anyone who is not an Australian or a New Zealander the poignancy of Anzac Day.

On the first anniversary of the landing, Letitia attended a moving evening memorial service at the Anzac Hostel, Cairo. After the formalities, she, along with her nursing colleagues and soldiers, visited the cemetery. Wreaths were laid and the graves of the two Australian nursing sisters, Louisa Bicknell and Norma Mowbray, were visited and their contribution remembered.[53] On her return to the wards Staff Nurse Moreton was called to the bed of a *...new patient...* and when she lifted the covers she found a very compliant donkey; the mascot of the Anzac soldiers.[54] She laughed and decided to leave it there as *...I never dreamed a little animal would lie there like that. I left it till the boys came back from the concert. You should have seen them laughing and running for me to see the fun, so I did not let on that I had left it there. It was 2 am before anyone settled down to sleep.*[55] At twenty-four years of age Letitia was already displaying the maturity and compassion of an indulgent but wise *...mother...* to her *...boys.*[56]

She knew that the heroes of military campaigns were not either dead or fit, strong, able-bodied men. Many First World War nurses witnessed true courage; not on the battlefield but later, in the hospital wards. They watched men, physically disabled or mentally ill, struggle to regain their identity and a sense of normality. What did Gallipoli mean for the eighteen year-old boy who was shot in the spine the day of the landing and was paralysed for the remainder of his life?[57] His ever-after story remains untold.

17 Australian Nurses in Europe 1914-16

...everyone might have an opportunity of paying a last respect to one who had come so far and who was among strangers – Maud McCarthy

The farmlands of France and Belgium were undergoing great changes in 1914-15. While Australian soldiers were enlisting, training and being transported to unknown destinations, the men and women of Europe were in the midst of battles on their doorsteps. The movement of troops through Belgium in October – November 1914 was slowed at Ypres as what was to become known as the First Battle of Ypres took place. It was here that an apocryphal event may or may not have taken place: The crucifixion of the Canadian Soldier. It was reported by persons unknown that an unidentified Canadian soldier was found crucified to a barn door at Ypres with German bayonets. While he was dying, Germans soldiers were seen mocking him. The incident has not been verified but it was repeated regularly at this early stage of the war. The horror of the incident incited hatred towards the Germans but especially by the Canadians. This had an effect on nursing contingencies when on 4May 1915 the incident appeared in the diaries of the British Matron-in-Chief, Maud McCarthy, who was organising staffing at CCS. She made *...arrangements to send all German wounded to the Hospital, for since the Crucifixion of the Canadian Sergeant Major it is not safe to have any Germans near the Canadians.* Ypres was not quickly decided so the trenches were dug and the stalemate began. The ugliness of the Western Front was entrenched and even the nurses knew it.[1]

Myrtle Wilson: The Western Front, Europe: 1915

Myrtle Wilson was one of a few Australian nurses serving on the Western Front in 1914. She was unable to join the AANS so paid her own fare to England, where she enlisted with the QAIMNSR on 13 May 1915. She was sent to France and served at 7GH, Boulogne during a particularly busy and trying time.

Myrtle Elizabeth Wilson: Origins: 1877-1915

Myrtle Elizabeth Wilson was the daughter of an English-born father, Andrew Stevens Wilson (1840-98), and a Scottish-born mother, Catherine McNaugton Craig (1841-1923), who were married in Victoria, Australia, in 1866. Initially, Andrew Wilson and his brother John owned and operated the Wilson Bros drapery business in Richmond (1865) but relocated to Brunswick Road, Fitzroy (Wurundjeri Country). The brothers operated from this location for nearly twenty years, starting the same year Andrew and Catherine were married. Their first two children were born in quick succession: James (1867), Andrew (1868) and Catherine Sarah arrived four years later in 1872. Catherine remained the only daughter and youngest child for five years until Myrtle Elizabeth (1877) was born, but the arrival of Lillian May (known as May) in 1878 heralded a year of mixed blessings because this same year Catherine, aged six, died.[2]

Myrtle Wilson spent her childhood in the suburbs of Melbourne. The family regularly moved house but mainly resided in the Fitzroy area. During hard economic times the family moved to Queensland where her father set up his own drapery business – one of eleven such businesses in Bundaberg. He took a calculated risk and established the only drapery business at nearby Gin Gin (Taribelang-Bunda Country), 28 miles north, where the discovery of copper was attracting new settlers. By 1895 Andrew Wilson was a Justice of the Peace, indicating that he had achieved a solid level of social standing.[3]

In 1893, when Myrtle was fifteen, she was a student at Mrs Boyles High School for Girls in Bundaberg, an establishment which catered for day students and boarders. Mrs RJ Boyle, an undergraduate of the London University, was ably assisted in her endeavours to 'finish off' the young ladies of Bundaberg with the assistance of Miss Ellwood (drawing), Miss Knipe (English), Madame Cavol who taught French and Mr Boyle who provided instruction in singing.[4] Myrtle excelled in languages and was awarded a special prize at the end of the year as well as a prize for the Upper Division (Form IV). Myrtle had a flair for the dramatic, being one of four young women who *…posed, first separately and then grouped in a tableau representing the four* *seasons. The effect was charming, and the young ladies stood firm at their posts, although the curtain was up rather an exceptionally long time.*[5] No doubt her performance and achievements would have been a source of family pride.

The death of Andrew in 1898, during a particularly harsh drought and economic depression, changed the family situation drastically. Andrew's sons continued to operate both drapery businesses. Despite having the *...respect and esteem of a large circle of friends in the district...*Catherine Wilson moved the remainder of the family to Redcliffe (Ningy Ningy Country), near Brisbane.[6] Myrtle completed her nurse training at the RBWH in 1910 and her younger sister, May, also qualified as a nurse. They shared the language of nursing – a language which is never forgotten and quickly revived whenever one nurse meets another.[7]

France: 1915

Once Myrtle joined the QAIMNSR she was invisible from Australian records but fortunately there are QA records of her service. While serving at 7GH in Boulogne she developed pneumonia and became seriously ill at which time she was sent to 14GH, Wimereux. She is first mentioned by Matron-in-Chief Maud McCarthy on 9 December 1915 *...Miss Wilson and Miss Donaldson, both very ill also.* Two days later she notes *...satisfactory reports received of all Nursing Sisters on serious list.* McCarthy was an Australian and despite her enormous workload she made regular checks on the wellbeing of sick nurses. While in Abbeville she wrote *...Miss Wilson, Australian, pneumonia, DI list – people in Australia, WO informed, and cousin in England.* This entry confirms it is Myrtle and her cousin was her geographically closest NOK. The next day *...Miss Wilson is no better.* On 23 December 1915 McCarthy recorded that she received a *...Wire to say Miss Wilson's condition critical...* but her last entry for that day noted *...Telephone message from 14 General Hospital saying Miss Wilson, Australian on Q Reserve, condition critical. Informed WO. Later to say she had died 7.30am.* Myrtle was 38 years old and her photograph at 7GH shows an Australian nurse in a QA uniform who died caring for allied soldiers. On 15 January 1916 the British Journal of Nursing recorded her contribution and sent *...sympathy to our Australian nursing colleagues.*

Funeral: Myrtle Wilson: 14 December 1915.

Maud McCarthy was dissatisfied with the organization of Myrtle's funeral. The next day she wrote … *Rang up early to find out when Miss Wilson's funeral was to take place. 2pm today, so I arranged to go, and asked 14 General to procure flowers for me if they had not already done so. Left at 11am. Raining incessantly. Arrived 1.30, had lunch, drove straight to 14 General, where I found Miss Fox had neglected to tell anyone in either the Boulogne or Wimereux area of the early date of the funeral, or the Australian Hospital. Not even the Assistant Principal Matron, so that she could have informed all Hospitals so that everyone might have an opportunity of paying a last respect to one who had come so far and who was among strangers. I was extremely annoyed. The rain was continuous. There were a great many officers, and not a dozen Nursing Sisters from the whole area. On return to 14 General the Assistant Principal Matron had arrived with flowers from some of the Hospitals, but did not know anything about the funeral.*[8]

Myrtle Wilson was the only Australian nurse to die during the European battles of 1915 while the AANS were in Egypt caring for the Anzacs. She is buried at Wimereux Communal Cemetery near the port of Boulogne, France.[9] Her sacrifice is recorded by the QAIMNSR and remembered by Australians. It was two days after Christmas that Mr GC Wilson …*was advised by cable to-day of the death in France of his sister.* Deaths at important times of the year often create a deep sadness which is long remembered.[10]

Sarah Furnifull: QAIMNSR: HS *Karoola*

In 1915 Sarah Furnifull … *was asked if I would be prepared, along with 19 other nurses, to fill vacancies in Queen Alexandra's Imperial Nursing Service as an Australian unit. I was happy to be part of this unit and we set sail in the hospital ship* Karoola. There is no evidence Myrtle Wilson was one of the nineteen other nurses. There are suggestions that Myrtle paid her own fare on the *Orontes* to get to England, where her cousin was residing, and joined the QAs in England. In contrast to the lack of information about Myrtle Wilson's war-time experiences, Sarah Furnifull wrote an excellent summary of her time with the QAs in The Australian Women's Weekly magazine in 1973.

Origins

Sarah was born in Albany, WA in 1887, the third child of eight, having six sisters and one brother. Her parents moved the family close to Kempsey (NSW, Dungutti Country) where they had a cattle station and Sarah *...lived a happy childhood.* Four of the daughters became nurses: Frances (AANS), Sarah Margaret (QAIMNSR), Jane and Annie. Frances trained at Royal North Shore Hospital and became good friends with Ada Thompson, who also joined the AANS.

Nursing

Sarah was sixteen when she commenced work at the Macleay District Hospital enjoying the camaraderie of the other three or four nurses and matron. Matron saw her potential and encouraged Sarah to make the life-changing decision of training in a larger city teaching hospital. She took the steamship to Sydney and commenced her four-year training at the Coast Hospital. Even during her time at Kempsey, Sarah nursed patients with typhoid. On completion of her training she was appointed the assistant matron of a tuberculosis clinic at Waterfall, NSW and later served the community of Berry (NSW, Dharawal Country) as the acting matron of Berry Hospital.

Sarah had extensive experience in infection control when she volunteered to join the AANS. This claim by a nurse who was asked to join an Australian Unit, leaves from Australia in an Australian hospital ship but wearing the QA uniform becomes intrinsically important to these twenty nurses. Sarah disembarked at Suez and boarded a train carrying typhoid cases to Cairo, during which time she began to incubate the disease. After a week in Cairo they boarded the *Nevassa,* which transported them to Naples where they embarked on the *Britannic.*

Sarah Furnifull: Typhoid: England

On arrival in England the Australian nurses were not happy to learn they were to replace English nurses who were in turn going to be sent to France. Unfortunately, Sarah developed symptoms of typhoid and spent three weeks in isolation at Rubery Hill Hospital, Birmingham. Once recovered, she and her colleagues approached the

Australian High Commissioner in London, Mr Andrew Fisher, who arranged for them to be transferred to France.[11] Sarah and her Australian nursing colleagues picked up their QA uniform and kit before sailing to Boulogne, France.[12] It is more than likely they were in the area when Myrtle Wilson died.

Volunteer Organisations Unite

When war was declared, the British Red Cross and St John Ambulance Association decided to put aside their differences and work together for the duration of the war. Queen Alexandra, President of the British Red Cross, donated £500 and called for donations.[13] A committee was formed and Lady Dudley, now estranged from her husband, was one of a number of aristocrats appointed.[14] Elizabeth McGregor, a RPAH trainee, was in Britain gaining further nursing experience. She volunteered with The Lady Dudley Field Hospital on 28 August 1914 but within a few months joined the British Red Cross. She was, more than likely, one of the first Australian nurses to serve on the Western Front. The Lady Dudley Field Hospital found it *...increasingly difficult to staff the hospital from voluntary sources and on 1 July 1916 it was taken over by the War Office, expanded and renamed the No 32 Stationary Hospital.*[15]

Elizabeth McGregor: Serbian Retreat: 1915-16

Elizabeth McGregor lived in central western NSW and was the fourth of five daughters born to John McGregor and his wife Jane (nee Smith). Her parents were Scottish migrants who married in Victoria before moving to Condobolin, NSW (Wiradjuri Country), in 1885.[16] John managed the *Micabil* and *Walloroi* properties for his uncle, William Campbell, while Jane, an ex-school teacher, educated her daughters at home. They were known in the district as *...the McGregor girls...* and could often be seen by their neighbours *...racing their horse and buggies at full gallop across the plains of their property.*[17] Elizabeth, who was known as Bess within the family, taught Sunday School at the local Presbyterian Church.[18]

The lives of the young McGregor girls changed dramatically when John died in June 1904 and Jane died in November of the same year.[19] The need for self-reliance enabled three of the sisters to pursue careers but they did not opt for teaching like their mother. Instead Kate became a masseuse while Elizabeth and her younger sister Helen (Nell) qualified as nurses at RPAH.[20] Elizabeth was the first in the family to go to Sydney to commence her training, 1907-12 and Nell joined her two years later in 1909. While Elizabeth was a competent practical nurse and a sound academic student, training at this time was hazardous and she had a break in service to recover from typhoid and scarlet fever.[21] In 1912 she was awarded her hospital nursing certificate and dispensing certificate and later acquired the important, ATNA certificate.[22] She travelled to England to gain nursing experience but nothing could prepare her for Europe in August 1914.

The Serbian retreat

Sister McGregor's stay in France was short-lived with The Lady Dudley Field Hospital as she joined the British Red Cross in October 1914. Her nursing expertise was tested that same month: She was sent to Serbia when the enemy *...crossed the Danube between 7 and 9 October.*[23] The German decision by Erich von Falkenhayn to overrun Serbia, thereby removing Russia's foothold in the Balkans and simultaneously opening an overland route from Berlin to Constantinople, meant that the young nurse from Condobolin spent the first year of the war amid a European winter of retreat and desolation. The situation worsened when *...on the 9th Belgrade fell to the Austrians once more...* while the Germans and Bulgarians enveloped the Serbs, forcing them *...to retreat either south towards Greece or South-West to Albania as the railway line to Salonika had also been cut.*

Wherever the Serbian Army went, so too did the civilian population. Children, the aged, the infirm and women nursing babies all fled an aggressive army in freezing conditions with the support of the Red Cross personnel. A retreat across the mountains to the Albanian coast was considered the best option. Eventually 140,000 Serbian soldiers were transported on allied vessels to Corfu and finally to Salonika; the army's original strength had been 420,000 men. Elizabeth nursed civilians and soldiers alike during the bloodshed and chaos of the Serbian retreat. As is often the case during war, the number of civilian casualties is not known; their misery and deaths reside on the periphery of historic battles.[24]

The sparse British Red Cross record of service of this amazing Australian nurse consists of two entries: Serbian relief from October 1914 until April 1916, followed by service in Corfu from May 1916 until June 1917.[25] Her contribution was recognised when she was awarded the Serbian Cross of Mercy *...for nursing the wounded and sick*.[26] An image of Elizabeth McGregor wearing the Red Cross uniform shows the face of an intelligent and resourceful young woman.[27]

Florence Farmborough: A British Nurse in Russia: 1915-16

In the absence of Australian nurses it is a British nurse, Florence Farmborough, who will provide insight into the allied offensive on the Eastern Front. Tsar Nicholas II was the emperor of the Russian Empire in August 1914 and Florence was in Moscow when war was declared. She kept *...her diary in notebooks and on scraps of paper ... but decades later, upon deciding to publish the work, she appears to have rewritten and augmented whole sections, such that it is impossible for the reader to know which parts were written contemporaneously with the events they describe, and which were later elaborations*.[28] The limitations of this primary source notwithstanding, her experiences provide a unique narrative and are included to that end only.

Florence Farmborough, aged twenty-one, obtained gainful employment as a governess in Moscow teaching English in 1908. She taught the daughters of a doctor and the family treated her as one of their own. When war was declared she and the doctor's two daughters joined the staff of the Lazaret Hospital as VADs. They were attached to the Princess Golitsin Hospital for wounded soldiers.

Red Cross Nursing

A Protestant, Florence believed God wanted her to nurse wounded soldiers and she was welcomed at a Russian Orthodox Church service for VADs. However, on learning that only a *...Red Cross Sister...* could go to the frontline she decided to undergo training. This involved learning the theoretical language in great detail and attending Red Cross lectures every evening for three hours. She learnt entire chapters parrot-fashion. Following the completion of six months' hospital work as a VAD and passing her Red Cross Society diploma, she was ready for war work.

Farmborough was a surgical nurse in the 10th Otryad of the All-Russian Zemski (Provincial) Soyuz. Once uniforms and clothes were purchased, she was dispatched by rail to care for Russian soldiers and refugees.[29]

Gorlice-Tarnów Sector: April – May 1915

The German objective was to relieve pressure on the Austro-Hungarian front and reduce Russia's offensive power. Their strategy was to break through the ...*Gorlice-Tarnów sector between the upper Vistula and the Carpathians...* which was an area that offered the German Army the least resistance and best penetration.[30] The Dardanelles Campaign was designed to divert the attention of the German and Austro-Hungarian armies from the Russian front. On 17 April 1915 Florence wrote in her diary ...*there is definitely something stirring on the Front.*[31] She was serving in a forward unit and found the ...*stream of wounded was endless.* Florence and her colleagues ...*dressed their severe wounds where they lay on the open ground ... firstly alleviating their pain by injections. And all the time the bombardment of Gorlitse was continuing with brutal ferocity.*[32] The German military leader, Mackensen, took advantage of the relatively easy advance in this sector by continuing the momentum until they dug in close to the Russian line, attacking in earnest on 2 May 1915. The element of surprise was catastrophic with 400,000 Russians taken prisoner.[33]

Retreat

Retreat was the constant refrain for the Russians and the nurses caring for soldiers in the advanced areas. Initially, the nurses thought they had been forgotten but when they were given the order to leave the wounded and their unit's equipment fear turned to incredulousness. Reluctantly they picked up whatever they could and fled from the advancing German Army while the voices of the wounded implored the nurses not to leave them. A military nurse's worst nightmare.[34]

Italy joins the Allies

Italy signed the Pact of London on 26 April, with a promise of territorial gains if victorious; war was declared on Austro-Hungary on 23 May 1915. This happened when the Ottomans were warding off the British invasion at the Dardanelles and the Germans were advancing on Russia. Italy's General Luigi Cadorna was of the view that Italians were *...morally unprepared for war.* He considered their individualism to be a hindrance and planned to remedy it with strict military discipline. Initially, he imposed his military power in the political sphere as he saw the war as ... *an opportunity to make peasants into Italians.* His earliest policy was to reintroduce ... *the Roman practice of decimation – the killing of every tenth man – for units which failed to perform in battle.* The General and his barbaric practice had a short but tragic reign during the early stages of the war.[35]

Ethel Cooper: Germany: 1915

It was a twist of fate and timing that saw Ethel Cooper providing diversionary activities to German soldiers. Her friend Dr Knopf was sympathetic to her plight and like many allied doctors he faced large numbers of German casualties with few human resources. Nurses and doctors in Germany were also keen to do their duty at the front. Cooper endeavoured to seek out allied soldiers who were POWs and offer comfort inconspicuously. The movement of civilians was controlled as early as November 1915 because *...there is not half enough food for the people ... the country is devastated beyond belief and the people are starving by thousands.*[36] The blockade had an effect on the German people early in the war but there was little sympathy for Germany at this time. An event had changed the perception of the allies, and indeed that of neutral countries, toward the Germans the previous month.

Edith Cavell: Belgium: 1915

Edith Cavell was an English nurse who worked in one of the few secular hospitals in Belgium, a predominantly Catholic nation, when the Germans invaded. She was given the opportunity to return to England but declined. Instead she continued to work in a hospital in Brussels and assisted the escape of more than 200 allied men once they had recuperated. On Wednesday 6 October 1915 she and a number of associates were taken to the Belgian Parliament House to stand trial for treason.[37]

Less than a week later, on 12 October 1915 at 7 am Edith Cavell was shot to death by a firing squad which consisted of two parties of German soldiers.[38]

No longer an ordinary nurse, her execution gave her martyr status which ignited a global groundswell of pride in nursing. The Australian Edith Cavell Trust Fund was established and money poured in from all sectors. She was hailed as a selfless and devoted nurse, and her death proved to be a propaganda triumph for the allied forces. Recruitment increased as news of the execution spread and hatred toward the Germans intensified.

18 Global Changes 1916-1918

> *...it was pitiful to see some of them, with legs off and arms off, and some fearfully burnt, face, arms and body. We even had destroyers up alongside discharging patients directly on board – Mary Clarke*

The impact of the war changed the political landscape of countries dramatically by late 1916 and continued until the armistice. A positive change for the allied forces occurred when the US Senate supported the entry of the USA into the war on 4 April 1917 and was overwhelmingly confirmed by Congress on 6 April 1917. However, civil disquiet in Russia throughout 1917 saw Russia withdraw from the allies formally in March 1918. Negotiations between Germany and Russia at Brest-Litovsk, then situated in Eastern Poland and under German occupation, concluded with a peace treaty on 5 March 1918. Today Brest-Litovsk is a city located in Belarus.[1] The Germans were no longer fighting on two fronts but had to face the energized allies who initially had US support financially and later, militarily.

An Irish revolt: April 1916

The Germans had also tried to provoke civil instability in Ireland by providing arms for a rebellion in 1916.[2] In Ireland, there had been a slim chance for Home Rule and it was hoped that the 'Irish Question' or 'The Troubles' would be amicably resolved.[3] However, the Sinn Feiners did not want Home Rule but preferred to be a separate nation, severing all ties with Britain. To this end, in Dublin, on 24 April 1916, Padraic (Patrick) Pearse proclaimed a provisional government of the Irish Republic.[4] The next five days witnessed a brutal response by the British forces and the term 'Easter Rising' entered the Irish lexicon.

At great personal risk to themselves, two remarkable and brave women, Louisa Nolan and Florence Williams, used their homes *...to shelter and nurse those wounded in the conflict.* Both were awarded the Military Medal for 'Bravery in the Field'.[5] Tragically, this was not the reward for the fourteen rebel leaders who were court-martialled and executed on subsequent days: Pearse was the first to be shot by a firing squad on 3 May 1916 at 3.30 am.[6]

Political revolt in Australia

Although the Easter Uprising was quickly quashed it had global ramifications. Irish Catholics were scattered around the world and many (like those living in Australia) were being asked to volunteer to defend the 'Mother Country'.[7] The Australian Prime Minister William (Billy) Hughes introduced a debate on military conscription. He was either in contempt of, or oblivious to, the implications of such a debate, which was in direct contravention of the spirit of his Labor Party policy platform.[8] Hughes spent a great deal of 1916 in Canada and England convincing the allies of Australia's commitment to victory at all costs.[9] On his return to Australia, Hughes argued that an additional 130,000 Australian men were needed by March 1917 and the conscription question should be put to a national referendum. A parliamentary majority approved the referendum question being put to the people, but twenty-seven Labor parliamentarians voted against it.[10]

Historian LF Crisp claims that Hughes had not contravened a written policy platform but concedes that five of the six States and the spirit of the Federal Labor Party were known to be anti-conscription. Crisp also claims, controversially, that Hughes could have introduced conscription without a referendum by claiming a *...moral mandate...* via normal parliamentary processes.[11]

Australian Conscription Referenda: 28 October 1916 & 20 December 1917

Despite being one of the few countries in the world which did not introduce conscription, soldiering was forced upon many Australian men by the blunt instrument of patriotism. The conscription debate was politically and socially divisive and some groups were not always trusted when they did volunteer. For instance, distrust of the Irish was not only centred on their political history but also their Catholicism. There is evidence of religious bias within the nursing profession generally and elements of the AANS.

Prime Minister Hughes pursued a 'yes' vote with a vengeance. Many unions tried to thwart his zealousness by appealing to the rank and file workers on the basis of class. Archbishop Daniel Mannix opposed Hughes on what many interpreted as sectarian lines because, he, an Irish Catholic, felt compelled to take up a public anti-conscription position following the Easter Rebellion.[12] Patriotism was often touted during these vicious public brawls which were supposed to be political debates. To be Irish and Catholic attracted public attention in 1916.

Voting Patterns

On 28 October 1916 Australians voted against the introduction of conscription. Those for were 1,087,557 and those against 1,160,033. This did not settle the question as the British asked Prime Minister Hughes to create a 6th Australian Division in 1917. There was a lag in recruitment as the reality of the Somme came home to the families of those serving in terms of the convalescing soldiers and a more critical media. Another military division would require the recruitment of 7,000 Australian men a month until the Division reached approximately 20,000 soldiers. A second referendum saw more controversy and ugliness on the home front with a more decisive defeat. Even the soldiers at the front did not support conscription. On 20 December 1917 Australians voted, once again, against the introduction of conscription. Those for were 1,015,159 and those against 1,181,747.[13]

The Labor Party moved to have the voting age of twenty-one years reduced to eighteen years in 1919 but this was not achieved until 1973 under the Whitlam Labor Government.[14] However, in 1943 the Curtin (Labor) Government gave the vote to servicemen serving overseas during the Second World War and for six months afterwards.[15]

AANS Vote

Australian sisters were required to vote on the conscription question. The opportunity to vote was not universally available to women and Anne Donnell (AANS) felt proud to be part of the only group of women permitted to vote on a national issue in England. The distinctive AANS uniforms with their scarlet capes attracted attention when Anne Donnell was holidaying in Ireland when a ...*young urchin...* peered into their carriage and *...then in a loud voice calls out "Suffragettes," and runs for his life.*[16]

White Australian women were among the first in the world to be given voting rights and the Australian nurses who were recovering from the effects of nursing men on the Western Front were in a good position to make a decision.[17] May Tilton had voted against conscription in 1916 because she was influenced by the opinions of the soldiers who did not want *...slackers or cold-footers...* in their regiment. However, the following year she decided for herself that conscription was necessary so she and her colleagues would not have to watch convalescing men be returned, all too soon, to the trenches when they should have been sent home.[18]

The war caused a hiatus in the momentum of the suffragette movement in Britain, and the British Prime Minister, HH Asquith, not only opposed votes for women but did not advocate universal suffrage because he believed ordinary men and women were likely to be swayed by the popular press. The media was not to be trusted – only the ruling class.[19]

The Battle of Jutland: 31 May – 1 June 1916

The Gallipoli campaign started in the Straits of Marmara and culminated in the land offensive of April 1915. A month prior to the Somme offensive the biggest naval battle of the war took place in the North Sea off the coast of Denmark, near Jutland. Scotland, Norway and Denmark were strategically placed to provide a relatively safe harbor for the British Grand Fleet and create a blockade against the Germans. Denmark and Norway were neutral countries but their dependence on Britain for supplies saw them as neutral allies.

On 31 May 1916 the British Grand Fleet was ambushed by the German High Seas Fleet: two hundred and fifty ships and 100,000 men were involved. The large dreadnoughts battleships had big armament and both sides engaged in a ferocious battle over two days. In terms of losses HMS *Lion* was damaged initially but when HMS *Indefatigable* and HMS *Queen Mary* had their ammunition magazines shelled the ships exploded. The British lost fourteen ships and the Germans eleven but it was the loss of souls that tells the tale of this battle: 6,000 Allied and 2,500 German.

Despite the high cost of lives it was considered a victory for Britain as they still had control of the seas, ensuring that the German blockade continued.[20]

Hospital Ships *Plassy* and *Grantully Castle*

Two hospital ships, the *Plassy* and *Grantully Castle* were in the area to provide support. British nurse, Charlotte Amy (Mary) Clarke, Queen Alexandra's Royal Naval Nursing Service, was aboard the *Plassy* and kept a record of the incident in her diary. Mary wrote on 31 May 1916 that the wounded were *...Crowded on the decks in most varied rig, we're the survivors from the poor lost ships. Then the men all looked cheery even at that hour one could hardly believe all that they must have gone through ...So they began to arrive, drifters by the dozen, six and seven deep on the port and starboard sides waiting to unload their sad burdens. Poor men they almost all had their faces and hands tied up. We started about 11am and by 12.30 had taken in over 100 and they said the worse ones, at least 90 cot cases, were still to come. We got them all into bed as quickly as possible, no easy job sometimes, and fed them with beef tea and the bad ones with brandy and left them to settle down a bit before we attempted their dressings.*

We washed up and snatched a little lunch as could then the bad cases began to come in. Poor things it was pitiful to see some of them, with legs off and arms off, and some fearfully burnt, face, arms and body. We even had destroyers up alongside discharging patients directly on board.[21]

The Zimmerman telegram: January 1917

While Russian leader Alexander Kerensky was focusing on winning the war at the front, the Germans saw an opportunity to win the war by creating social revolution in Russia. A country fighting against itself has no energy to fight an outside threat. The German Foreign Minister, Arthur Zimmerman, saw an opportunity to incite unrest in Russia with a view to negotiating a peace. This would enable the diversion of German and Austro-Hungarian troops to the Western Front. Zimmerman had made a serious diplomatic miscalculation in January 1917 when he dispatched a telegram to the Mexican President inviting him to join Germany when America entered the war, with a promise of *...the return of Texas, New Mexico and Arizona,* *which had been conquered by the United States in the middle of the previous century.* Zimmerman also showed remarkable prescience when he sought assistance from Mexico to persuade Japan to desert the allies *...and attack America in the Pacific.*[22] The coded telegram was intercepted, deciphered and eventually made its way to the desk of President Wilson.

Undeterred, Zimmerman persuaded the Kaiser to smuggle the Bolshevik' leader, Lenin, from exile in Switzerland back to Russia; Lenin *...crossed Germany in a sealed train...* and arrived in Russia on 16 April 1917.[23] Kerensky's Provisional Government wanted to win the war and reinvigorate the political system of Russia from a position of strength. The Bolsheviks saw the war as imperialist in nature and wanted a social revolution.

The idea of a social revolution within an army is a paradox. Discipline is an essential component of military success but how this is enforced has an enormous bearing on the loyalty of the soldiers to their leader. Kerensky introduced a number of changes, including the abolition of capital punishment in the army. He decreed that officers would not use the condescending term 'thou' when addressing their soldiers but would instead use the less patronizing term 'you'.[24] It could be argued these were small concessions in a Great War but the ripple effects were dramatic and gave Lenin an opening for fomenting disquiet amongst the troops.

USA enters War with Germany: 6 April 1917

German submariners gained infamy on 7 May 1915 when they fired a torpedo at the *Lusitania,* sinking it off the coast of Ireland. Eleven hundred civilians, including Americans, perished. Sea travel required courage during the war because all manner of vessels - transport, troop, hospital, passenger ships - quickly sank when a sea mine was hit or a torpedo made contact. Loss of life was often heavy. Apart from the danger, the logistics of transporting hundreds of thousands of men and women across the seaways during a global war saw neutral countries suffer. President Wilson took another two years before committing troops to the European war despite the sinking of American ships by German submarines. It was the German preparedness to entice Mexico into war with the USA which convinced the

American people that Germany was not interested in peace, only victory.[25]

The Russian Revolution: 1917: Florence Farmborough

While the Australian nurses in Europe endured the worst of the major offensives on the Western Front, others were trapped in the middle of dramatic changes. Language was a barrier to effective nursing, especially when caring for POWs and refugees. Soldiers were fearful when they were nursed by female doctors and nurses whom they could not understand. Florence Farmborough had an excellent command of the Russian language but in May 1917 she was pleased to find *...an English hospital in Podgaytsy, run by a group of English nurses, under the leadership of an English lady doctor.* She could speak to them in her mother tongue and feel the camaraderie of that experience, but because she was just a young VAD the only work she was given was to soothe the wounded soldiers. Given Farmborough's experience of nursing during the Russian retreat of 1915 and the offensive of 1916, this was rather a demotion. However, her limited nurse training as a VAD became apparent when she acknowledged '*the medical terms they used were Greek*' to her.

Nevertheless, she was able to reassure the wounded Russian soldiers who *...betray a certain anxiety when they find themselves at the mercy of nurses whose language they cannot understand*; they begged her not to leave them alone with the English and Scottish nurses.[26] The Scottish Women's Hospitals were often found in the forefront of battle after reputedly being told by the War Office in 1914 *...that all that was required of women was to go home and keep quiet.*[27] Fortunately, they chose not to do either and the unit was a remarkable resource which was often found in non-English speaking parts of Europe.

A Russian revolt: March 1917- March 1918

In January 1917 Florence Farmborough was granted leave to visit her dying friend Dr Usov and attend his funeral in Moscow. During her journey and visit she was struck by *...discontent among the masses.* Farmborough was disturbed to find that *...sabotage was the order of the day...* as industrial sites were burnt and railways destroyed. These actions benefited the enemy armies, and a few months later she recorded the words ...*The Tsar has abdicated...* and later that day heard that it had been necessary to ...*cleanse the Court of pro-German satellites.*[28] The initial uprising began in March 1917 and the Tsar was forced to abdicate the following month.[29] Alexander Kerensky became head of the Provisional Government and the anarchists at the time believed this marked a new era of reform.[30]

On the Russian Front there was no confidence in the competence or fairness of military leaders.[31] Like most people of influence, Kerensky was an exceptional orator and he persuaded the front-line soldiers to stay loyal to Russia and obey their officers. For instance, on 13 May 1917 Florence Farmborough was at Podgaytsy when Kerensky addressed ...*tightly-packed masses of soldiers.* At first she thought ...*he looked small and insignificant ... less than his 36 years and his beardless face made him even younger.* However, the great orator waited in silence and then unleashed his power and ...*his eloquence literally hypnotized...* the crowd. That day Kerensky spoke of victory in war and sowed the seed of freedom as he addressed ...*free men of a Free Country.* The Russian soldiers took him at his word and they started to claim their right to choose whether or not to go into battle.

The following month Farmborough was working outside Bojikov when she observed first-hand what freedom amongst the oppressed looked like. A meeting was in progress and soldiers were openly critical of the tactics of their commanding officer and ...*demanded that blankets be distributed among the troops without delay, and all disabled soldiers receive special compensation.* She asked the salient question ...*Since when had our soldiers acquired the right to denounce their Commanding Officer in public?* The answer was obvious; since Kerensky declared they were free men in a free country. This meeting was resolved when news of a dramatic victory by the Russian 8th Army reached the soldiers and the ...*revengeful feelings smoldering among the soldiers seemed suddenly to melt away.*[32] Just as their animosity quickly melted away, so too did their resolve to make good the gains, so ...*when the German reserve counter-attacked, the Russian forces, eager for peace, melted like snow.*[33]

Russia signs Armistice with Germany: 25 December 1917

Finally Lenin and the Bolsheviks seized power from the Provisional Government and Russia signed an armistice with Germany in December 1917. After a number of false starts, hostilities ceased in March 1918.[34] Despite the collapse of this front, which gave the Germans the impetus for the Big Push on the Western Front in early 1918, the blockade was still effective. Florence Farmborough finally reached Moscow on Christmas Day 1917 after a distressing train journey leaving her colleagues in the Red Cross Unit. She found Moscow to be in the grip of *...winter and famine.* Sadly, her Russian friends were educated, wealthy citizens and they suffered at the hands of the Red Guards. Intellectuals, women and members of the church fared badly under the new regime and Florence was given a food ration which entitled her to either two potatoes or two ounces of bread per day - her reward for years of nursing Russian soldiers in dire circumstances.

It was soon announced that foreigners would be *persona non grata* and it was necessary for an English VAD to go home. Finally she, along with a number of British citizens, was transported in a goods train across Siberia in winter. They endured freezing conditions and visits from Red Guards, but she still *...felt like a coward...* because she had forsaken her Russian friends in their distress. Finally, after 28 days in the goods train the party of refugees arrived at Vladivostok on 28 April 1918, where they saw one of four cruisers anchored in the harbor flying the Union Jack. For the first time in a long time Florence Farmborough felt safe because she was nearly home.[35]

The mother of Tsar Nicholas II, the Dowager Empress Maria Feoderovna, refused to believe her fifty year old son, forty-six year old daughter-in-law and their five children had been murdered. She died in 1928 still clinging to hope she would see them again. For eighteen months the dowager empress sold her jewellery and lived on the charity of her Danish and English relatives. In April 1919 she and her family were sheltering uneasily in an insecure environment at the imperial palace of Livadia near the resort of Yalta. Their fate was uncertain until the British battleship HMS *Marlborough* arrived to take her to Malta. She refused unless all her family and servants were permitted to board. Hence, the end of the First World War saw the largest contingent of Romanovs leave Russia —never to return. They were scattered throughout Europe with the Dowager Empress settling in her native Denmark with her nephew King Christian X in power. Marie was British Queen Alexandra's sister and while they remained close their lives were dramatically changed by the First World War.[36]

19 Establishing Australian Hospitals and Casualty Clearing Stations in Europe and England 1916-1918

Madame Curie was often found educating nurses about the practical aspects of x-ray technology on the Western Front -
Guy Williams

The Battle of the Somme commenced on 1 July 1916 and the British Commander-in-Chief General Sir Douglas Haig optimistically …*sought and believed in a breakthrough.* The French Commander-in-Chief, Joseph Joffre, and the British Commander of the Fourth Army, BEF, Henry Rawlinson, correctly foresaw the Somme to be …*an attrition battle.* It proved to be a fast-flowing stream of wounded, gassed and dying soldiers.[1]

AGHs in Britain and Europe 1916-19

Today, it is difficult to imagine the natural development of 48 general hospitals and 19 stationary hospitals to deal with millions of casualties. In 1914 these hospitals had a capacity of 10,000 beds, which expanded to …*80,000 and 90,000 in 1917-18, and 95,000 at the time of the Armistice.*[2] The staff establishment and plant of the three main AGHs were transferred to France from Egypt in 1916 and Australian CCSs (numbered one, two and three) were established on the Western Front. Auxiliary hospitals (numbered one, two and three) were relocated to Britain and were essentially used as 'clearing centres' for the implementation of the six months' policy.[3] That is, CCS nurses were rested every six months because the workload was excessive. The complex infrastructure needed to cater for thousands of casualties necessitated a policy of moving the units only when absolutely necessary.

Table 1: The primary location and role of Australian hospitals in Europe and Britain (1916-19)

Hospitals	Location, Date and Role of Hospitals
1 Australian General Hospital	**Rouen, France. 16 April 1916 - 30 Nov 1918.** 1AGH with capacity for 1,300 beds during 'Big Push' from March to Aug 1918 including one-third in Nissan type huts and the remainder in marquee tents. **Sutton Veny, England. January 1919 until RTA.**
2 Australian General Hospital	**Marseilles, France. 1 April 1916 - 2 June 1916.** Tented hospital received the sick from transports. **Wimereux, France. 2 June 1916 - 26 February 1919.** 2AGH with capacity for 1,900 beds at the time of the Big Push (March to Aug 1918) including 1,300 beds in huts and 600 in tents.
3 Australian General Hospital	**Previously known as Kitchener War Hospital, Brighton, England. October 1916 - April 1917.** **Abbeville, France. 9 May 1917 - 23 May 1919.** Mainly surgical cases and high number of fractures. 3AGH had capacity for 1,500 beds at the time of the Big Push (March to Aug 1918) but admitted over 1,900 soldiers. Half of admissions were nursed in huts. Successfully utilised the labour of No.196 POW Coy (100-200 POWs) who provided a substantial labour force for the last 18 months of the war.
1 Australian Auxiliary Hospital (AKA Harefield)	**Previously known as Harefield Convalescent Hospital, England. 1916-19.** 1AAH had 1,000 beds and dealt with immediate and reparative surgery including specialised medical treatment such as fitting artificial limbs. 1AAH was designed to move soldiers from the acute stage to rehabilitation or convalescent care. Soldiers who could return to the front were enabled to so and those who needed more rehabilitation/convalescence were often transported back to Australia.
2 Australian Auxiliary Hospital (AKA Southall Gardens)	**Previously known as the St Marylebone (Orphanage) School in Southall, Middlesex, England. 1916-19.** 237 bed facility but later added Beaconsfield School increasing to 470 beds. Initially a clearing station for 1AAH but later dealt with large numbers of amputees. Developed expertise fitting artificial limbs and by 1917-18 was specializing in the treatment of amputees.
3 Australian Auxiliary Hospital (AKA Dartford)	**Infectious Diseases Hospital, Dartford, Kent. Oct 1916-19.** A 1,400-bed facility which specialised in nerve surgery and the treatment of psycho-neuroses including shell-shock/ PTSD
No. 2 Command Depot (AKA Weymouth)	**Weymouth, England.** Repatriation centre. An 8,000 bed facility where soldiers who were considered to be unable to return to the front due to psychiatric issues awaited transport home.

ACCS in Europe 1916-19

When the three ACCS left Australia in 1915 there was no provision for nursing staff. In Europe, initially five and then seven nursing sisters were attached to the personnel establishment of CCS in early 1915. However, by the time the offensive in Flanders was underway in 1917 a system of 'surgical teams' was adopted. In effect, one surgeon, one anaesthetist, one theatre sister and one theatre attendant created a team which was located at the nearest hospital but was ready at a moment's notice to go to the forward line and work in the operating theatre of the CCS.

It must be remembered that CCSs did not exclusively treat surgical cases; a wide range of cases were received and treated at the stations. Furthermore, 1 ACCS and 3 ACCS were detailed as 'Corps Rest Station' in 1917-18, which indicates that the units responded to the changes in battle conditions being endured by the soldiers. The number of cases treated at a CCS was nominally 200 but in reality the figure was closer to 1,000 which created enormous pressure on every team member.[4]

Table 2: The following flow chart is copied from the notes of Major PA Stevens (AAMC) 'Working Scheme of Casualty Clearing Stations' [5]

Entry	Triage	Process	Outcome	Exit
	Medical		Evacuated	
	Resuscitation			
Admissions	Preoperative	X-Rays Operating Theatre	Post-operative & Evacuation Wards	Evacuated
	Chest	Ditto	Ditto	Evacuated
	Minor Wounds	Ditto	Ditto	
	Gas			Evacuated

The operating theatre needs to be a quiet, relatively peaceful environment to enable the surgical team to work quickly and efficiently. This reduces both the time the patient is under anaesthetic and the risk of adverse events during the post-operative period, such as infection. In a CCS, apart from the sheer volume of cases, the teams operated close to the front-line. The danger and the horrendous noise was ever-present.

Table 2 shows that soldiers suffering from medical conditions or who had been exposed to gas were immediately evacuated while the remaining cases underwent a surgical response. There is no mention of the 'moribund' or 'dying' ward where soldiers, who had no hope of recovery, were placed. Nonetheless, nurses make mention of it and they found this placement and that of the resuscitation ward particularly harsh and particularly sad.[6] The absence of any mention of an 'intensive care unit' (ICU) is because the first ICU in NSW (Prince Henry Hospital) was not established until 1962.[7]

Madame Marie Curie's Portable X-rays

Each of the units had four departments: command and administration; clinical (including X-ray and pathology); Quartermaster and pharmaceutical (including transfusions and infusions). While mobile X-rays were utilised by 1ACCS at Gallipoli and on Lemnos, a portable X-ray unit was not available during the Battle of the Somme, which created great hardship for staff and poor clinical outcomes for the soldiers. Marie Curie provided portable x-ray machines to assist surgeons who had to make quick decisions about the need to amputate a limb or identify the extent of shrapnel penetration throughout the body of a patient.[8] For instance, by February 1918 all soldiers who had an obvious fracture were X-rayed before surgery at 2ACCS. Madame Curie was often found educating nurses about the practical aspects of x-ray technology on the Western Front.

The Morgue on the Western Front

A pathology department, which was not officially required, tended to be a small room which was set aside for the purpose of post-mortems in CCS. This idea was promoted because it encouraged medical staff to continue their ...*study*. Consent, permission and ethics were all relative terms amid the corpses of CCSs in the First World War.[9]

Table 3: The location/date of establishment/role of Australian Casualty Clearing Stations in Europe (1916-19)[10]

Location and Date	Role and Battles
No 1 Australian Casualty Clearing Station (1 ACCS)	
Estaires: 17 May 1916 - May 1917.	Supported Fourth Army, the Somme (1916).
Bailleul: 19 May 1917 - June 1917.	Flanders offensive (1917). Casualties from Battle of Messines (June 1917). Bailleul bombarded and number of casualties at 1ACCS (including AANS nurse Rachel Pratt, MM). Moved to Oultersteene to avoid further shelling.
Oultersteene (9 June 1917)	Supported Fifth Army, Arras (1917).
No 2 Australian Casualty Clearing Station (2 ACCS)	
Trois Arbres, near Steenwerck: 17 June 1916	Within 10 hours of opening dealt with 900 casualties from Battle of Fromelles. Supported Second Army, Messines (June 1917). Five miles from the front-line and sustained direct hits. During June, July and August 1917 treated 16,357 cases (including 1,077 gassed soldiers). 3rd Battle of Ypres (20 Sep - 10 Nov 1917).
No 3 Australian Casualty Clearing Station (3 ACCS)	
Gézaincourt, near Doullens: 14 October 1916 - 9 February 1917	Battle of Beaumont Hamel. In first 48 hours 1,516 men admitted and 1,400 evacuated.
Edgehill: 9 February1917 - 7 April 1917	Endured atrocious conditions during Battle of the Somme winter 1916-17.
Grévillers, near Bapaume: 7 April 1917 - July 1917.	Casualties from Lagnicourt & Bullecourt.
Branhoek railway siding adjoining Ypres-Poperinghe road (14 Aug 1917) but following severe shelling was moved five miles behind Poperinghe to 'Nine Elms' (until March 1918).	Supported Fifth Army, Ypres (July 1917).
Euskirchen, on the Rhine (occupied Deaf and Dumb Institute): 19 Dec 1918 - 27 Apr 1919.	Supported Second Army during the British advance.

Table 3 provides some level of detail about the location and role of the three ACCS

which operated on the Western Front (1916-19). At first glance it may appear 2 ACCS acted more like a stationary hospital than a CCS.

Bluebirds: *Kanowna* to Egypt: July 1916

There were many ATNA qualified Australian nurses spread throughout England and the Europe from 1916 to the end of the war. One group joined a Red Cross contingent courtesy of a horseracing group.

The Bluebirds were an Australian Red Cross contingent sponsored by the Australian Jockey Club. It financed twenty qualified Australian nurses to serve overseas. The Bluebirds sailed on the *Kanowna* in July 1916. Unlike the AANS there were no marriage restrictions. A number of nurses who had served with the AANS and been required to RTA when they married were pleased to be able to continue their war service. Two such cases were Elsie Cook and her friend Fraser Thompson, AANS, who married while on service overseas and were required to resign. Their service was terminated in May 1916 on their RTA and they sailed on the *HS Kanowna* a few months later destined for France where they *...served with the British for the rest of the war.*[11]

November 1917: Training Nurse Anaesthetists

However, being a member of the AANS was preferred by the civilian trained nurses. It gave them a level of protection in a very dangerous part of the world. It also gave them unique opportunities. On 10 November 1917 Elsie May Tranter (AANS) was serving in France and noted in her diary that *...there is a scheme afoot for army nurses to be trained as anaesthetists so as to free medical officers for medical and surgical work. To this end, two hundred and fifty volunteers have been called for from amongst all the nurses on service. I have given in my name and hope to be accepted.*[12]

Elsie Tranter and two of her AANS colleagues, Mary Aitken and Beulah McMinn, were fortunate to be selected for training because Dr Neville Howse (DMS AIF) *...refused absolutely to participate in the scheme for training nurses for this duty, which was fairly extensively employed in the BEF, following American precedent.*[13] Within a few months these nurses were being described as *...the three Australians who give the* *dope*... and sling ...*the slumber juice.* The number of Australians who managed to complete their training is not recorded in the official history but ...*all countries are represented – Great Britain, Canada, South Africa, United States, New Zealand and Australia.*

McMinn and Tranter both trained in Melbourne while Aitken was a Queensland nurse. McMinn and Aitken were both 26 years old when they enlisted in 1915. Tranter, being slightly older, found the return to study difficult and often related to the idiom ...*It is hard to teach an old dog new tricks.* She was thirty years old when she enlisted in 1916.[14] McMinn and Aitken worked together on Lemnos before being transferred with their unit to Abbassia (Egypt), Brighton (Britain) and finally to Abbeville (France).[15] Tranter was transferred from Melbourne to England in 1916 and was sent to 26 GH in France for her first taste of military service. Strangely enough she contracted a rather mundane but nonetheless serious condition, measles, a few months later.[16]

Mary Violet Aitken (AANS) was of slight build. While nursing on Lemnos she suffered from paratyphoid and during her later tour of duty in France she survived influenza. Beulah McMinn had dysentery and later tonsillitis while in Egypt and suffered from anaemia in France. The two nurses were promoted to 'AANS Sister' in 1917 and were MID in 1918.[17] Tranter was promoted to 'AANS Sister' at the end of 1918. It was when the three nurses were serving together at 5 Stationary Hospital that they were selected for additional training in anaesthetics.

New York Presbyterian Hospital: France: January 1918

They arrived at the American unit, New York Presbyterian Hospital, about 20 miles from Le Havre, on 16 January 1918. They were made very welcome by the Americans ...*who are truly charming people and have such quaint sayings.*[370] On their first day they were given instruction on the use and administration of anaesthetics by Miss Penland who, apparently, was Dr Mayo's anaesthetist in America. The two-month course was followed by an examination which, if passed, enabled the nurses to administer anaesthetics unsupervised in CCSs. The training consisted of operating theatre nursing, the supervised administration of anaesthetics and lectures.[371] The administration of general anaesthetics was an enormous responsibility for nurses and they found the work *...very interesting but it seems as if it will be a long time before we know enough or have sufficient confidence to stand alone.*[18]

Australian born Maud McCarthy was the BEF Matron-in-Chief and she visited the nurses, noting they were *...brave to have undertaken this anaesthetic work*. After her visit and on completion of an examination on 16 March 1918, the 200 trained nurse anaesthetists were despatched to CCSs throughout France.[19]

Australian Nurse Anaesthetists on the Western Front: 1918

During the next few months the three Australians served at 29 CCS (near Amiens) and 3 Canadian Stationary Hospital (Doullens). Within days of her arrival Elsie Tranter gave 20 anaesthetics in one night – in future this was to be a very quiet night.[376] A few short weeks later she had given 31 anaesthetics (supervised) and on occasion the nurses gave short, unsupervised anaesthesia to patients in the wards who had to endure painful and complicated dressings. After surgery the nurses visited the patients *...to see how they recovered ... and to learn from them how to make the administration easier and more pleasant for them.* By the time Tranter was ... *learning about re-breathing apparatus...* she had administered 49 anaesthetics and had been training for just over one month. Despite the failure of the Australian medical military leadership to embrace the concept of nurse anaesthetists, the soldiers (including Australian) on the Western Front benefited from the American-led initiative.

The operating theatre on the Western Front was not a pristine surgical suite. Elsie Tranter was about to administer an anaesthetic to a Tasmanian soldier on the Western Front when *...His Majesty the King and Sir Douglas Haig ... came into the theatre but did not stay very long ... as there were two cases of gas gangrene, I think His Majesty was glad to get away to the outside air.*[20] The ... *unpleasant odour* ... of gangrene is not easily forgotten. The smell permeates the pores of your skin and the stench lingers within your nostrils for days. The smell is also horrific for the sufferer, whose limb is dying, sloughing in front of them.

A startling contrast to how the responsibilities of nurses changed once the war was over is demonstrated by an incident in a suburban public hospital in Sydney. In the 1950s the matron was ...*not impressed*...when a doctor decided to teach nurses how to record the blood pressure of a patient; she claimed if a patient was ill enough to require a blood pressure reading, the patient was ill enough to require the presence of a doctor.[21] Life for a nurse was very different on the Western Front thirty years previously.

20 Australian Army Nursing Service in Europe and England 1916-1918

... claims of brothers must be considered before those of sisters unless there are good and sufficient reasons ... why they should be ignored – Deceased Soldiers' Estate Act, 1918

In April 1916 Australian units began to arrive in France. Nurses from 1 AGH accompanied these units. Several weeks later, 1 July 1916, the Battle of the Somme commenced and allied forces endured unimaginable horror and hardship. The AIF also spent several weeks near the ruined village of Pozières, where they suffered terribly during the Battle of Fromelles, where an allied diversionary attack had taken place. The end of 1916 brought with it the war's most severe winter of trench warfare. This was also the year of the first conscription debate and the politics at home was ugly.

Although the trenches of the Western Front were much maligned, they provided protection against the onslaught of firepower, the ferocity of which had not been experienced in previous wars. Trenches were also ideal homes for rats, which caused disease, spoiled food, took up precious space and impinged on the soldiers' rare chance of sleep. They thrived and consequently multiplied when offered a corpse from which to feast and the surrounds of the trenches were full of them. Soldiers on all fronts endured the misery of louse infestations. The European winters, especially 1916, brought added misery to the men as they tried to keep frostbite, trench foot and gangrene at bay.[1]

Gangrene occurred on all war fronts but those who served on the Western Front were particularly susceptible. The Belgian and French countryside was well cultivated and manured prior to the war so when soldiers dug into the soil they also dug into a host of bacteria.[2] The causative organism of gas gangrene, Clostridium, was particularly virulent and resulted in many amputations and deaths until two French doctors, Carrel and Dakin, developed a technique to clean the infected areas within a wound.[3]

Carrel and Dakin Technique

Basically, the procedure involved the removal of all foreign bodies, if possible, around the wound site. An incision of sufficient length to irrigate every section of the infected area was made. A number of Carrel tubes were inserted to provide maximum irrigation coverage in the wound. The internal wound was then irrigated, via the tubes, with an aqueous solution of chlorine compounds of sodium known as Dakin's solution.[4]

On arrival in France, nurses were required to attend lectures on the administration of the Carrel-Dakin treatment.[5] The nurses generally considered the method to be effective and Sarah Furnifull worked with Carrel and Dakin at Le Havre.[6] Her hospital service was extraordinary and she spent a week touring all the French hospital teams with a doctor educating staff on how to implement the treatment. She went on to work at Camier near Etaples, a CCS during the Somme, and later on train duty, which was particularly hazardous. It was not until near the end of 1917 that Sarah Furnifull, who had only recently recovered from typhoid, finally received a period of well-deserved leave in England.[7]

Pearl Goodman: Wartime Demotions

The staffing problem was compounded when returning soldiers were admitted to specialist military hospitals. Some senior civilian nurses joined the AANS, enduring demotion and the uncertain prospect of overseas service, to nurse returned servicemen. For example, Pearl Goodman was appointed acting Matron of Cairns Hospital in far north Queensland when Miss MacDonnell vacated the position for overseas duty. However, it was not long before the local newspaper, the *Cairns Post*, reported on 13 October 1915 that ...*Matron Goodman relieved of duty to go to the front. Given an additional £20 bonus to mark appreciation of work done since relieving Miss MacDonnell previous Matron.*[8] Acting Matron Pearl Goodman became a staff nurse,

AANS, when she enlisted in 1 MD in October 1915. The position of Matron of Cairns Hospital was once again vacant. Staff Nurse Goodman was on home service at 6AGH for a week and was transferred to 13 AGH, Brisbane, where she worked from 28 October 1915 until 29 December 1916.

Known as *Pearly* to her family, friends and colleagues, she was a small young woman weighing 57 kgs and just 154 cm tall with grey eyes, fair hair and complexion. It is easy to imagine her slight frame carrying the heavy serge uniform of the AANS and her young face framed by the large material veil with the small but distinguished scarlet cape around her shoulders. Her religion was listed as being either Baptist or Anglican.[9]

Pearl Goodman: France: 1917

Pearl Goodman enlisted with the AIF on 12 November 1916. She boarded the *Themistocles* in Sydney and spent the better part of the first two months of 1917 heading for Plymouth. She arrived 3 March 1917 but her stopover in England was short-lived as she was transferred to France on 12 March 1917. She had nursed the casualties of Gallipoli at home but was about to face the reality of war nursing at close quarters.

Pearl was posted to 7 GH where she remained on staff for four months. On 17 July she was transferred to 38 BSH and a month later made her way to 36 CCS where the scale of casualties was overwhelming. After seven months of service in France, including two months with a CCS, she became ill and was admitted to 14 SH, Boulogne, on 22 October 1917. She returned to 36 CCS on 3 November but only lasted another two weeks before her tour of duty was cut short when she was diagnosed with *…TB lungs*. She returned to England on HMHS *Jan Breydel* and remained at Southall Gardens Hospital (2 AAH) until she was RTA on the *Kanowna* on 16 December 1917.[10]

Pearl Goodman: Tuberculosis (TB): Medical Examinations

In London on 11 December 1917 Pearl Goodman was medically examined by an AIF doctor and found to have tuberculosis in her right lung.[1395] She had served with the

AANS for two years and while in France had contracted pneumonia, but that infection never seemed to subside and as a consequence she *...has never felt well since this illness.*[1396] The Medical Board recommended her return to Australia on a hospital ship and be nursed in a cot. In the opinion of the examining doctor her disability was caused by military service and was contracted under circumstances that she had no control over.[11]

Pearl returned to Australia on the *Kanowna.* She disembarked in Melbourne on 13 February 1918 and then proceeded to Sydney. On 5 March 1918 she was once again examined by an AIF doctor at 4 AGH, Sydney, who decided her disability originated prior to enlistment. He claimed that she had *...pneumonia at Brisbane 4/12* [four months] *before leaving for the front. Pt has had a constant cold with very slight expectoration since arriving in England. Now has given positive TB sputum.* The questions on the AIF medical history form were prefaced with the requirement that the *...Medical Officer will carefully discriminate between the man's unsupported statements on his case, and recorded evidence furnished by his documents, military and medical.*[12]

There is no supporting evidence in Pearl Goodman's service record that she had TB prior to enlistment but unfortunately her *Certificate of Medical Examination* was not completed when she joined the AIF. Therefore the Australian doctor retrospectively diagnosed, in the absence of any supporting evidence, that she had TB not pneumonia prior to her transfer to France in December 1916, which was two years prior to his examination of Pearl.

The routine medical certificate, like many of the male-based Army forms, was not likely to alert an examining male doctor to any medical problems specifically encountered by female nurses. For example, it is unlikely that Staff Nurse Goodman suffered from *...marked varicocele with unusually pendent testicle...* or *...traces of corporeal punishment.*[13] However, if the examination had been completed, the presence of TB may have been diagnosed by simply listening to her chest with a stethoscope.

Tuberculosis

It was a French doctor, René Théophile Hyacinthe Laënnec (1781-1826), who first developed the idea of listening to the sounds of the chest via a long rolled-up sheet of paper instead of the ear-to-chest method which had reputedly been used since the days of Hippocrates. By 1821 his treatise was translated into English and the use of the stethoscope became the normal practice in medical circles. Laënnec did a great deal to identify the presence of pulmonary tuberculosis in the lungs and tragically he died of the disease. [14]

TB represented a serious public health problem in the early twentieth century and every effort was made to increase public awareness through health promotion and disease prevention initiatives. The examining doctors would have heard the crepitations in the lungs caused by scarring if advanced TB had been present.[15] The standard medical and nursing texts focus on the volume of sputum expectorated by the patient and detail the process for measuring sputum before incinerating the infected material.[16] Pearl Goodman only produced a small amount of sputum during the initial stages of her diagnosis while in London – this was unusual for TB patients.[17]

Often the onset of TB is symptomless because the body's immune system is able to cope with the first infection. A chest X-ray may reveal a scar on the lung and this may be the first evidence that the person has been previously infected. Chest X-rays (CXR) were available but not routine at the time of the First World War and there is no reference to a CXR in any of the three medical reports on Pearl Goodman. In March 1918, when she was examined at 4 AGH in Sydney, it would have been very difficult, especially in the absence of a CXR, to ascertain when she was first infected with tuberculosis.

Despite the lack of evidence about the date of infection, it is likely that the type of TB was of a particularly virulent form because she was very ill by the time she returned to Australia. There is no suggestion in any of her medical reports that her overseas service did not exacerbate the progress of the TB. Prior to the research and development of antibiotics, the treatment for TB was very limited. Much later streptomycin, isoniazid and para-aminosalicylic acid (PAS), either singly or in combination, were found to produce improvements in TB patients.[18] The only course of treatment available to Pearl Goodman was a 'rest cure'.

After she was examined at 4 AGH she was transferred to the *Malahide Sanatorium* at Pennant Hills where she was re-examined on 10 September 1918 by order of the Principal Medical Officer. Her condition was not improving and it was recommended that she remain at the sanatorium and continue her rest cure. She was discharged from the AIF on 2 October 1918 but remained on a pension. Five months after her discharge on 8 March 1919 the *Cairns Post* recorded under the headline 'Nurse Deceased' that Pearl Goodman had died after she *...contracted pneumonia, which developed into consumption, and her death took place in a Sydney Hospital, where she had been some considerable time.*[19]

'Actual next-of-kin'

Pearl Stella Goodman was born around 1887 in the parish of Millthorpe near Orange, NSW. At the time of her enlistment both her parents were deceased and her sister, Frances Helena Tait (née Goodman), who was residing at Federal Farm at Forrest Reefs, NSW, was her next-of-kin.[20] Pearl left her entire estate (valued at just under £274) to another sister, Caroline Irene Joy Goodman, who lived in Sydney.[21] Unlike Frances, Caroline was unmarried, which may account for Pearl's decision to bequeath her entire estate to her. Furthermore, when Pearl served overseas she deferred part of her pay, which soldiers and nurses often did if they had dependent relatives at home.[22] Two of Pearl's brothers also enlisted with the AIF and returned safely home; her eldest brother had migrated to the USA.

Pearl's eldest sister, Frances, was her designated next-of-kin. She never disputed the terms of Pearl's will but was distressed when the Army would not forward Pearl's medals to her.[23] This situation caused a great deal of angst within the family after Pearl's death because the *...instructions under the Deceased Soldiers' Estate Act, 1918 demand that the claims of brothers must be considered before those of sisters unless there are good and sufficient reasons as to why they should be ignored.*[24] There was a great deal of letter writing between the Army and Mrs Frances Tait but in the end the eldest brother wanted Pearl's war medals. It seems particularly incongruous that the Army required Pearl Goodman to nominate a next-of-kin at the time of her enlistment and then dismissed her wishes. However, correspondence from the Army to Pearl's eldest brother shows that the Army wanted to give the medals to Frances Tait but the difficulty for the Army officers was that the procedure was a statutory requirement not a discretionary one. Sadly, the brother wanted the medals and Frances was informed that as the eldest brother he was the *...actual next-of-kin...* so the Victory Medal and British War Medal were forwarded to him. They were sent to him in the USA on 28 April 1922.[25] Frances Tait received no medals but she had the opportunity to care for and visit Pearl while she slowly died.

For some time, a notation with the Central Army Records Office and a small obelisk outside the Cairns RSL club in north Queensland was the only official references to Pearl Goodman's sacrifice. This situation has since been amended and her name, rightly, appears on the AWM Roll of Honour.[26]

21 First Australian General Hospital (1AGH) in Europe and England 1916-1918

The men who were digging graves stood to attention while we breathed a prayer beside a loved one. There were only three rows of new mounds in the cemetery where to-day, there are thousands. – May Tilton

The First Australian General Hospital (1AGH) had its in origins in Queensland. Formed in August 1914 the personnel and plant departed Brisbane aboard *Kyarra* on 21 November 1914. The staff cared for soldiers suffering from physical injuries, diseases and shell-shock in various buildings throughout Cairo. When 12 BSH was relocated to Sutton Veny in Wiltshire, England, in April 1916 the 1 AGH took over its location at Rouen, France and remained there until 1919.[1] It was a tented hospital located on the Rouen racecourse, amongst a community of other military hospitals. A patchwork of facilities made up of huts, tents and any other cover that could be requisitioned for use as a hospital. There were more than one hundred AANS nurses attached to 1 AGH and they were sent to different units by their matron, Miss Findlay, until a suitable site was established for their tent hospital. Once organised, there was cause for celebration as the AANS staff rejoined their unit and colleagues.

Mary Stafford: 1 AGH: Rouen: April 1916

Mary Stafford sailed with her unit, 1 AGH, on the *Salta,* disembarked at Marseilles in April 1916 and after a delay finally entrained for their journey to Rouen. The nurses found *...a nightmare – it was terribly cold – we travelled from Egypt very light, in accordance with orders. Some of us without even a rug, and it was bitterly cold on the train. We stopped occasionally for food, but the rush was so great you could hardly get it ... We could not get a wash the whole time; 2 nights and three days. At Rouen the British Red Cross* *people at the station took us in, and fed us, which was a God-send. It was 3 p.m. and we had had no breakfast or lunch. We were put in busses and went from Hospital to Hospital, trying to get taken in.*

Mary Stafford & Leila Smith: No 24 & No 15 Ambulance Train: Western Front: 1916

Mary Stafford, who had recently recovered from influenza, was sent to an isolation hospital at Etaples for a month before joining the staff of No 24 Ambulance Train.[930] Train duty in France was unlike Egypt or England because the nurses lived on the ambulance train for three months at a time. Leila Smith served on Princess Christian's No 15 train which formed a small community of...*cooks, carpenters and men for all sorts of duties...* and the *...kitchens were two, one at each end, one for personnel and one for patients ... running to different places; never confined to one route. We were attached to different armies; we never knew when or where we were going.*[2]

Once her stint of train duty was completed, Mary Stafford was assigned to 3 AGH at Le Tréport, where she served from 16 August 1916 until February 1917, and later returned to 1 AGH at Rouen. During the intervening time she suffered another bout of influenza from 9 to 15 December 1916 and was sent to London to convalesce until she was medically cleared in early January 1917. Stafford's tour of duty with her original unit was short-lived when after five months at Rouen she returned to England, where she spent most of July and August of 1917 at 1 AAH and 2 AAH.[3]

1AGH Rouen: Louise (Louisa) Riggall, VAD

Another person who was an integral part of the 1 AGH administration was Louisa Riggall from Victoria. Born in 1868, she was an accomplished artist who studied in Victoria and Paris. When war was declared she joined the VADs and was sent to Egypt on the RMS *Moldavia,* serving with 1AGH. In 1916 she sailed on the HS *Salta* and eventually the 1 AGH was stationed in Rouen, France. Her ability to speak French fluently was an enormous help to the nursing staff and soldiers. Her administrative skills included *...managing hospital supplies...buying gifts for soldiers to send home...arranging entertainment for convalescents.* Louisa tragically died from a brain haemorrhage on 31 August 1918 and her sacrifice is recorded on the AWM commemorative roll. Her loss was felt by many.[4]

Hilda Knox (1 AGH) and Edith Moorhouse (2AGH): to France via 14 AGH, Egypt

The move to Europe wasn't an easy transition for all nurses, especially those caught up with transport duty. Before the 1 AGH transfer to Europe, Staff Nurse Knox was promoted to Sister on 1 December 1915. She, along with Amy King and Valerie Woinarski, were attached to the *Argyllshire* for transport duty back to Australia on 3March 1916 and their unit relocated to France in April.[5] Once the repatriated soldiers were safely home, Sister Hilda Knox was eager to return to her unit, now in France. Similarly Edith Moorhouse was waiting in Australia after transport duty separated her from 2 AGH.

Edith Moorhouse: 14AGH: Cairo: 1916-17

On 19 August 1916 Edith Moorhouse and Hilda Knox embarked on the *Karoola* for a return journey to Egypt as part of the 14 AGH staff establishment, arriving at Suez on 20 September. They hoped for a transport duty to England so they could easily get to France and join their respective units. Tragically, within a month of Edith's arrival in Egypt the sad news reached her that her cousin, Leslie, Captain Moorhouse, had been killed in action on 1 October 1916.[6] He was one of the many young Australian men, 29 years old, to die during the Battle of the Somme. Edith was devastated by the news.

Hilda Knox and Robert Knox: 14AGH: Egypt: 1916

While in Australia waiting for another transport duty there were a number of family changes in the Knox household. Hilda's younger brothers Robert, Francis and James had enlisted with the AIF in medical units. No doubt Mary and James Knox enjoyed a respite from worry about their daughter in the months from April to August 1916 while she remained in Australia.

Sister Knox and her younger brother, Private Robert Knox, joined the 14 AGH contingent and departed Melbourne aboard the *Karoola* on 19 August 1916. The Knox family farewelled Hilda, a mature and experienced 32-year-old military nurse, and Robert, a 23-year-old bank clerk. Nurses tended to spend as much time as possible with their soldier brothers because they made excellent chaperones. Hilda now had two brothers in Egypt and young Robert settled into the routine of a busy hospital.

A Missing Soldier: Robert Knox

On Boxing Day 1916 Robert was granted leave from 5pm until 10pm. He left Abbassia with Private Darcy but at the tram station they parted company; Robert Knox went to Cairo while Private Darcy went to Heliopolis. Apparently, they did not know each other. The next morning Robert was reported absent, over-staying his leave. A general description of the young man was relayed to the hospitals in Cairo and the military police. Robert was of slight build, dark like his sister and in keeping with his upbringing he was a teetotaller. In the past he had never over-stayed his authorised leave and had spent his time in Cairo strolling around the Ezbekia Gardens, as opposed to visiting the notorious brothel district.

Two long weeks passed with no news but finally Robert's body was found in the River Nile on 9 January 1917. His body was viewed at the Government Hospital, Benha, and positively identified against his medical records, identification disc and uniform, which included the unit colours of 14 AGH (chocolate diamond with green cross-bar). His belt and boots were missing. A post-mortem indicated that Robert proceeded to Cairo where he was hit on the back of the head before he fell or was pushed into the river. He had been in the water for at least eight days.

The death of Robert Knox was viewed as suspicious by the court of inquiry but it was decided not to pursue the matter and not to divulge the results of the inquiry.[7] Robert's parents were informed that their son had 'drowned', but it would have been difficult to keep the details of Robert's death secret from Hilda and her brother.[8] Robert was buried in the Greek Cemetery at Banha, Egypt, on 9 January 1917 and he was re-interred after the war at Tel-el-Kebir Military Cemetery.[9] Hilda spent her thirty-third birthday, four days after Robert went missing, worrying about his fate and not knowing he was already dead.

Edith Moorhouse(2AGH) and Hilda Knox(1AGH) to France: 1917

Matron Creal, 14 AGH, was an exceptional Australian nurse: A strong leader and caring individual who was a staunch advocate for her nurses. It may have been the death of Hilda's brother and Edith Moorhouse's cousin that prompted her to enable Hilda and Edith to serve on the HS *Essequibo* en-route to England. Two weeks after Robert's burial Hilda, her grief still acute, left Alexandria on 16 January and finally both nurses arrived in France on 8 February 1917.

Hilda Knox: France: 1917

Hilda was attached to 11 BSH at Rouen three days later. On the morning of 17 February 1917 she awoke with a headache and stayed in bed. Matron Allen organised for a doctor to see her and analgesia was ordered and given. By 4pm she had lapsed into unconsciousness and it is likely that at this time a diagnosis of cerebrospinal meningitis was made. At least her physical suffering was short-lived. Her records suggest there was an element of panic in the decision to transfer Hilda to the larger 8 BGH because she was dead on arrival. She died somewhere between 11 BSH and 8 BGH in Rouen, France at 7.15pm on 17 February 1917.

At her funeral the next day at St Sever Cemetery a detachment from 1 AGH formed part of the mourners and she was once again reunited with her original unit.[10] The funeral was attended by 100 rank and file, officers from all hospitals and her nursing colleagues. A squad of 30 men fired a volley of shots over her grave and then a trumpeter sounded the Last Post. Her parents received notification of her death within three months of their son's death and still had to deal with the anguish and uncertainty of having two other sons serving overseas. Matron Allen wrote to her parents …*Miss Knox only came to me on the 11th, and in that short time we had grown very fond of her, she was so sweet*…while the chaplain told them that …*Every one that knew Hilda loved her. She was the most popular girl in the unit, and so utterly unspoiled by it – sweet and gentle and unselfish.*[11] There is little doubt that Hilda Knox had truly fine attributes.

1AGH Reinforcements: *Essequibo* to England: August 1916

Edith Moorhouse and Hilda Knox were not the only HS *Essquibo* 1 AGH reinforcements in August 1916. It was a peripatetic lifestyle and the best a nurse could hope for was to remain with some of her AANS colleagues throughout the war and occasionally return to their unit before once again being sent to another area of high need.

Elsie Grant and May Tilton: England: 1916-17

On 20 August 1916 Elsie Grant and thirteen of her colleagues departed Egypt and nursed 600 patients aboard the *Essequibo* en route to England. After some service in England, Elsie along with May Tilton and two other Australian nurses, Jane Hall and Ivy Ripper, were set to enjoy a Cook's Tour of Wales, Scotland and the Lake District. Disaster struck days before their planned twenty days recreational leave when May developed three unsightly boils on the left side of her face. Her friends refused to let her report to headquarters in case she was put in hospital and missed her chance of leave. A number of contingencies were put in place for a few days until May's face healed. They made the most of their precious rest and relaxation leave.[12]

Elsie Grant and May Tilton: France: 1917-18

Elsie's Cook's Tour ended on 4 May 1917 when she and Sisters Heard, Ripper and Hall were sent to Le Havre, where they also nursed wounded German POWs.[13] Sister Agnes Cullen Jones (AANS) found the German POWs were *...the greatest ... at bearing pain one could imagine. He seldom flinches. They are only children some of them.*[14]

At this time, Elsie Grant met up again with May Tilton on 4 August 1917, three years after the war commenced, near Brandhoek. All places outside the hospital grounds were out of bounds but May Tilton, accompanied by three colleagues including Elsie, sought the grave of her much loved cousin Norman Ellsworth, who was reportedly buried on the road towards Dickebusch. After a walk in knee-deep mud two of the nurses went back but Elsie and May continued on their quest and they *...almost despaired of finding the place, when, by a miracle, Sergeant B – appeared, crossing a field ... when he could not persuade us to return, he went with us to the grave. He was* *carrying a wooden cross which he had made to place there. The men who were digging graves stood to attention while we breathed a prayer beside a loved one. There were only three rows of new mounds in the cemetery where to-day, there are thousands.* The shared grief of two Australian nurses with soldiers digging the graves of their mates creates a poignant image. Experiences forged in war remain foreign to civilians who have never experienced such levels of intimacy.

3ACCS: Nine Elms (near Ypres): October 1917: Elsie Grant

Soon after this event and following her promotion, Sister Elsie Grant spent 1917 working in the CCS operating theatre. On 2 October 1917 she was recalled to 3 ACCS which at the time was located at Nine Elms, six miles from Ypres. It was at this spot that some Australian nursing sisters …*passed some Australian troops on the way to the line. Elsie Grant recognised her brother's battalion colours, jumped out of the fast travelling ambulance in her excitement, and ran back along the line of marching troops. The next moment brother and sister were clasped in each other's arms. He brought her back and put her back in the ambulance. She was nearly distracted, seeing him marching up to the never-ending thunder and lightning of the guns. He laughed at her fears and said he would be down to see her the very first chance. But he never came. It was their last farewell.*[15]

Allan and Elsie were close in age, she was the youngest and he was just two years older.[16] The Roll of Honour reads '*Allan Herbert Grant (2 Lt) 40 Battalion The Ypres (Menin Gate) Memorial Belgium*' but, sadly, there is no space for the words 'much loved big brother of Elsie'.[17] Elsie never recovered from this loss. Sister Grant continued nursing the casualties of the battle that had taken the life of her brother but by December 1917 it was decided by the matron that she and May Tilton needed a rest.

22 Second Australian General Hospital (2AGH) in Europe and England 1916-1918

The Somme to be ...*a magnificent river, but somehow when one looks at its beauty, one shudders and remembers ... it is the bloodiest battlefield in the history of the war* – *Agnes Cullen Jones*

The Second Australian General Hospital (2AGH) originated in NSW and staff were recruited from 2MD (NSW), 4MD (South Australia) and 6MD (Tasmania). The personnel and plant departed Sydney aboard HMAT *Kyarra* on 28 November 1914. Matron Nellie Gould, who had departed a month earlier with six other nurses, met the contingent and took up her new role as a military leader on 21 January 1915. The locations of 2 AGH included Mena House and Ghezireh Palace totalling 1,500 beds. In April 1916 2AGH was transferred to Wimereux ad arrived on the eve of the Battle of the Somme. Nellie Gould, now in her late fifties and a nurse leader of two wars, was about to face her biggest trial.

2AGH: France: 1917

It is somewhat surprising to discover that nurses found aspects of the landscape truly beautiful. Agnes Cullen Jones (AANS) found the Somme to be ...*a magnificent river, but somehow when one looks at its beauty, one shudders and remembers ... it is the bloodiest battlefield in the history of the war*. Nature had provided the most beautiful of all decorations for the graves of the Somme casualties ...*cornflowers, poppies, marguerites, tiny forget-me-nots, and lily of the valley*. She recorded that those who were buried under the ...*acres of land marked with its little wooden crosses...* were better off because they were finished with the ...*heart scalding that those left behind are suffering*.[1] Tragic to think of a young woman believing so many young men were better off dead than alive but it was, after all, France 1917.

Edith Moorhouse: 2 AGH &1 ACCS: 1917-18: France

Following the death of her cousin, Edith Moorhouse served with 14 SH in Rouen from 9 February until 26 September 1917, at which time she re-joined 2 AGH. This was, no doubt, a joyful reunion, as nurses felt a keen allegiance to their original unit in the same way as soldiers. However, Edith's path had crossed many times with Hilda Knox so hopefully she was able to be a mourner at the funeral of her colleague. Edith was granted leave and spent two weeks in England at the end of January 1918 before returning to 2 AGH in Wimereux for another six months. This was a particularly harsh time for the civilians, soldiers and nursing/medical units on the Western Front. Decisive battles were being fought and the front line was forever changing.

Moorhouse was given another two weeks leave to London at the end of August. On her return to 2 AGH (29 September 1918) was transferred to 1 ACCS for a few days before again returning to 2 AGH. The first of October 1918 was the second anniversary of Leslie's death and was bittersweet because Edith was promoted to sister AANS.

Sister Moorhouse became ill at 1 ACCS two days after the armistice on 13 November and was diagnosed with influenza. Her family was notified three days later reporting she was *...seriously ill.*[2] She was transferred to 39 Stationary Hospital but her condition worsened and she died of pneumonia on 24 November. Leila Smith (AANS), a colleague and most competent and experienced nurse at 1 ACCS, noted that it was *...during this night duty that the late Sister Moorehouse* [sic] *took ill but would not give in until she could not move, and it was too late to save her precious life.*[3]

The Tyson family

Fanny and Theresa Tyson both joined the AANS in May 1915 and travelled to Egypt as part of the 1 AGH reinforcements on separate ships. As previously stated, it was not unusual for a family to have more than one daughter on overseas service during the First World War.[4] The Tyson family had two daughters overseas and their only son, Charles, also joined the AIF in 1916. When he sailed the following year he was just eighteen years old.

Fanny Isobel Catherine Tyson was known to her AANS colleagues as 'Topsy' Tyson.[5] Correspondence suggests it was a term of endearment and may have originated as an early family nickname. Theresa and Fanny Tyson were only a year apart in age. Theresa was born in Hay (NSW, Nari Nari and Wiradjuri Country) to John and Theresa Tyson, Fanny (1890) and Charles were born in Balranald (NSW, Mutthi Mutthi, Ngiyampaa & Barkinji Country).[6] The family moved to Victoria and Theresa and Fanny trained at Bendigo Hospital from 1911 to 1914 (Dja Dja Wurrung and Taungurung peoples of the Kulin Nation). Theresa, being a year older, completed her course of training in August while Fanny finished in October; they both successfully completed the RVTNA examination. Theresa gained experience as a deputy matron of a private hospital and Fanny continued to nurse at her training hospital.

Once enlisted with the AANS, Fanny Tyson embarked on HMAT *Wandilla* in Melbourne on 17 June 1915. When she arrived in Egypt she was sent to the Egyptian Artillery Barracks, which had been converted into a 420-bed infectious diseases hospital known as 4 Auxiliary Convalescent Depot.[7] As was often the case in infectious hospitals, the nurses became the patients and on 11 November 1915 Fanny was herself admitted for mumps. A month later on 16 December she was well enough to return to duty.

Fanny Tyson: 1 and 2 AGH: France

Originally she had been part of 1 AGH reinforcements and after a stint with 2 AGH in Egypt, was eventually transferred to 1 AGH. She sailed from Alexandria with her unit, which included her sister Theresa and Mary Stafford, on the *Salta* in April 1916. They arrived at Marseilles a week later. While they awaited the re-commissioning of 1 AGH in Rouen, Theresa and Fanny were once again separated; Fanny to 6 BGH and Theresa to 5 BGH until 22 April 1916, when they both finally joined 1 AGH as preparations for the first Battle of the Somme were underway.[8]

There are no adjectives to describe the conditions the soldiers and those caring for them endured at this time. Suffice to say Staff Nurse Fanny Tyson deserved her first leave from 3 to 22 February 1917 after ten months continuous service at Rouen. Whether by luck or design, Theresa had leave a few weeks earlier but they had one week overlap in England.

Fanny returned to 1 AGH, still located at Rouen, and the steady stream of casualties kept her occupied until April 1917, at which time Theresa developed diphtheria and had to be transferred to 25 SH for isolation nursing. Fortunately, Theresa's condition stabilised and she returned to 1 AGH where she was promoted to AANS Sister on 4 September 1917.[9] Unfortunately, the two siblings rarely worked together from June 1917 until October 1918. During the Somme nurses were sent wherever they were needed at short notice.

The movement of the allied forces in 1917 was matched by the German advance in 1918. Fanny Tyson served in two of the more harassed units; 2 AGH and 2 ACCS. The conditions at 2 ACCS were of hardship and endurance due to extremes in weather, which caused a lack of usable water and an abundance of mud, rain and slush. The CCS was erected wherever the constantly moving 'front-line' ended up. The construction of the infrastructure depended upon transport delivering duckboards which were used to construct usable paths between the tents/marquees. Unfortunately, these pieces of wood often commandeered for more urgent use before they reached the CCS. Squelching through the mud, while moving from area to area, was a serious hardship for the CCS staff. The Battle for Messines Ridge (1917) saw 2,300 cases go through 2 ACCS in 19 hours so the pressure on the staff was enormous. One of those in the thick of battle was the future husband of Sister Minnie Kate Porter.

Sister Minnie Kate Porter: ARRC: 2AGH: 1916

Minnie Kate Porter had sailed with the first contingent aboard the *Kyarra* in 1915 and remained with 2 AGH. As we know she served with distinction on the *Gascon* as it rescued soldiers from Gallipoli. Minnie Kate returned to 2 AGH where she nursed Lieutenant John Ebenezer Donaldson, who was suffering from paratyphoid in January 1916. It is not known if they knew each from Sydney Hospital, where John Donaldson had been a resident pathologist. Whether he completed his residency before the war is unclear but he joined the 19 Battalion, AIF, not the AAMC. They were engaged soon after they met at 2 AGH and his will was changed to favour Minnie Kate on 1 April 1916. At this time Minnie Kate was promoted to AANS Sister and sent to France with 2AGH.

Sister Minnie Kate Porter served with 14 BGH (Boulogne), 14 GH and 2 ACCS while in France. However, her life changed when Captain Donaldson was shot on 11 August 1916. When notified of his wound, Minnie Kate was accompanied by one of her friends, Sister Sophie Durham, to see him. Maud Kellett noted that everyone was *...awfully sorry for the man. Everyone says he was such a good fellow, a Sydney man.*[10] Captain Donaldson and Sister Minnie Kate Porter had a deathbed marriage. Widows were allowed to continue nursing in the AANS but Mrs Donaldson elected to return to Australia via England and meet her new in-laws. While it is impossible to know how she was received by her in-laws she did later re-enlist as Sister Katherine Minnie Donaldson and joined 14 AGH on 27 October 1917. She served under Rose Creal until 1919 when she RTA, nursing on the HMHS *Delta*. She had endured and survived influenza in 1919, but not all nurses were so fortunate.[11]

Fanny Tyson: Western Front: 1918

In early 1918 the German advance toward the strategic town of Amiens was imminent. Like May Tilton and Elsie Grant, Fanny Tyson was assigned three weeks leave in January 1918, which she spent in Cannes, and once rested she returned to her unit at the front. It was after the armistice on 10 December 1918 that she was finally promoted to Sister Fanny Tyson, AANS: A military nurse veteran of more than three years who was aged 28 years.[12]

Armistice

Luck and superstition played a part in the psyche of soldiers, even when the war was over. For instance, Sister Elsie Tranter, now a proficient anaesthetic nurse working in the operating theatres of the Western Front, was also a brunette. Apparently this made a difference to her Scottish patients, who believed that on New Years Eve (1918) if a *...dark haired woman "first foots" they will have luck.* Elsie

Tranter obliged her soldier patients and ...*well supplied with cigarettes*... she set off in the snow to visit them.[13] It would appear her competence was matched by her empathy.

Fanny Tyson spent the early months of 1919 in England nursing convalescing Australian soldiers at 1 AAH and 2 AAH. On 19 April she was ...*marched out to Fovant Street AANS*... with a ...*very bad headache*... but the reason for her illness was not known. Many nurses who had served in CCSs experienced severe headaches. The constant noise and images of the Western Front were not easy to leave behind.

Fanny Tyson died at 8 pm on 20 April 1919; Theresa and Charles were by her side at 1 AGH, Sutton Veny.[14] It took three days for the cause of death 'cerebral haemorrhage' to be reported and was most likely confirmed by autopsy, as a request for permission was made and a three-day delay in burial was unusual at this time.[15]

On 23 April 1919 the coffin of Sister Fanny Tyson was conveyed to the graveside on a gun-carriage and six Australians supported the pall. She belonged to the Church of England and was buried with full military honours. Her young body was placed into a ...*separate single grave in virgin soil*... in consecrated ground in the military section (plot 85) of the St John the Evangelist Churchyard, Sutton Veny. When her body was lowered into the ground, Theresa and Charles were present as was 'Mr Fry (a friend)' - one can only speculate about his loss and grief. The Army and AANS were well-represented and there were numerous floral tributes to young Fanny Tyson. Finally,...*the last post was sounded and volleys fired over the grave*... and her life and death were finalised.[16] She was the last AANS nurse to be buried on foreign soil – until the next war. The parents of 'Topsy' Tyson may have had solace in the attendance of their son and daughter at her deathbed. They were assured that she had indeed died and that she was buried appropriately.

23 Third Australian General Hospital (3AGH) in Europe and England 1916-1918

... felt she couldn't give in – died, one might say at her post, for she was on duty the day previous and died of pneumonia the next day ... She was buried in our peaceful corner with our own hero boys – Anne Donnell

The Third Australian General Hospital (3AGH) originated in NSW and staff were primarily recruited from 2MD (NSW) with later reinforcements from 4MD (South Australia) and 3MD (Victoria). The personnel and plant of the 1000 bed hospital departed Sydney aboard RMS *Mooltan* on 5 May 1915. Matron Grace Wilson led the nursing staff of 3AGH for the entire war. She did spend time in England from September 1917 to April 1918 when she was temporary Matron-in-Chief during Evelyn Conyers period of leave.

The locations of 3 AGH included Lemnos, on the Greek Island of Mudros, during the Gallipoli Campaign. Then to Abbassia Army barracks on the outskirts of Cairo from early 1916 until the unit was transferred to Kitchener War Hospital, Brighton from October 1916 until May 1917. It was transferred to Abbeville, arriving in readiness for the Battle of Messines. Grace Wilson was one of the most respected and decorated nurses of the First World War and would later make a significant contribution during the Second World War. The arrival of 3 AGH in France was a great trial.

Matron Grace Wilson: 3 AGH: England & France 1916-18

Grace Wilson and her 3 AGH staff proceeded to England and on 5 October 1916 they took over the Kitchener War Hospital at Brighton, Sussex.[1] The buildings were old and the nurses arrived in time for a very cold winter where they nursed the casualties of the Somme. Wilson and her nurses enjoyed some *...very happy and busy months at Kitchener.*[2] Finally, 3 AGH was transferred to Abbeville, France, in May 1917 where they remained for the next two years.

Ruby Dickinson: 3 AGH: Origins

Ruby Dickinson was born in Forbes (NSW, Wiradjuri Country) on 8 July 1885 and her sister Adelaide was born a few years later in 1882.[3] When Ruby was twenty-six years of age her father, William, died and when war was declared her mother, Julia, was living at 'Arizona' in Almora Street, Mosman, NSW, where she remained throughout the war.[4] Ruby completed her training over a five-year period at Lister Private Hospital in Sydney from February 1906 until 1911. Once registered with ATNA on 7 April 1911, she gained experience private nursing until February 1913 and then became Head Nurse at Gunnedah Hospital in north-west NSW. A few months later she was appointed Head Nurse at the nearby Narrabri Hospital.[5] Dickinson arrived in time to work in a new facility because on 20 August 1912 the old Narrabri Hospital was *...doused in petrol and lit at a given signal ... to get rid of any germs which may have collected over the years.*[6]

Staff Nurse Ruby Dickinson enlisted with the AANS on 26 July 1915. She was a woman with a fair complexion and when she was thirty years of age she had a slight build, weighing just 57 kilograms despite being 167 centimetres tall. She embarked in Sydney on the *Orontes* on 31 July 1915 as a member of 3 AGH and served on Lemnos during the Gallipoli Campaign. Although 3 AGH was transferred to France via England in early 1916, Staff Nurse Dickinson remained in Egypt until 17 July 1916, at which time she departed Cairo 'in charge' of HT *Seang Choon.* The ship arrived in Melbourne and Ruby once again left Australia for transport duty aboard the *Anchises* on 24 January 1917 bound for England.

Ruby Dickinson: 3 AGH: England and France: 1917

On arrival she commenced duty at 3 AAH, Dartford in Kent on 12 April 1917. The hospital consisted of seventy-five huts built along a central roadway and was heated by steam with a covered throughway.[7] It was sometimes referred to as the Orchard

Hospital because there was a *...fine apple orchard adjoining the hospital.*[8] Ruby wanted to rejoin her 3 AGH colleagues, who had become a close-knit community since the shared experiences on Lemnos.[9] Unfortunately, while at 3 AAH she became ill with a severe pain in her left ear which was diagnosed as otitis media. Eventually the pain subsided when a thick, yellow discharge finally drained from her ear. However, a ruptured tympanic membrane was diagnosed when she continued to suffer from severe tinnitus (ringing in the ear) after the pain had subsided. The condition was sufficiently serious to warrant two more hospital readmissions but Ruby rejoined her unit, 3 AGH, in France by 10 October 1917.

Matron Miles Walker: 3 AAH, England & 5 BSH: Dieppe: 1917

Dickinson was under the capable care of Nellie Miles Walker who, in October 1916, attained the rank of Matron 3 AAH, Dartford.[10] The common stereotype of the First World War nurse - the ministering angel - is used reluctantly but seems to be the most apt in describing Miles Walker. The pedestrian term - kindness - gains in strength when placed in the context of allied hospitals in France during the war. Photographs of her convey her gentle nature. Miles Walker was later appointed matron of 5 BSH, Dieppe, on 11 July 1917 and Staff Nurse Leila Brown (AANS) found it to be *...another British Hospital staffed by Australian sisters. It was a small Stationary Hospital and took mostly local sick and injured – it being the principal port for the landing of war materials, there were frequently accidents. Here we were billeted in a charming house and had everything one could wish for to make life happy. We had a 'Tommy' as cook and you could not have recognised army rations in the excellent dinners he served up every night. Here for the first time I worked the hours generally set in Australian Hospitals ... one whole day per week off duty, and alternate long and short days. There was a golf course nearby and I was able to play quite often, there was also a tennis court built us by a French Baron who owned a house close to ours and if we brought visitors to the house ... Miss Mills-Walker* [sic] *who was Matron welcomed them and made the atmosphere quite that of a home.*[11]

Battle of Messines: June 1917

A month after they arrived in June 1917 the Battle of Messines took place. While it was considered to be one of the better organised battles from a medical viewpoint, the extent and type of casualties were a shock to the nurses. The effect of mustard gas on the soldiers was particularly cruel. Nurses of 3 AGH had not witnessed such distress in their soldier patients before, because gas was not used as a weapon at Gallipoli.[12]

Gas attacks and shell-shock

Although 5 BSH sounds like a home away from home, it was there that a number of experienced war nurses sought refuge from the unrelenting demands of work in the CCSs of France. Nursing soldiers who had endured serious burns to their face, respiratory tract and eyes from mustard gas was extremely challenging. Anne Donnell recalled *…the expressions on those dear boys' faces as they come pouring in with their frightened, anxious, hunted look, combined with the suffering of fear, pain, and shock. Those who could see led queues of bandaged blind, each one placing his hands on another's shoulders, and thus feeling the way.*

German Advance: 30 November 1917

This incident occurred during the German advance on 30 November 1917 and Anne was so distressed by the mutilated bodies of the *…Guards, the Grenadier, the Irish, Scotch, Shropshires, and many other…* that for one of the first times in her years of work in a CCS she found herself *…going to the marquee flap to hide the tears that will gather, and ask for strength to control a distorted face, and go back.* During military and medical catastrophes such as those faced by the nurses on troopships during the Gallipoli Campaign and nurses in CCSs in France, they were given an enormous amount of autonomy to administer pain relief, which basically consisted of morphia. In the situation Donnell found herself in it is hardly surprising that given she was *…free to use my own discretion in giving morphia or stimulants, and you may be sure I was ever ready to use either, when I thought it was the least bit necessary.*[13]

May Tilton found the nights in a CCS to be a continual rush but *…one night discovered* *a Lancashire lad of eighteen crying in pain. He whimpered "no one has been near me and I am in pain." I brought him some nourishment and a sedative, made him as comfortable as possible, and found time to sit beside him until he fell asleep. Holding my hand in both of his, he whispered, "You are good to me. I feel lovely now". He died before morning.*[14] This description of the tragic death of a child-man is made bearable by the narrative of a nurse who has a perfect understanding of what it is to be a nurse.

Emma Cuthbert (AANS) found it difficult to keep her emotions in check at 6 BSH, France, in December 1917 nursing men who had endured a gas attack, because ...*the boys came in quite blind with enormously swollen eyelids ... and the eyes discharging freely'*. She noted '*the patient is burnt over the face and body with huge blisters...* and the ...*burns are very painful ... & frequently the patient is unable to speak above a whisper.*[15] The treatment was rudimentary as nurses, like Donnell and Cuthbert worked ...*hour after hour, putting cocaine in those poor smarting eyes, then sodi-bicarb. pads and a bandage.* Nurses were also at risk of being affected by gas when stationed at advanced CCS posts in France. Anne Donnell was sleeping soundly on New Year's Eve 1917 when she ...*was awakened suddenly at the early hour of 2.30 am with the sound of close shelling, and quickly detected a faint sweetish scent like pineapple ... I jumped up, as did most of us, and got dressed, shivered and shook and coughed, and I thought I never should manipulate that mask.*[16] The mask was a heavy and awkward piece of apparatus but at least it offered the wearer some hope of protection.

The Shock of Mustard Gas: July 1917: Europe

The USA declared war on Germany on 6 April 1917 and this had an immediate impact on the war in Europe. Mustard gas was first used in July 1917 by the Germans in an attempt to break the stalemate. The allied Field Marshall Sir John French claimed it was illegal because it caused victims to ...*die a painful and lingering death.*[17] However, it did not take long for allied chemist James B Conant (USA) to agree to lead a research team on the development of gas and chemical warfare agents because he ...*did not see ... why tearing a man's guts out by a high-explosive shell is to be preferred to maiming him by attacking his lungs and skin.*[18] However, a gas attack had an enormous impact on the mind of the soldier as he ...*saw, first of all, a white smoke rising from the German trenches to a height of about 3 feet. Then, in front of the white smoke appeared a greenish cloud, which drifted along the ground to our trenches, not rising more than about 7 feet from the ground when it reached our first trenches.*[19] It is hardly surprising that they ...*were more frightened than hurt*... and that when the physical effects of the gas had abated ...*there was left an emotional disturbance like a mild attack of shell-shock.*[20]

Effort Syndrome or Disordered Actions of the Heart (DAH): Western Front: 1917

There was an increase in the incidence of Disordered Actions of the Heart (DAH) on the Western Front (1917) when chloropicrin and phosgene (lung irritant gases) were used against the allied forces.[21] Emma Cuthbert noted that ...*in some cases the 'Gas' has affected the heart*...which indicates the cardio-pulmonary side-effects of the gas were known to the nurses at the time.[22] However, due to the suggestive nature of the syndrome when soldiers were grouped together it was decided to rename DAH to 'Effort Syndrome' (29 May 1918) because there was no evidence that it was cardiac in origin. Therefore, affected soldiers received ...*ordinary graduated Command Depot training*...and were not treated as special.[23]

Diagnosing cowardice

A differential diagnosis of a psychosomatic as opposed to a physical condition had dire consequences, and indeed proved fatal for a number of soldiers during the war. During the First World War the British War Office Committee had a policy of ...*Informed Common Sense*... whereby after a brief period of rest the soldiers were made aware of the ...*facts*... intrinsic to their diagnosis. The medical officer and staff were required to use ...*energetic persuasive methods*... but acknowledged that a number of patients may not respond because their ...*personality was of a low grade and strongly anti-moral.*[24]

Casualties were generally divided into three categories: physical wounds, illness and mentals. Physical wounds were obvious and a man with a gaping wound in his stomach or a limb missing was beyond reproach as a coward. Illness was more difficult to evaluate and soldiers and nurses alike would stay at their posts while suffering from the effects of typhoid, dysentery, cholera, pneumonic influenza and malaria; often until it was too late to receive treatment.[25] Shell-shock was a grey diagnostic area and depended upon the sympathetic diagnosis of the attending medical officer. As the war continued and the number of shell-shock casualties increased, the Army came to the conclusion that medical officers were not being sufficiently objective in their diagnosis.[26]

For example, a British medical officer was asked to visit a youth in the trenches on the Western Front who *...had been classed as normal by all who knew him, and had always come up to scratch...* but the doctor found him *...gibbering...* while sitting on his *...cramped bunk, leaning forward, gripping hard an upright with both hands. In most of the bunks were men who stirred as they slept. Some woke but did not complain of the boy's shouting*. The doctor concluded that the boy was an *...undoubtedly intelligent child*; his age was not known. The treatment consisted of a morphia injection so the boy could be transferred down the line but a less sympathetic doctor may have interpreted the symptoms as 'fear,' which at the time was not too distant from cowardice.[27] The non-judgemental acceptance of the young soldier's mental instability by his comrades suggests the boy had previously proven himself in battle and his mates were in a position to empathise. Maybe they knew it could happen to any one of them under the circumstances.[28]

However, when a man was considered to be a coward and was looking for a way to avoid his duty he was held in contempt by his comrades, so even if he was found not guilty by a court martial *...he'll probably get shot by his own mates the next time...* he goes over the top.[29] The British used public executions as an example to other soldiers who were tempted to behave dishonourably, that is, supposedly cowardly.[30] The Commonwealth Defence Act and Regulations did not include the death penalty for military crimes, so Australians under British command on the Western Front could be tried and sentenced to death but the punishment could not be enforced without the approval of the Australian Government. Fortunately, this was never forthcoming.

25 BGH: Hardelot: Maud Kellett: July 1917

Following a number of administrative problems with the AANS and British nursing units, the Australian nurses were brought together to make up three central British units. The nurses resented leaving their forward posts where they believed they could do the most good for their boys. Maud Kellett was appointed matron of the largest hospital, staffing one hundred, 25 BGH at Hardelot, France, on 10 July 1917.[31] Despite the high level of military activity on the Western Front at this time, 25 BGH was more a convalescent hospital than an acute facility. Hence many nurses who had been recalled from CCSs felt their expertise was being wasted.

Skin Hospital: 25 BGH

The 25 BGH specialised in the treatment of skin diseases including psoriasis, eczema and scabies.[32] While the cases may have been relatively easy from a physical viewpoint because the men only had skin conditions, it must be remembered that the system of discharge at the time meant that the men in 25 BGH were going to be sent back to the front. The general and stationary hospitals usually sent the soldier back to a British convalescent camp as a 'sitting case' by ambulance. From here he would return to duty at a depot in France, where the final decision was made to either send him back to the front-line or (if more convalescence was needed) to Britain (*Blighty*) for further treatment.[33] This situation placed a great deal of pressure on the doctors and nurses who reported on the patients' recovery.

Matron Kellett: RRC, MID (1916 &1919), CBE, FN Medal

There is little doubt that Kellett was an interesting personality who amused nurses with her penchant for acronyms and abbreviations as well as her obsession with her pristine uniform. By the end of 1916, Kellett had left Egypt for England where she was appointed Matron of 2 AAH where Marion Hall (AANS) reported for duty to find *...Kellett reigning there*. During the Somme offensive 1 AAH at Harefield was inundated with casualties, necessitating the requisition of St Marylebone Orphanage school located at Southall in the western suburbs of London. 2 AAH was opened on 4 August 1916, the second anniversary of the war.[34]

Her idiosyncrasies aside, Maud Kellett had a distinguished military career and was MID a number of times (1916 and 1919), awarded the RRC (1919) and appointed a Commander of the British Empire (CBE) Military Division in 1919.

Kate Porter: 25 BGH: Hardelot, France: 1917

A number of nurses like Kate Porter were once again under the influence of Matron Kellett who had been assistant matron to Rose Creal during her training years. Kate Porter was promoted to AANS Sister in April 1917 after service in Egypt with 1AAH and 1 AGH in France since March 1916. She endured a couple of weeks in hospital in April 1917 when she contracted measles but was soon back to work. As was the policy, Kate Porter had two fortnight furloughs during her time is in France. So, like many nurses with her war experience, she was a competent military nurse who was keen to take on more serious cases. By December 1917 the pressure of mounting casualties necessitated the disbursement of nurses to other units and Kate was sent to 53 CCS on 22 March 1918.

Meanwhile her parents had been incorrectly informed she had married and was returning to Australia, creating confusion and no doubt distress, until the marriage of Minnie Kate Porter was clarified. When Kate Porter returned to the front she was attached to 3 AGH, Abbeville, under the leadership of Nellie Miles Walker and later Grace Wilson. Kate more than likely recorded her feelings in her trusted diary. Sadly we will never know what she wrote because in April 1918 she was evacuated with her unit from Rouen as the enemy approached and she left with only the clothes on her back.[35]

Matron Nellie Miles Walker: 3AGH: The Big Push: 1918

Both May Tilton and Anne Donnell had served with Nellie Miles Walker at a time of heightened angst. At a leadership level, the most challenging situation for Miles Walker occurred when she was matron of 3 AGH in Abbeville during the German advance in early 1918. German General Ludendorff wanted to avail himself of the opportunity for a breakthrough on the Western Front which the withdrawal of Russia from the allied forces presented. Conversely, the revitalization of the allied offensive with the USA entry into war in April 1917 coupled with the helplessness of the Austro-Hungarians, who were enduring a famine, put pressure on the enemy positions. The Germans decided to retreat, reform and then push through on the Western Front.

In March 1918, 3 AGH received orders to act as a CCS as the enemy advanced to Amiens – an important strategic location for the allies to resist the 'Big Push' by the Germans.[36] Number 3 AGH was inundated with 1,800 casualties. The German Army advance saw Matron Miles Walker's 1,500-bed general hospital turned into a 2,000 bed CCS practically overnight.[37] Her concern for her nurses was paramount and she kept in contact with some of her nurses who were constantly being sent to forward areas as the front line continually changed.[38] The nurses found this time particularly difficult as they were bombed each night, so rest was near impossible.[39]

Grace Wilson returns to 3AGH: Big Push: April 1918

Grace Wilson had been in England serving as the acting Matron-in-Chief while Evelyn Conyers was on leave. Wilson returned to her unit on 23 April 1918 and although the prescribed staff establishment of 3 AGH consisted of four head sisters, twenty-eight sisters and fifty-eight staff nurses, she dealt with the avalanche of casualties with a staff of one head sister, fifteen sisters and twenty-four staff nurses. Matron Wilson led her nurses through one of the more trying times of the war because they not only had soldier patients to attend to but *...every three weeks makes an influx of Medical cases, as the Hospital receives all local sick in rotation with the other two Hospitals in the area.*[40] As has been the case in so many wars the locals suffered.[41] The French villages, which were being devastated as the Germans advanced towards Amiens at an alarming rate, contained French citizens who were now refugees.[42] Australian nurses were Nightingale-trained and they cared for all people irrespective of nationality, creed or religion. Despite this pressure, her nurses found her *...to do her best in all our interests and I believe she had a very uphill task of it.*[43] Another nurse identified Matron Wilson's ability to *...understand many things without having to be told – and she was very human too.*[44] This is exemplified in her attention to the health needs of her nurses and her attempts to monitor their workload when the task seemed near-impossible. Kate Porter continued to nurse the never-ending casualties until the Armistice was declared.

During the 1918 German offensive the role of 25 BGH changed dramatically, as it acted as CCS during August and September 1918.[45] The nurses were pleased to be working without time off because they were doing real war work, not just skin management.[46] Sister Kate Porter was granted two weeks furlough in Paris before 25 GH ceased to be operational in February 1919. She returned on the *Medic* as nursing staff from England on 10 April 1919 and arrived home to her family on 1 June 1919.[47]

Ruby Dickinson

Although the influenza pandemic did not, purportedly, start until October 1918, Anne Donnell found the first six months of 1918 to be …*our busiest time, too, the influenza swept over us, involving extra work for those who kept well. When the worst was over more help came, but I shall always think that it came too late and at the price of life; for Sister Dickenson* [sic] *– a dear comrade who was with us at Lemnos and who felt she couldn't give in – died, one might say at her post, for she was on duty the day previous and died of pneumonia the next day at Southwell Gardens. It was a sad shock to us all. She was buried in our peaceful corner with our own hero boys.*[48]

Ruby Dickinson continued to endure bouts of ear infections and continuous tinnitus. She was sent back to England and in between intermittent admissions to Southall Gardens Hospital she served at 1 AAH for six months.[49] On the morning of 23 June 1918 she was once again admitted. Her observation chart was prepared for the period 23-25 June but only one entry was made of her temperature on admission, which was 102°F and she died the same day.[50] Ruby was buried two days later on 25 June 1918, just a week before her thirty-third birthday.

Staff Nurse Ruby Dickinson's funeral was well attended although a gun carriage was not available her body was transferred by ambulance. She had a military funeral and was laid to rest at the Harefield Parish Churchyard in consecrated ground. Her coffin was described as being in 'good condition'. The list of people who attended was impressive, with no fewer than nineteen wreaths being laid in her memory. Wreath number ten is particularly touching being from …*Ward 40 (her own patients)*

No.1 AAH. Just as nurses had a tendency to lay claim to 'their patients' during the war, the reverse also occurred.[51] Her mother later wrote ...*it has been a source of much consolation to me to know how and where she was laid to rest.*[52] Many mothers during the years of 1914-19 had no such consolation.

Ruby Droma Dickinson

As previously mentioned Ruby shared her name with another AANS nurse and the brother of Ruby Droma Dickinson was notified that his sister had died of pneumonic influenza.[53] A tragic mistake was identified and both families were notified of the error: One family bereft and the other relieved. Ruby Droma Dickinson was born in Geelong, Victoria on 3 April 1885 and returned home to her family on the *Norman* on 4 July 1919.[54] When she arrived home there was one family who felt they had been given a reprieve from grief.

24 2 ACCS and a Night of Valour on 22 July 1917

...could hear nothing for the roar of planes ...I seemed to be the only living thing about – Alice Ross-King

Sergeant Clair Whiteside was one of the 5,533 casualties from the 5th Division, AIF at Fromelles. He was shot in the head by a sniper and as he made his way back to a dressing station he found it ...*interesting, though none too pleasant, speculating whether you are going to get the full effects of a shell, a mild earthquake or merely a ton or two of dirt on top of you ... a most unpleasant side of warfare, lying out on a battlefield – wounded, maybe perfectly helpless with no chance of aid being given to you. It must be bitterly cruel to the man nearly out to it.*[1]

The number of official cases of shell-shock appears conservative compared to the level of reference to the condition in the diaries and letters of soldiers and nurses. This may have been due to the behaviour of the victims being so unusual and that it prompted comment from those around them. Until June 1916 there were fifty recorded cases of shell-shock in the AIF on the Western Front but by the end of July the incidence had increased to 376; the first Battle of the Somme commenced on 1 July 1916.

This influx resulted in the Army forming diagnostic centres which dealt with the condition along ...*scientific lines.*[2] For instance, Dr Springthorpe established a clinic at 3 AAH, Dartford, for Australian soldiers suffering from war neuroses, who were awaiting transport back to Australia. K. Laity (AANS) claimed the main form of treatment was to ...*try and amuse them, to make them forget.*[3] Given the reality of the Western Front this was a difficult nursing care plan to implement. Unfortunately, the results of the treatment were inconclusive but the research did demonstrate the need for reform in the area.

However, the success of Major J B Lewis, who treated a variety of neuroses at No. 2

Australian Command Depot (Weymouth), and others who contributed to statistical analysis of syndromes which had previously been discounted as 'mental' problems, assisted in changing the viewpoint of the medical and nursing professions about the legitimacy of psychiatry and psychology.[4]

Shell-shocked nurses

Shell-shock was not the exclusive domain of combatants – the service records of AANS nurses are littered with diagnoses of 'debility' or 'neurasthenia' which was defined as *...debility or exhaustion of the nervous system; a functional disorder with severe depression of vital forces.*[5] Australian nurses like Mary Dwyer and Anne Donnell who were stationed in CCSs on the Western Front endured constant night air-raids where they *...thought our last hour had arrived.*[6] Anne Donnell, while on leave in London for 'debility', makes the simple statement that *...I long sometimes to breathe again...*, which is suggestive of an anxiety state. There is little doubt her experiences in the CCSs of France were anxiety provoking.[7] May Tilton had a somewhat different experience after the war when *...suddenly, I felt something happen to my brain. It seemed to expand, as though a tight band was suddenly lifted from it. I will never forget the experience or the relief.*[8]

Facing the enemy

Just as it had been for the Russians and their nurses, including Florence Farmborough in 1915, the approach of the Germans was a terrifying prospect for the nurses. They were, as ever, reluctant to leave their patients, who dreaded the idea of being captured. The CCSs and AGHs began to meld during the shelling at Hazebrouck. Mary Dwyer (AANS) recorded that the order came for their *...immediate evacuation, we left about 2 o'clock by a London bus, luggage inside and Sisters on the top. It was a pathetic sight to see the civilians carrying their personal belongings in a barrow or bicycle and leaving their homes.*[9] During the retreat, nurses like Edith Simpson (AANS) were supposedly *...evacuated 25 at a time to Hardelot and Boulogne...* but the continual bombing of infrastructure and the close proximity of the Germans created an atmosphere of organised chaos.[10] Miles Walker and Wilson did not lose any of the 3 AGH nurses during the retreat, although one BCCS was captured; patients and medical officers were taken as POWs.[11] The number of soldiers who died during the retreat is inestimable but the noise, pain, fear and absence of a normal hospital infrastructure compounded the misery of their deaths.

As at Gallipoli, Casualty Clearing Station (CCS) refers to a system of triage (evaluation) and emergency first aid close to the battle.[12] There were no nurses on the Peninsula; 3AGH at Lemnos was the closest nursing unit to the front in 1915. The inclusion of female nurses in the personnel of CCS was initially controversial but their expertise, especially in the operating theatres, made their presence invaluable in Europe.[13]

Casualty Clearing Stations: Staffing Disputes

The Australian DMS, Neville Howse, implemented a policy of leave every six months but the British Matron-in-Chief, Maud McCarthy, was a strong critic. She claimed it was difficult to introduce relief nurses to forward zones without causing unnecessary destabilisation of the units and a number of Australian nurses preferred to stay in the advanced CCS.[14] Regular leave was not universally welcomed by nurses because it was difficult to readjust to war conditions on their return.

An Extraordinary Nurse Leader: Ethel Sarah Davidson

Ethel Davison was one of those ordinary nurses who had an extraordinary capacity to solve problems under pressure. While the following experiences of the nurses who were awarded military medals show outstanding bravery and resolve to protect their patients at all costs, they were under the command of nurse leaders who required such resolve.

Born in 1872 at Payneham (South Australia, Kaurna Country) she had a tragic early life. Her father, William Davidson was a Master Mariner, who had three grown sons and three grown daughters when he married a second time, to Elizabeth Green. Ethel was five years old when her family, including two young brothers and a baby sister were drowned when her father's brigantine, the *Emily Smith*, was wrecked off Kangaroo Island. Ethel was not with her family at the time so she spent her childhood with her half brothers and sisters. There is no information about her education until she trained at the Adelaide Hospital. Once she graduated in 1897 she undertook District Nursing and Private Nursing with time spent on the Control Board of Health.[15]

Ethel joined the AANS in 1904 and enlisted on 26 September 1914. She sailed on the *Shropshire* with Evelyn Conyers, where they most likely met for the first time. Her service in Egypt included being in-charge of the pneumonia ward at the NZ Hospital, Abbassia, where she worked alone for just over four months nursing sixty patients. In preparation for the Gallipoli casualties she was transferred to Mena House and from August 1915 until January 1916 she was Acting Matron 3 AAH, Cairo. For her service at this time she was MID and ARRC.[16] In June 1916 she reverted to Sister AANS and went to England for six months with the Medical Section of the AIF HQ. Her remarkable administrative skills were evident during this period of flux as Australian nurses travelled to France for service. Ethel Davidson ably supported Evelyn Conyers as her secretary from July 1916 – February 1917. However, Davidson wanted to get back to war work, so Clarice Dickson (RRC) took over the position of Secretary to the Matron-in-Chief in 1917.[17]After a small stint at 1AAH, Harefield, Ethel Davidson was attached to 2 AGH, Wimereaux and after a month, in March 1917, she was Acting Matron of 2 ACCS, Trois Abres, near Steenwerck. The reality of this location is evident in the following pages and it is not difficult to imagine the workload of Ethel Davidson, aged 45 years. She recalls in her narrative that the first eighteen hours during the Battle of Messines saw 2,800 patients admitted and four hospital trains with five hundred in each went out. In July 1917 she was sent to 38 BSH Calais before being transferred to Italy, where she established the Genoa Hospital Corso Torino. She was in-charge of thirty-five Australian Sisters and five English VADs with RAMC officers caring for Tommies but after the Armistice they had 250 Austrians admitted. She was acting matron until her rank was confirmed in January 1918. For her service at this time she was MID and RRC. It was on 3 June 1919 she was appointed CBE in the King's Birthday Honours, making her one of the most highly decorated nurses of the war.

After the Armistice Matron Davidson returned to England and was appointed matron of 2AAH, Southall until she RTA and was demobilized at 4 MD on 5 December 1919. She did not rest for long and was appointed matron of the Military Hospital in Keswick, Adelaide where she remained until her retirement in 1933. She was also President of the Returned Army Nurses' Association of South Australia (1922-26). Ethel Davidson died on 21 April 1939, after three months' illness, at her home. The people of Adelaide mourned her passing and she was described in as *...a woman of outstanding character.*[18]

2 ACCS: Trois Arbres, France

It is difficult to convey the reality of war. Impossible to imagine the strain on nurses who could hear the explosions, feel the earth rumble under their feet as they faced soldier after soldier with horrific wounds. Nurses setting up operating theatres in tents while trying to observe aseptic techniques amongst the mud. During June, July and August 1917 the staff treated 16,357 cases, including 1,077 gassed soldiers.

It is easy to think of a CCS as being a relatively small group of canvas tents making it easy to manage casualties arriving straight from the battleground. In fact, 2ACCS had operating theatres, x-ray facilities, mortuary and wards. Connection of these marquee style tents was via duckboards which were often inundated with mud making transfer of patients hazardous. However, importantly, 2 ACCS was located not too distant from a railway line and only five miles from the front line. The railway made it a target to some extent but usually it was safe from attack because it was a clearly marked health facility. The staff of 2 ACCS were used to stress and pressure when we consider that within ten hours of opening, the staff dealt with 900 casualties. The unit was well established at Trois Arbres near Armentières where staff cared for the casualties from the Battle of Fromelles (June 1916) and a year later supported the Second Army at Messines (June 1917).[19]

2 ACCS: Trois Arbres near Armentières: 22 July 1917

Dorothy Cawood, Mary Jane Derrer, Clare Deacon and Alice Ross-King had all trained at different Australian hospitals. Sisters Cawood, Deacon and Ross-King embarked on the *Kyarra* in 1914 and Staff Nurse Derrer was a 1915 *Orsova* reinforcement. Alice Ross-King, who was attached to 1 AGH since her enlistment, was on loan to 10 SH (St Omer) and from there was sent to 2 ACCS (Trois Arbres) the following month. The other three nurses were primarily attached to 2 AGH.

During the evening of 22 July 1917 Sister Alice Ross-King was on duty, walking along the duckboards, when two bombs hit ACCS at about 10.30 pm. One fell at the back of ward C.5 which Ross-King referred to as *...Gilmore's tent - which was 3 marquees joined together, with about 46 stretchers in it.* Lt Col J Ramsay Webb reported that it left *...a hole in the ground about 15ft in diameter and 6ft deep in the centre.* When the explosion hit, Ross-King raced ahead and the next thing she knew she was in the crater and had to scramble out on hands and feet through clay and blood. Sister Clare Deacon was off duty when the bombs fell but she along with Staff Nurse Mary Jane Derrer and Sister Dorothy Cawood rushed to the ward to help patients escape the burning ward. Ramsay Webb describes the damage in the 2ACCS unit diary, recording that Ward C5 was made up of *...4 small hospital marquees arranged in a square. Of these one was completely destroyed and the three others rendered unfit for service. Some equipment was destroyed. The mortuary is also wrecked, the roof and two sides being blown out.* Ross-King shouted for help but *...could hear nothing for the roar of planes ...I seemed to be the only living thing about.* Nonetheless she soon realized her patients were in peril and she joined her colleagues as they entered burning tents to save their patients. *The second bomb dropped outside the southern boundary of the Camp near the Cemetery.* The death toll was two patients and two orderlies killed with fifteen of the already traumatized soldiers, once again wounded. Unfortunately, the 3rd Battle of Ypres (20 Sep - 10 Nov 1917) saw more bombing of CCS as the front line became less defined.[20] These four remarkable nurses were awarded the Military Medal for *......great coolness and devotion to duty.* They were the first AANS nurses to be given such a distinction.

Alice Ross-King (MM, ARRC, MID, FNM): Origins

Alys King (1887-1968) was born in Ballarat, the daughter of Archibald Ross King, a storekeeper, and his wife Henrietta. Alys used the more common spelling Alice from an early age. The family moved to Perth but tragedy struck when her father and two brothers drowned in the Swan River. Henrietta and her daughter returned to Melbourne, where Alice was educated. Alice Ross trained at The Alfred and eventually became acting matron before taking charge of a private hospital in Collins Street. She remained a competent theatre sister.

Despite her outstanding civilian experience, she joined the AANS as a Staff Nurse and hyphenated her name to Ross-King to differentiate herself from another nurse with the same name. She left Australia in November 1914 and served at 1 AGH but was soon transferred to work in Suez at an evacuated orphanage which was now operating as a clearing station. In late 1915 she was detailed for transport duty back to Australia but returned to her unit and served with 1AGH from April 1916 to January 1919 at Rouen. A month after being awarded the Military Medal she received the ribbon the following month from General Sir William Birdwood. By December of that same year she was MID and the following May (1918) she was awarded the ARRC. After the war, on her return voyage to Australia in January 1919 she met a Sydney doctor, Theodore Appleford, who in time became her husband. Alice Appleford returned to full-time duty training VADs in 1942 when Australia was under threat from a Japanese invasion. She achieved the rank of major in the Royal Australian Army Nursing Corps (RAANC) and was appointed Senior Assistant Controller for Victoria. In 1949 she was awarded the Florence Nightingale Medal by the International Red Cross for her work during the Second World War, which included extensive support of women. On 17 August 1968 Alice Appleford died at Cronulla, NSW, and was buried at Fawkner Cemetery, Melbourne. She was survived by her four children but her husband had predeceased her by ten years. The Alice Appleford Memorial Award is presented annually to an outstanding member of the RAANC. This award serves to perpetuate her memory and recognises the significant contribution she made to nursing generally and military nursing in particular.[21]

Dorothy Cawood (MM, MID): Origins

Dorothy Cawood was born on 9 December 1884 in Parramatta (NSW) and trained at the Coast Hospital, 1909-13.[2] She was a 2AGH original who embarked on the *Kyarra,* serving in Egypt and was promoted to AANS Sister in December 1915. Dorothy served on various transport ships until she was sent to France and resumed service with 2 AGH at Wimereux.

After her service with 2 ACCS where she was awarded the Military Medal, she served at 38 SH in France and was MID. She was transferred with her unit to Genoa, Italy in November 1917, 38 SH was under the matronship of Ethel Davidson. Agnes Cullen and Dorothy Cawood were two of the twenty-seven nurses, collected from Abbeville Nurses' Home and transferred to Genoa on the No 21 Ambulance Train. Cullen found the scenery beautiful but aspects wanting, including sufficient provision of food for the journey.

On arrival in Genoa 38 SH took over Cristoforo Colombo Boys School and Matron Davidson soon had an excellent 520 bed hospital in operation. The 11 GH was set up in the Miramare Hotel and included twelve beds for sick nurses. Cawood was admitted to 11 GH for a week in early 1918 suffering from tonsillitis. Ethel Davidson wrote a reassuring letter to her mother detailing the mildness of her illness and mentioning her daughter is *...a most excellent nurse- one of the very best Australia has sent out.* Dorothy recovered and returned to 38 SH but did manage a months' leave in the UK August 1918. She returned to 38SH a few months before the cessation of hostilities on 11 November 1918. After the war she waited for transport home while caring for sick and wounded soldiers, many suffering from influenza. Dorothy had seven days leave in Rome in January 1919 before returning to England. On arrival she served at 3 AAH (Dartford) and 2 AAH (Southall); she RTA in July 1919 aboard HMHS *Soudan* and was discharged in September.

Like most military nurses, Dorothy had no time to rest because she had to earn a living in the midst of a pandemic in Australia. She worked at the State Hospital in Liverpool, NSW but it was the David Berry Hospital in Berry on the south coast of

NSW where she cemented her civilian career, as a matron from 1928-43. In 1944 she retired to her old family home in Parramatta where she remained until her death on 16 February 1962.[22]

Clare Deacon (MM): Origins

Clare Deacon was born in Tasmania on 13 March 1890. Her parents, William and Ellen, had five children but Clare lived with her aunt and uncle in Burnie for a number of years before training at Hobart Hospital. She enlisted with the AIF on 13 November 1914 and travelled on the *Kyarra* with Dorothy Cawood as part of 2 AGH but was allotted to 1 AGH in Egypt. Promoted to AANS sister in December 1915 she was transferred to England in mid 1916 where she served at 3 AAH before being reunited with 2 AGH in France. On 1 February 1917 she nursed in France when in June she was transferred to 2 ACCS. A month later, when the bombs hit Ward C 5 (Gilmore's tent), Deacon was off duty but she immediately raced into the burning marquee to save her patients. On 26 August 1917 Sister Clare Deacon MM returned to 2 AGH at Wimereux and was sent to UK for leave. It was during this leave she reputedly received the MM from King George V at Buckingham Palace.

She returned to 2 AGH until January 1918 when she was sent to Croydon War Hospital and later 2 AAH. From there she RTA working on HMAT *Osterley* in April 1918 and was discharged soon afterwards. Clare continued to nurse and married James (Jock) McGregor, a dentist, in 1922. They settled in Crows Nest near Sydney and did not have children. Jock Died in 1941 and Clare died suddenly from meningitis on 7 August 1952 at home.[23]

Mary Jane Derrer (MM): Origins

Mary Jane Derrer was a Queenslander born at Mackay on 3 February 1892. She qualified as a nurse from Mackay Base Hospital in the year the war commenced and worked as a sister at the local Lister Private Hospital before joining the AANS in early 1915. She is often referred to as Mary-Jane but her signature clearly shows a non-hyphenated spelling. Mary Jane is also referred to as a Staff Nurse but she was promoted to Sister prior to her second tour of duty on 25 September 1918. She sailed on the *Orsova* arriving in Egypt and attached 2 AGH serving at Mena Convalescent Depot.[24]

Seven months later she was on her way to France, disembarking at Boulogne for duty with 2 AGH at Marseilles and later 14 SH, Wimereux. She served in France from June 1916 until December 1916 when she was sent to 2 ACCS. Compared to the other three nurses, she was young and had relatively little military nursing experience. However, she was the only Staff Nurse of the four nurses who were awarded the MM on the night of the 22 July 1917 but Mary Jane had the most experience at 2 ACCS. Six months in this ACCS was harrowing for a young woman in her twenties who had been away from her original unit for seven months at the time of the bombing.

After the bombing she also had 'special leave' to England from 18 August to 1 September, where she most likely received her MM from King George V at Buckingham Palace. When she went to return to her unit in France the 'authorities' decided she was unfit for further service. No information or medical record was filed with her service record but she was allowed to have her name on the register for further service. This was not uncommon for soldiers and nurses who suffered from 'shell-shock' or PTSD. The stigma was removed by not recording the diagnosis. If Mary Jane did have PTSD she recovered quickly. She RTA on HMAT *Beltana* in October 1917, performing nursing duties on the way home and nursing at Kangaroo Point Military Hospital in Brisbane before she re-enlisted for service in India on 9 November 1918. Before Sister Derrer MM disembarked in Bombay (present day Mumbai) the war was over. She served with 34 WGH, 18 BGH and 19 BGH.[25] She remained there for a year after the conclusion of the First World War and was one of a number of Australian nurses who were utilized during the war on the Indian and Afghanistan border, despite the absence of approval to participate from the Australian Government.[26] On 9 November 1919 Sister Derrer RTA from Bombay via Singapore aboard SS Kashgar. After the war she married a widower, Dr Gallagher, who had two children, and they increased the family by another three.

These four ATNA nurses, who trained at different Australian hospitals, came together on one night in France and displayed extraordinary courage during particularly heavy bombardment.[27] They were the first AANS nurses to receive a MM but they were not the last.

25 The Valour Continues at CCS

... served with the British Red Cross Society at Mons and Gallipoli and in Serbia and was awarded the Military Medal... German airmen swooped to the height of 20 feet and fired at her with a machine gun – Westralian

During and after the war a number of Australian nurses went to Buckingham Palace to receive awards and occasionally medals. The Military Medal was awarded to non-commissioned officers for ...*Bravery in the Field*... and to ...*women for devotion to duty under fire*. Seven AANS nurses serving in CCS in France received this award. There were another two Australian nurses who received the MM: Eileen King received the British MM while serving with QAIMNSR and Louise Dorrington, who served with the French Flag Nursing Corp, was awarded two MM, one from France and the other from Serbia.

The Military Cross (MC) was instituted on 31 December 1914 for commissioned officers in the Army ...*in recognition of distinguished and meritorious services in time of war*.[1] Australian nurses were nominally officers from 1916, however, they were not considered to be members of the Army but part of the AAMC. It is interesting to note that Captain (Dr) Hugh Kingsley Ward (1887-1972) was quite correctly awarded the MC in France for continuing to care for his patients after he was wounded. There is little doubt he was a member of the AAMC. Much has changed since 1915, especially for servicewomen, but none has been awarded the MC despite their expanded role in military action.

Rachel Pratt (MM): 1ACCS and 3 AGH

Rachel Pratt was born near Heywood, Victoria, on 18 July 1874. She was over the acceptable age as a trainee when she commenced her training at Ballarat Hospital on

18 January 1909. Therefore, she reduced her age from 35 years to 31 and qualified in August 1912.[2] Her experience at the Royal Women's Hospital in Melbourne was extensive from October 1912 until May 1915, when she embarked for overseas service as part of the staff of 3 AGH. The unit, under the able leadership of Grace Wilson, finally arrived in Egypt and after the war Pratt recorded her nursing experiences on Lemnos.[3] After the evacuation of Gallipoli she stayed with 3 AGH at the Abbassia Army Barracks (December 1915 - September 1916) until they were transferred to France. She was assigned to 1 ACCS and it was here that she was badly wounded by shrapnel when it lodged in her lungs on 4 July 1917. The next day she was promoted to sister AANS and was awarded the Military Medal.

She was hospitalised following the bombing raid and in October 1917 she was transferred to 2 Australian Convalescent Hospital (Weymouth) and later to 1 AAH and 2 AAH before returning to Melbourne in October 1918. She was discharged from the AIF in April the following year. Despite suffering chronic bronchitis from her war injury, she continued to work and in 1927 she went into a partnership - a rest home in East Malvern, Melbourne. The rest home was sold in the mid-1930s and Pratt went to England for a holiday. When she returned she lived in various locales and finally purchased a home where she settled until her death at the Repatriation General Hospital on 23 March 1954. She was cremated with Anglican rites.[4]

3ACCS: July 1917: France

A few months later in October 1917, nurses at 3 ACCS were also under fire and threat. During an air raid on 3 ACCS, when everyone else was running for cover, Sister Alicia Mary Kelly (AANS) was found by a Padre sitting next to a patient holding his hand. When asked why she had not run away she replied that she could not leave her patients. She was awarded the Military Medal by King George V at Buckingham Palace on 16 October 1917. Her award was a popular choice with her colleagues, including May Tilton.[5]

Alicia Mary Kelly (MM, ARRC): Origins

Kelly (1885-1942) was born in Ireland and trained at the Melbourne Hospital. She served with 1 AGH in Egypt and was promoted to sister on 3 April 1917. Sister Kelly had extensive experience in a number of locations in Egypt and Europe as well as on transport duty from August to December 1915 on the *Euripides* during the Gallipoli Campaign. When 1 AGH was transferred to France she served at 29 CCS, Rouen (December 1916 - 31 July 1917) and then at 3 ACCS.

From August 1917 to March 1918 she was attached to 3 AGH and then served another protracted tour of duty on transports (March 1918 - May 1919). On 1 January 1918 she was awarded the ARRC and promoted to sister-in-charge of the transport on her return voyage to Australia after the war.

During the post-war period she married an ex-Light Horseman, Arthur Chipper, and they settled into a farming lifestyle in WA. Mrs Chipper retired from nursing for health reasons and they had no children. However, despite poor health she returned to nursing during the Second World War as matron of the Old Women's Home at Guildford. Alicia Mary Chipper (nee Kelly) died of pneumonia, aged 57 years, and was buried in the Anglican section at Karrakatta Cemetery (WA, Whadjuk Noongar Country).[6]

Elizabeth Pearl Corkhill (MM): 38 BCCS: France: July 1918

Elizabeth (Pearl) Corkhill had a long and remarkable life, of which the four years of war were a relatively small part.[7] Born on 11 March 1887, on the south coast of NSW in the small community of Tilba Tilba (Yuin Country), she was the daughter of William and Frances Corkhill. William, a farmer, was also a remarkable photographer. His collection of photographs of Tilba Tilba's early years are of such quality they are held at the National Library of Australia. Pearl was more than likely acquainted with Narrelle Hobbes (AANS) who was nine years her senior and also grew up in the area.

Pearl Corkhill trained at Burilda Hospital, Summer Hill (NSW, Gadigal Country) and embarked for overseas service with the AANS in 1915. She was attached to 1 AGH but was lent to Choubra Infectious Disease Hospital from August 1915 until

January 1916. Pearl was sent to France with 1 AGH but on arrival was attached to 2BGH at Le Havre for two months before rejoining 1 AGH at Rouen. While in France she served at 1 AGH and occasionally 3 AGH, but it was between June and August 1918 that she saw service at 38 British CCS near Abbeville.

In July 1918 air raids targeted the area but she continued to care for patients without any apparent regard for her own safety and was awarded a MM. In a letter to her mother she reported that she had been awarded the MM because she had been on night duty a few months earlier when a bomb had been dropped on the hospital. She was at a loss as to why she would receive a medal for taking care of her patients under the circumstances.[7]

In the presence of Queen Mary, she was presented with the Military Medal by King George V at Buckingham Palace prior to returning to Australia in 1919 on the *Ceramic.* Pearl shared her concern about the presentation with her mother because her mess dress was worn out and she would have to find the money for a new one. Amidst the chaos and carnage of the Western Front, Pearl embroidered a white linen cloth which can be viewed at the Australian War Memorial.[8] She was certainly able to keep her nerves at bay.

Pearl RTA in March 1919 and was discharged but she continued to nurse in Australia and overseas until 1951. Like many returned nurses, Sister Corkhill continued to nurse war veterans at Randwick Military Hospital and she later became Matron of the Soldiers Limbless Hospital at Vaucluse. Eventually she returned to her childhood home to care for her ageing mother, and took on the position of senior sister at a Bega District Hospital. In 1961 *...Sister Corkhill, as she was always known...* retired to Akolele overlooking Wallaga Lake. She remained active and rode horseback at Cooma Centenary Show when she was 88 years old. Pearl was living independently until just prior to her death aged 99 years.[9]

Eileen King: MM, RRC: QAIMNSR

Amy (b. 1882) and her sister Eileen King (1884-1943) were the daughters of the Queensland Auditor General, T M King. They reputedly trained in England but when war was declared Amy joined the AANS and Eileen joined the QAIMNSR.[1445]

Eileen King served in Egypt, on Lemnos and on transport duty but was in France when she sustained serious wounds from a bomb which directly hit the tented field hospital where she was working. Despite a section of her thigh being seriously damaged she *...managed to get her wounded out of the burning tent. Soldiers who knew her described her as one of the bravest women they had ever met.*

During the war Eileen King was awarded the MM and RRC and her sister, Amy, was MID twice and received the ARRC.[10] Their brother R M King (MLA) was appointed Deputy Premier of Queensland during the Moore Government.[11] After the war, Eileen nursed between Australia and England, but it was during the next world war that she was presumed lost at sea when the *Melbourne Star* was sunk on its return voyage to Australia in 1943.[12]

Louise Dorrington: French Flag Nursing Corps:

One Australian nurse who was given the distinction of being awarded two Military Medals (Serbian and French) was Louise Dorrington. She completed her training at Adelaide Children's Hospital (1897-99) and gained experience at Wakefield Street Private Hospital. She then moved to WA before travelling to England.[13]

The Nursing Profession in France (1870- 1922)

Considering the advancement of Australian nursing by 1914, it is worth reflecting on the situation in France. The French Third Republic (1870-1940) had abandoned the Catholic model of nursing. In 1901 many Catholic Nursing Sisters, who worked in the civilian and military sector were dismissed. Within the military sector, they were replaced by unqualified and unsuitable orderlies and it soon became apparent to the public that the quality of nursing was poor. In 1907 qualified female nurses were able to serve within the military but the numbers were low due to the lack of civilian training programs. There were only forty nurses recruited in 1908.

Dr Anna Hamilton established a Protestant training school in Bordeaux along the lines of Nightingale's scientific method. Unfortunately, there were only eight such schools when war erupted on their homeland, so the French were ill-equipped to deal with the mass casualties emanating from the Battle of the Frontiers. In August

1914, in one day, they lost 27,000 men. The French Red Cross had a presence but provided volunteers, not qualified nurses.

Grace Ellison was a wealthy Scots journalist who was living in France in 1914. She saw the shocking situation and suggested to the head of the French Army Medical Corps that *...three hundred British nurses ...*be recruited. However, those who volunteered for the FFNC were not qualified so she asked Mrs Bedford Fenwick for advice. Fenwick was a proponent of nurse registration in Britain and the editor of the British Journal of Nursing so she had sufficient influence to decree that only trained nurses could join the FFNC.

Members of the FFNC were not volunteers but professional paid nurses with a six monthly renewable contract. They were paid £40 with board. Lodging and travel were paid by the French Government, which suggests that the British paid the salary and the FFNC was referred to as a British unit. The British War Office was annoyed that Fenwick was directing their nurses to another military unit, even if it was allied. On 24 October 1914 only eight nurses were recruited and the following month another sixteen joined. Levels peaked by April 1915 with 108 trained nurses, but the numbers dwindled as the war continued and there were only 48 remaining in November 1918. Louise was not one of the remaining 48 as she had by this time joined the American Red Cross.

When war was declared Louise Dorrington was working at the Middlesex Hospital, but when her offer to join the AANS was declined she joined a British unit, the FFNC. Her sister Amy was also ATNA qualified and joined the AANS. Amy Dorrington saw service in France but it is not clear if their paths crossed.

Role of FFNC in France

The FFNC were stationed at seventeen different sites throughout France but it was at the St Union Hospital in Bergues where the biggest trial occurred. A typhoid epidemic resulted in the nurses providing support to civilians and refugees as well as the soldiers. This endeared the Corps to the French people and its reputation grew. During a particularly harsh bombardment when a hospital was destroyed *...forcing patients and nurses to shelter in caves underneath...* the nurses displayed courage and compassion. Louise is likely to have been the only Australian but Canadian and New Zealand nurses enlisted, some of whom sadly died during their service.

Interestingly the success of the FFNC was considered to be down to the *...Scots, Irish and Colonial Nurses ...* rather than those from the London teaching hospitals. The reasons for this are not known but Ellison wrote *...The most successful of our nurses have been those who have the patience of Job, wrapped up in a keen sense of humour*. That may explain it.

Louise Dorrington: American Red Cross

Louise Dorrington later joined the American Red Cross and saw extensive service in Europe including Poland, during the Bolshevik uprising, and Czechoslovakia as well as France. She worked in the field of child welfare after the war, in England and South Australia. Details regarding Louise Dorrington's service in both the FFNC and the American Red Cross are scant as she was an Australian nurse doing war work within foreign units. It must have been a somewhat isolating war for Louise in many ways, although there is little doubt she would have met up with many Australian nurses during her service.[14]

Nurse Morrison: Unidentified MM

The service record of Maud Morrison (AANS) includes a cable which relates to a report of the death of Nurse Morrison at a nurses' hostel in London from influenza on 23 October 1918. Maud Morrison did contract influenza in England but it was in February 1919 and she recovered.[15] Christina Morrison (AANS) who was in England in May 1919 following two years of service in India also contracted the disease but she too recovered.[16]

The *West Australian* newspaper reported on 11 December 1918 an incident which occurred on 6 October 1918 where *...one of the latest sufferers from the brutality of Hun airmen is Nurse Morrison, formerly of the Adelaide Hospital who served with the British Red Cross Society at Mons and Gallipoli and in Serbia and was awarded the Military Medal. While she was crossing between two wings in a hospital in France, German airmen swooped* *to the height of 20 feet and fired at her with a machine gun, wounding her three times in the arm. Nurse Morrison is now convalescent.*[17] Nurse Morrison did not train at the Adelaide Hospital but she may have been a VAD, making her historical footprint even more difficult to uncover.[18] The *Daily Mail* reported her death a few months later from pneumonia, but there is no reference to her in the Commemorative Roll nor is there any mention of another Australian nurse being awarded the Military Medal. Her identity remains a mystery but her bravery cannot be doubted.

26 Nursing the Australian Light Horsemen in Egypt 1916-1919

Had the Transcaspian troops possessed one quarter of the pluck of these nurses… observed one British officer sourly…*then it would have been a fine army- Peter Hopkirk*

News from the front in mid 1916 included the Battle of the Somme on land; the Battle of Jutland on sea and the death of Field Marshal Horatio Kitchener (Earl) when his transport, the cruiser HMS *Hampshire*, struck a German mine and sank off the Scottish Orkney islands. Kitchener was on route to meet with the Russian Tsar. Although publicly mourned, his death on 5 June 1916 was considered by some to be a relief, as he failed to ensure effective communication between the Cabinet and Army leaders. After Kitchener's death, the wartime finance minister, David Lloyd George, was appointed War Minister in the Asquith Government. However, there was continued mutual suspicion between the Cabinet and the BEF leaders as Lloyd George continued to push for a concentration of troops in Salonika. Kitchener was popular and believed in a volunteer army but after his death the government pushed through conscription. The Easter Uprising and the death rate on the Somme resulted in the formation of a Coalition Government in July 1916. Finally, in December 1916 Herbert Henry Asquith resigned and David Lloyd George became the Prime Minister of Britain in December 1916, remaining in the position until 1922. Asquith continued as the Leader of the Liberal Party but failed to support his successor at every turn.[1]

AANS Leadership Review and Changes: 1915-1919

In 1915 Major General Richard Fetherston, Director-General of the AAMC, was commissioned to investigate the controversy at 1 AGH between Bell and Ramsay Smith. Following the investigation, one of Fetherston's recommendations was the creation of a number of leadership positions within the AANS, with a view to improving the overall management and ultimately the conditions for the nurses.[2] He was so impressed by the quality of the nursing care delivered on Lemnos that he offered the position of Principal Matron of AIF, Cairo, to Matron Wilson.[3] Wilson refused the offer because she did not want to leave her nurses, who were enduring such trying conditions on Lemnos.[4] Following her refusal Fetherston appointed Miss Evelyn Conyers as Principal Matron, AANS, Egypt. Despite a limited number of AANS personnel in England at this time, Fetherston also appointed Acting Principal Matron Jessie McHardy White to the position of Principal Matron, AANS, England.

Appointments Confirmed 1916

An over-arching position, Matron-in-Chief, was established and was responsible to the DMS. Furthermore, a number of 'principal matron' positions were created. In April 1916 Australian soldiers were transferred to France, so AIF HQ was established at Horseferry Road, London. It was at this time the first Matron-in-Chief of the AANS, Miss Evelyn Conyers, was officially appointed. She was answerable to the DMS and had responsibility for the AANS in England, France and Egypt. The following month, Miss Ethel (Tracey) Richardson was appointed the Matron-in-Chief of the AANS in Australia and was responsible for AANS nurses in Australia, on hospital ships and travelling on sea transports. She was located in Melbourne as part of the staff of the D-G.[5] After the appointment of Evelyn Conyers it would appear Jessie McHardy White was no longer required at AIF HQ. She was returned to Australia on HMAT *Marathon* for 'retirement', with her discharge from the AANS, 3 MD, dated 24 September 1916.

Personal letters and postcards of AANS are littered with references to their leaders, positive and negative. However, it cannot be overstated that the choice for the two Matron-in-Chief positions attracted a great deal of controversy within the ranks. It is also true that some leaders accept the challenge and grow into the position: Evelyn Conyers was such a leader.

Matrons-in-Chief

One of the more significant accomplishments of Hester Maclean and Nellie Gould was their ability to facilitate the transfer of the experiences and competencies of the civilian-trained nurse to the military sphere. A number of excellent nurse leaders developed administrative, management and leadership skills during the war including Mabel Thurston (who became the NZANS British-based Matron-in-Chief) and Maclean (who remained the New Zealand-based Matron-in-Chief).[6] Ironically, in 1916, when it was finally decided to appoint a Matron-in-Chief as the most senior nurse in the AANS, it was New Zealand-born Evelyn Conyers who was selected for the position.

AANS Matron-in-Chief: Evelyn Conyers

When Conyers was officially appointed Matron-in-Chief on 12 January 1916, Olive Haynes (AANS) was at 2 AGH (Mena House) and was disheartened because *...Nobody seems to do much but growl. Think they're overworked or something. It seems the lectures have stopped and Miss Conyers is Matron-in-Chief.*[7]

The experiences of Conyers in Egypt enabled her to make decisions based on the practical needs of the nurses but she was a stickler for discipline; many leaders were of the view that adherence to rules and regulations would promote the professionalism of the AANS. In Egypt she gained valuable experience as an operating theatre sister, night superintendent and as Acting Matron of 1 AAH (Luna Park, Cairo). The climatic conditions were extreme and *...the thermometer hanging in the ambulance registered 117 degrees. It was the first time in Egypt's history, I think, that white women had worked through the heat of the day. But there was no time for nurses to take the usual siesta between noon and 4.00 pm.*[8]

Prior to leaving Egypt and before her appointment, Miss Conyers enjoyed a meal with some colleagues on 28 December 1915. Sister Alice Kitchen, who a few months previously had been on duty on the *Gascon* during the Lone Pine offensive and had come to the conclusion that *...this is a dreadful war. More like wholesale murder...* was also present.[9] She had a moment to put the immediate horror behind her and enjoy *...dinner at the Continental with Col. Springthorpe, Major Hurley, Major Simmons and Sister Conyers. We had a little coffee cup as souvenir to be produced at the return dinner when "we shall all meet again at home".*[10] They all had much to endure before their reunion dinner.

Evelyn Conyers was based in Horseferry Road, London, and the Australian position was given to Ethel Tracy Richardson who was based in Melbourne. To complete the intercultural mix of First World War nurse leaders, the most senior nurse of the British Expeditionary Force was Australian-born Maud McCarthy.

The appointment of leaders at this level was not without controversy. Conyers was a respected civilian nurse but she held a comparatively junior rank within the AANS when she was appointed the first Matron-in-Chief. During the 1890s, Evelyn Conyers migrated to Australia and commenced her training at the Melbourne and Children's Hospitals in Victoria. Once qualified she gained leadership experience as a matron and was a founding member of the RVTNA in 1903. She was an original member of 3MD and held the rank of 'sister' when she sailed with the first contingent in 1914.[11.]

The rationale for not appointing Nellie Gould to the Matron-in-Chief position is not clear, but her age and declining health may have been contributing factors; she was 10 years Conyers' senior. Given Gould's experience in the NSWANSR and the AANS, she may have had a reasonable expectation that she would be appointed and there is evidence that she was interested in taking up the position, but there is also evidence that she was not politically astute or universally liked.[12]

Greece and Salonika

Despite Greece allowing the islands of Lemnos and Mudros to be used during the Gallipoli campaign for the establishment of 3 AGH and troop transfers it was not officially an ally. Greece and Serbia had a treaty to become allies in the event of Serbia being invaded by Austria. However, Greece was reluctant to honour the treaty, given that Serbia was also being invaded by Germany and Bulgaria, which created an enormous risk to the Greek people. However, when the Serbs retreated to Greece they were not repulsed. The Premier, Venizelos, convinced his King that if the allies provided 150,000 men Greece should honour its pledge to Serbia. The King eventually agreed to allow predominantly British and French troops to operate from Greece.[13]

The Australian Light Horse: The Middle East: 1916-1918

Australian soldiers were not involved in the Salonika campaign but they were about to make history in Egypt as they moved towards Beersheba. One of the most efficient military campaigns in history occurred in Palestine in 1918 when Allenby successfully achieved a triple dislocation of the Turkish Army.[14] In short: *...to cut an army's lines of communication is to dislocate its physical organization. To close its lines of retreat is to dislocate its morale. And to destroy its lines of 'inter-communication' – by which orders and reports pass – is to dislocate it mentally, by breaking the essential connection between the brain and the body of the army.* It is also recognised that the battles of 1917 contributed to the success of the final conclusion in September 1918.[15] The jewel in the campaign's crown was Jerusalem.

Harry Chauvel: Military Experience

Like Nellie Gould, Harry Chauvel saw service in the South African Campaign. He was part of the Queensland Mounted Infantry and later a commander of a composite force of Queensland, British, Canadian and South African horsemen. This period was an important grounding for Chauvel, who later led the Desert Mounted Corps consisting of Australians, New Zealanders, British Yeomanry and Indian Cavalry.[16] Harry Chauvel was on his way to London to *...act as Australia's representative on the Imperial General Staff at the War Office...*and on arrival, he requested deployment to France. His fate was sealed when he inspected Salisbury Plain while in England and recommended the Australian and New Zealand contingent go to Egypt to train, as the conditions in England were far from satisfactory. He was later informed that he was to command the mounted force of an Australian division of infantry and a Lighthorse Brigade. He met up with his soldiers in Egypt following the evacuation of Gallipoli in December 1915.[17]

Rose Creal: Principal Matron of 2MD

Rose Creal was a founding member of ATNA (1902) and became Principal Matron of NSW (2 MD) in October 1915, replacing Gould who had left for overseas service the previous year.[18]This position was an adjunct to her main duties as matron of SHSEH which, like all civilian hospitals at the time, was feeling the effects of nursing staff shortages.[19] PM Creal, AANS, was responsible for interviewing nurses prior to their embarkation. She was acutely aware that many of her trainee nurses would ultimately end up being part of the AANS and their first post-graduate experience would be in a war zone. When Rose Creal left Australia she was entrusted with establishing 14 AGH in Egypt in readiness for Harry Chauvel's casualties.

Rose Creal and Harry Chauvel Biographies

When the First World War was declared Harry Chauvel and Rose Creal were decidedly middle-aged. They were born in the same year, 1865, in NSW but their early years were quite different. Chauvel, the grandson of a retired Indian Army officer, grew up with a love of horses on the family cattle station near the Clarence River in Northern NSW. In his early life he enjoyed being the amateur jockey at race meetings but eventually settled on a military career. Chauvel, who attended school at Toowoomba and Sydney Grammar, was not known as a scholar but he was a keen reader of military history. Chauvel was a quiet, some have suggested shy man, who *...won favour with the men of Anzac by his quality as a soldier.*[20]

Rose Creal won favour with the military officers, her nurses and the soldiers for her competence and empathy: two extremely positive attributes for any nurse leader. The early life of Rose Creal was harsh but typical of those living in the gold mining districts of Australia. Rose had the good fortune to train at the SHSEH under the guidance of two outstanding nurse leaders, Matrons McKay (1885-91) and Gould, but it was the latter who had the most significant influence on her life.[21] Within two years of completing her training Rose Creal was appointed Gould's deputy matron. This may, in part, explain why Creal also developed a keen interest in military nursing. When Gould resigned in 1898, Creal became acting matron and her appointment was confirmed in February the following year. Therefore, within eight years of commencing her training she was matron of one of the most prestigious hospitals in Australia.

Rose was thirty-four years old when she was appointed matron, the same age as her mother at the time of death during childbirth. They had vastly different lives due to the developing professionalism of nursing and the autonomy it gave women like Rose.[22] Before her brilliant career as an author took off, Stella Miles Franklin worked as a probationer at SHSEH during Rose Creal's matronship and left an excellent analysis of the character of Matron Creal.[23]

Leadership of Chauvel and Creal

At a character level Creal and Chauvel were similar. They were absolutely committed to the health and welfare of their nurses and soldiers respectively. To a point they were disciplinarians but never bullies. To his great credit Chauvel has been described as *...a man of infinite patience ... he was never in a hurry to win expensively today that which could be won cheaply tomorrow*. Although he was criticised for caution, the results speak for themselves as he and his horsemen took vast swathes of land with battle casualties described as *...trifling*.[24]

At an administrative level, Creal had the double task of keeping the two Australian Matrons-in-Chief, Tracey Ethel Richardson in Melbourne and Evelyn Conyers in London, fully informed. She was also responsible for chaperoning white Christian women in a religiously diverse country as they cared for thousands of men.[25] Rose Creal was a pragmatist; she had seen enough of life to know rules and regulations are important but not at the cost of personal humanity. Privately, Creal found solace in her *...little puppy dog...* which slept on the end of her bed.[26]

Principal Matron Rose Creal: 14 AGH Abbassia, Cairo: 1916-1919

Rose Creal officially joined the AIF in 1916 during the nurse leadership flux. She signed her attestation papers on 14 August 1916 and within five days embarked on the *Karoola* in Melbourne. She was assigned to the position of matron of 14 AGH before she left Australia.[27] On 21 September 1916 she, accompanied by nine sisters and twenty-one staff nurses, arrived at the Egyptian Army Barracks to take over from 3 AGH. Matron Creal had been led to understand that when 3 AGH vacated the building all the equipment would remain, but instead, she arrived to find the staff packing it up. The Red Cross Society came to the rescue and provided quilts, screen covers, pillow slips, extra sheets and pyjamas etc.[28]

The 14 AGH was located at Abbassia, a suburb on the outskirts of Cairo, for the duration of the war with an annex established at Port Said in 1918. The building structure of the barracks was suitable as a large military hospital because it had originally been commissioned by Napoleon Bonaparte and was erected during his occupation of Egypt from 1798 – 1799.[29]

The design had its limitations with no gas or water supply in the wards. Ironically, a hot water service was available in a number of the rooms but not the wards. The wards were spacious, well-ventilated and clean, but the lack of water made the ablutions of a busy surgical ward very difficult. The downstairs wards had asphalt floors which were easily broken and a shortage of basic equipment such as ward linen, surgical appliances and instruments made life burdensome for the nurses.

Rose Creal was known as a relentless worker who had equally high expectations of her nurses. Nonetheless, she took care of their needs and was sometimes referred to as Ma(tron) Creal. The sisters' quarters were situated opposite the hospital and consisted of three buildings: One was used as an officers' mess, while the second was set apart for the night staff. The day staff took the main building, which had a beautiful old garden attached. The rooms were comfortable and staff nurse Bessie Annie Taylor, who later served in France, proved herself to be a very capable Home Sister who was responsible for taking care of the nurses.[30] The Home Sister position was introduced at SHSEH when the Nightingale Wing (nurses' home) was first established. Catering for the nurses' meals was undertaken by contract and cost each nurse 3/- per day, which was sixpence a day more than the allowance. It was not uncommon for the nurses to be out-of-pocket, no matter where they were stationed.

Casualties & Staffing Levels

On arrival at the Egyptian Army Barracks Rose Creal found the staff levels grossly inadequate for the proposed 1,040 bed hospital. Grace Wilson (matron 3 AGH) allowed one sister and twelve staff nurses to remain with Creal's unit as a temporary measure because the 200-300 hundred patients had increased to 600. The burden on the staff was substantial. Eventually, on 24 November 1916 an additional three sisters and eleven staff nurses arrived from England.[31]

Kaiser-i-Hind reinforcements

Further reinforcements were slow in arriving compared to the speed of admissions. Jessie Tomlins and Dora Mearns were two of sixty AANS nurses who responded to a specific request of the British Government in July 1916. There were no hospital ships available at the time so the nurses were sent to Egypt as first-class passengers on the mail ship *Kaiser-i-Hind* (Empress of India) departing Sydney on 9 December 1916.[32] On 10 January 1917 the nurses arrived in Alexandria, where Jessie, who trained at SHSEH, caught a train with her colleagues to Cairo. The nurses were a welcome sight for Matron Creal who was waiting at the station.[33] Jessie Tomlins was exactly where she wanted to be —with her old matron and close to her two brothers, Fred and Will, who were Light Horsemen.[34]

It has been claimed that some 250 members of the AANS worked at 14 AGH, but it is likely that these figures include those nurses passing through Egypt while awaiting further transport duty.[35] Bed numbers of 14 AGH oscillated in response to the movement of troops as they moved through the desert.

Battle of Romani: 3-4 August 1916

Before Rose Creal arrived in Egypt, Chauvel had made a name for himself as a remarkable tactician. The competence of the Ottomans in the desert was clear when they attacked outposts near Ogharantia and Katia in June 1916. Chauvel quickly realized access to water was paramount for any success in the desert. The Battle of Romani (3-4 August 1916) was one of the more significant for Chauvel as the Official Historian claims ...*the simple truth is that, so far as leadership went, Chauvel won Romani single-handed.* Chauvel set up defence posts and protected wells around Romani to ensure the Australian, New Zealand and British soldiers maintained a reasonable water supply.[36]

Rania MacPhillamy & Ronnie MacDonald

As the allied troops moved toward Katia and El Arish, Ronnie MacDonald had been ...*too miserable knowing the suffering*...his sexual indiscretion had caused his fiancée Rania MacPhillamy. However, after the success of Romani she sent a birthday gift of tobacco and a cable to him. He reached for the chance of reconciliation and wrote to his *...dear broadminded little girl...* with new enthusiasm and optimism for their future. Accompanied by his mate, George Edwards, in the advance party, Lieutenant Ronnie MacDonald was shot in the head by a sniper. The next day George Edwards returned to bury his friend and he sent Ronnie's spurs and badges to Rania.[37]

On 8 August 1916 Rania and Ronnie's future was over. They were not alone. In total the enemy casualties at the close of 5 August were estimated at 5,250: 1,250 dead and 4,000 wounded. Another 3,900 men were taken prisoner.[38]The Australian and allied losses were 1,130 with only a few men being taken prisoner.[39] The impact of those losses on those at home was incalculable.

Taking Gaza in three Battles: 26-27 March 1917

Initially, the tactical change from a defensive position to an offensive one centred on securing Gaza. British Commander-in-Chief, General Sir A J Murray, and the British Eastern Force commander, General Dobell, failed to appreciate the complexity of desert warfare during the two initial battles. At a military level the first Battle of Gaza, 26-27 March 1917, was a missed opportunity and the second on 19 April 1917 was an unmitigated failure. During the First Battle of Gaza, when victory was within reach General Dobell, *...decided to postpone the offensive without giving a day for the resumption.*[40]

Second Battle of Gaza: 19 April 1917

The enemy forces were well prepared for the second offensive and General Dobell ordered the troops to make another frontal assault. The cost, for no gain, was outrageous with 6500 allied casualties and 2,000 enemy casualties. Rose Creal's nurses saw the results in the wards and noted the soldiers fared much worse after the second battle.[41]

Adele Brennan's war was centred on caring for the veterans of the European battles in England. She remained at the 5 Northern General Hospital, Leicester for two years and during that time undertook rudimentary training as a VAD. The hospital reached a bed capacity of 1,870 with only 218 trained and 163 untrained staff so she and her colleagues were never short of work. She was a woman with an open and interesting face who appeared proud to be wearing her VAD uniform.[42] Her brother William and his regiment were still in Palestine and during the Second Battle of Gaza he was promoted to Lieutenant. On that same day, 19 April 1917, he was shot in the chest and head. He died the next day.[43] Adele continued to work tirelessly until the end of the following year, with the Armistice signed, she died on 24 November 1918 from *...septic pericarditis following influenza.*[44] Peace eluded the Brennan family when their heartbreak doubled.[45]

Third Battle of Gaza: The Battle of Beersheba: October 1917

The soldiers, including Chauvel's Anzac Mounted Division, lost confidence in Murray and Dobell. The British government saw a need to replace the leadership of the Palestine Campaign. This time they chose well. They were respectively replaced by General Sir E H Allenby and General Chetwode. A plan was devised to establish troops around Gaza via Beersheba.[47] The third Battle of Gaza, also known as the Battle of Beersheba, commenced in October 1917 and was a resounding success for the allies and Chauvel's light horsemen in particular.[47] The Battle of Beersheba was a strategic and morale-boosting turning point for the allies and was due, to a large measure, to the firm and fair leadership of Allenby.[48] One of the wounded was Will Tomlins who, fortunately, found himself at 14 AGH under the care of his sister, Jessie, where he made a complete recovery.[49]

Port Said Annex of 14 AGH: 1918

Australian Matron Jessie Ross Gemmell had been en route to Salonika with the fourth Australian contingent, when she was instructed to take charge of 31 BGH, located at the Suez Canal Company Workshop during the Battle of Beersheba. [1192] Success at Beersheba saw the troops move quickly through Palestine and the Sinai and the 14 AGH needed to be closer to the ever-changing front line. In late 1917 and early 1918, Rose Creal was to take over 31 BGH and make it an annex to 14 AGH. She had to mothball a major hospital in Cairo and establish another 120 miles (200km) away. The troops were transported by boat, when possible, to Alexandria making the transfer more comfortable.[50]

The nurses found 1918 in Port Said more difficult and many suffered from influenza and other contagious diseases. Rose Creal was also responsible for the nurses who were coming back from Salonika in a very poor state of health. She requested seven additional nurses, taking her complement from ninety-three to one hundred in October 1918.[51] The request was refused and 14 AGH admitted more than 10,000 medical cases and 2,800 surgical cases during 1918.[52] The surgical cases were mainly the result of battle wounds while the medical cases included malaria, dysentery and influenza.[53]

Concluding the Campaign

By 20 September 1918 Chauvel and his men had pressed on to Megiddo to establish advanced Corps HQ. Like Monash in France, he was meticulous in his planning and once the plan was in place there was nothing for it but to wait. The Official Historian, while referring to Chauvel, claims that *...through the long advance, which was to be carried up to Aleppo, nearly 400 miles away, his complete calm, his old-fashioned courtesy to all ranks, and the quiet, even almost languid, tone in which his rapid decisions were expressed in orders, gave his staff and his fighting commanders a steadying touch of inestimable value ...Every leader felt the serene and unpretentious little man at Corps Headquarters, who had led the mounted work unbrokenly from the Canal, was an organiser of victory.*[54]

Charlotte (Chassie) Berrie: 8 January 1919

As the Australian and allied troops moved through Palestine and pressed forward to Megiddo, Chassie Berrie kept working. Unlike her training hospital and *Mooltan* (May 1915) colleague, Agnes Corfield, who died early in the war, she remained on loan to QAIMNSR for the entire war. By the time the Armistice was declared she was in the forward area of Belah, and three months after the peace she was transferred to an American hospital where she died. It had been a long and hard war in the desert for the young woman and it ended with a quick death from influenza. On 8 January 1919, aged 32, she died in the holiest of cities, Jerusalem.[55]

She was buried far from her native Queensland at the British War Cemetery (then in Palestine, now in Israel) which *...stands on the northern end of the Mount of Olives, to the east of Mount Scorpus ... the Garden of Gethsemane is only a little way from it in the hollow, and from the cemetery you can see the site of Cavalry. There are 2,180 soldiers and airmen of the United Kingdom lying there, and 143 soldiers from Australia and 34 from New Zealand. There is one woman's grave in those white ranks, that of Nurse Charlotte Berrie.*[56] An unnamed friend wrote *...she was a marvelous nurse ... the only woman buried with full military honours among many of the troops she looked after so faithfully. She truly gave her life on active service.*[57]

The last word on the contribution of the nurses of the 14th AGH comes from Chauvel who noted that *...no words which to tell of the service of the splendid band of Australian nursing sisters who, under the inspiration of ... Rose Creal, matron at the No. 14 General Hospital, greeted the battered men from the front as they reached hospital and nursed them back to strength, or softened the close of their soldier life.*[58] A week before Charlotte Berrie died, on 1 January 1919, Rose Creal was awarded the RRC...*in recognition for her valuable services with the British forces in Egypt.*[59]

27 Australian Nurses on the British Salonika Front 1917-1919

This damnable country, enervating and malaria-sodden, soul-blasting and mind demoralizing ...we have paid her toll in deaths, ruined constitutions and broken spirits-
Gladys Walter

The Australian troops were not welcome in Greece but their nurses were. Canadian and British Hospitals were established and by 1917 the QAIMNS nurses were exhausted. Australia was requested to provide nursing support and it has been estimated that 340 - 390 AANS nurses served in Greece making up twenty percent of the nursing workforce on this front. The AANS were mainly situated around Salonika where they provided nursing care to British soldiers and Bulgarian POWs.

Campaign Overview

The following summary of the British Salonika Front sets the scene as to why Australian nurses were sent to a location where Australian soldiers were not. Wakefield and Moody write... *After withdrawing from Serbia in November 1915, Allied forces took up defensive positions around Salonika, assuming that Bulgaria forces would try and advance into Greece. The expected invasion never took place. Instead, the Bulgarians dug in along the Greek-Serb border from the coast of Albania to Lake Doiran and the Bulgarian border. In 1916, Allied troops in Salonika advanced against the Bulgarian defensive line. The British Salonika Force (BSF) took up positions at Doiran and advanced into the Struma Valley to the east, driving out Bulgarian forces during September. The French, supported by Russian, Italian and later Serbian troops, captured the strategic town of Monastir in November 1916. In April 1917, the Allies launched a major offensive. The main thrust was made by French and Serbian forces to the west, with the British launching a diversionary attack at Doiran. Both these attacks failed, and the campaign settled down to stalemate until September 1918, when Serbian forces broke through the Bulgarian lines. Bulgarian resistance quickly crumbled and on 30 September an armistice came into effect.*[1]

Australian Nurses in Salonika, Greece: 1917 -1919

Principal Matron Jessie McHardy White led the first of four contingents of

Australian nurses to Salonika.[2] She had held the position in England and it would seem the position and title followed her to Salonika. There is a lack of clarity as to whether Rose Creal was a Principal Matron or Matron. She was the most senior nurse leader in Egypt when 3 AGH left for France. In reality Rose Creal had overarching responsibility for the Salonika nurses when they arrived in Egypt before being transferred to their unit. While in Salonika Jessie McHardy White was responsible for the AANS nurses and she had the power to repatriate and promote them, as did many matrons. When they became ill they were returned to Egypt for review by a medical board and often recuperated at 14AGH under the care of Rose Creal. She was also responsible for AANS nurses who were in transit on hospital ships and stopped at Suez or Alexandria en-route to Britain, Europe or back to Australia. There is no doubt that the responsibilities of both remarkable leaders were far-reaching.

Principal Matron Jessie McHardy White: Biography

At the time of her two enlistments her Christian names were Jessie McHardy and her surname was White. Her parents were John Williamson and Mary (née McHardy), Scottish farmers and Jessie was born in 1870 at Yarra Glen in Victoria. She married Thomas James White, a bookkeeper from Fitzroy in 1893, who tragically died only three years later. They had no children. Jessie decided to become a nurse.[3]

Nurse Training: 1896-1901

Jessie joined The Alfred as a probationer in December 1896 and was RVTNA qualified in February 1900. She immediately joined The Women's Hospital as a pupil midwife and qualified in March 1901. Thirty-one years old, Jessie went onto administer a private hospital by 1906 and had joined the AANS reserve.

War Service 1914-16: Egypt and England

When war was declared she enlisted and was known as Jessie McHardy White throughout the remainder of her career. The use of a nurse's middle name was not unusual when a nurse had a common surname, such as White, and wished to differentiate herself. This was especially the case for nurse leaders. She embarked on HMAT *Benalla* as part of 1AGH in November 1914. Her leadership skills were noticed by those in authority and she served as matron 2 AGH, fleetingly, during the Jane Bell controversy.

Salonika Contingents: June 1917 to June 1918

The four contingents were made up of nurses from different States with the first mainly consisting of 3MD nurses and the second from 2MD. PM McHardy White embarked on the RMS *Mooltan,* which left Sydney in June 1917 with 215 nurses onboard. She was followed by Matron Beryl Campbell with 52 nurses on the *Wiltshire* in August. The third and fourth contingents were made up from composite States, but the third contingent was led by Matron Ethelda Runnalls Uren from 4MD. She remained in the position until 1918 when she had to RTA and was replaced by Matron Christense Sorenson.[4]

The fourth contingent of forty-one nurses led by Matron Jessie Ross Gemmell arrived in Egypt in October 1917 and was held back at a British Hospital to care for the soldiers who were in readiness to capture Gaza via Beersheba.[5] PM McHardy White vented her anger at Matron Gemmell for not standing her ground and refusing to stay in Egypt but this would have been a very difficult call for a young nurse leader who was obliged to follow military orders. However, this fourth contingent finally regrouped and reached Salonika in April and June 1918.[6]

Salonika: Location and Role

The first contingent went to 66 BGH, which was a tent hospital at Hortiach located twenty km from Salonika. It later moved to 52 BGH, a hut hospital, at Kalamaria in November 1917. The second contingent went to 52 BGH while the third started at 60 BGH, Hortiach. Finally, when the fourth contingent arrived it was sent to 42 BGH, another tent hospital at Kalamaria and later moved to Uchata. The weather was extreme so during the summers there was movement to Hortiach which was located high in the hills towards Bulgaria. To escape the snow in winter the nurses moved closer to the coast near Lembet.[6] When Edith Jackson (AANS) arrived she found makeshift tents erected near stagnant and filthy ponds of water, perfect breeding grounds for the malaria-carrying mosquito.[7]

Nursing in Salonika: Ione Nowland

PM Creal was well aware that service in Salonika was harsh because perfectly healthy nurses were returning to Egypt enervated and ill. They were often RTA from 14 AGH after a medical discharge. For instance, Gladys Walter, who was born in Brisbane and completed four years training at SHSEH, arrived in Egypt on the *Mooltan*.[8] She and another SHSEH trained nurse, Ione Nowland were destined for Salonika. They were joined by Gertrude Munro (Munnie) who left India and spent twenty days in Egypt before embarking on the hospital ship *Manitou* on 4 August 1917.[9] Nurses like Nowland mistakenly believed service in Salonika would ensure a more rapid transfer to Europe, as many thought Egypt, Salonika and India were merely outposts of the real war.

Gertrude Munro: India: 1916-17

A Victorian born in Ballarat, she trained at the local hospital with another AANS nurse, Blodwyn Williams. Munnie was thirty-four years old when she enlisted with the AIF for British Indian Service on 16 August 1916.[10] After spending three months at Cumballa War Hospital, Bombay, she was transferred to the Deccan War Hospital at Poona, where Jessie Gibson also served. The prevalence of deadly snakes in India caused the Australian nurses some concern, especially when they found them in their rooms. One AANS sister was bitten at the Deccan War Hospital but fortunately survived.[11] After seven months' service Munnie was sent to Egypt while she awaited transfer to Salonika.

Gertrude Munro: Salonika:1917-18

On arrival in Salonika, Munnie was appointed temporary head sister on 1 September 1917. She enjoyed the respect as well as the affection of those with whom she worked.[12] She was described by a British matron as …*the type of nurse who would be a comfort to any nursing administrator. She was skilled in her profession, a reliable domestic manager, and a lovable woman.*[13]

Gertrude Munro was admitted to 42 BGH on 1 October 1918 suffering from the effects of malaria and influenza. She was nursed by infection control nurses but Matron McHardy White or one of Sister Munro's friends was always in attendance during the ten days of her illness.[14] This knowledge may have been of some comfort to her mother Emma and father Alexander. Cruelly, she endured two of the more difficult placements, India and Salonika, for two years and then died a month before the Armistice.[15]

She died on 10 October at 12.10 am and was buried the next day, in the Church of England section of the British War Cemetery, Mikra (grave 591), with full military honours. [16] Munnie was the only Australian nurse to be buried in Greece but she was not alone: During wartime a cemetery is rarely a lonely place. Although Gertrude Munro was buried in a distant land, her life was recorded and remembered in Ballarat with the inclusion of her name on the honour rolls of the Queen's Church of England Grammar School, Alfredton State School, St Peter's Church of England and the Ballarat Hospital.

Nursing in Salonika: Gladys Walter

Gladys Walter was interviewed by Maud Kellett after the war in England. She provides a matter of fact description of her wartime experiences to her much senior nursing colleague. However, in a letter to an unidentified colleague she is more direct and honest. She writes how …*two years have altered one's opinion. God's garden is not here! This damnable country, enervating and malaria-sodden, soul-blasting and mind demoralising, is like the harlot who with false graces and charms, lures to destruction. And we have paid her toll in deaths, ruined constitutions and broken spirits.*[16]

In January 1918, Gladys Walter left Salonika and was reviewed by a medical board at 14 AGH. She had endured a number of episodes of appendicitis and was invalided back to Australia where she had six months' leave, including three months off for her surgery. Appendicitis was not an easy operation at this time because the risk of sepsis was ever-present. Fortunately she recovered and was en route to Egypt when the Armistice was declared. [17] Although there was …*great rejoicing on board…*

the ship continued to Egypt and she was loaned to the British hospitals for relief nursing of influenza patients. Gladys Walter returned to her original unit, 14 AGH, where *...there were a lot of mixed infectious cases ...but most were awaiting transport to Australia.*

It is worth reiterating the reality of just getting to this part of Greece from Egypt during a world war. The trip often took four days. However, Susan Arnold (AANS) recalls the second contingent only took 48 hours to reach Salonika by sea, sailing on the admiralty ship HMS *Osmanieh*. However, the *Osmanieh* was torpedoed on the next trip with many casualties. Ellen Riordon (AANS) supported what Gladys Walter learnt when she was invalided back to Egypt and the trip took *...14 days to do the 4 days journey from Salonica to Egypt, as the Bulgarian planes tried to bomb the ships. We had to stay in Malea for some time, as the "Goeben" and the "Breslau" threatened to shell the harbour. As we were on our way to Alexandria, we saw the wrecks of the "Osmanieh" and the "Aragon", and the bodies of some of the victims floating about. Several English Sisters, and V.A.D.s were drowned, and 200 soldiers were among the victims.*[18]

Nursing in Salonika: Ione Nowland

Ione Nowland did not endure the hardships of Salonika easily and returned to Egypt with 'nervous debility' twelve months later. Matron Creal and her closest friend, Jessie Tomlins, who trained at Sydney Hospital could not believe the change in the young woman. She was well cared for by her colleagues but her recovery was slow. Often convalescent nurses who were 'RTA' due to illness were required to work on the transport home, but her condition was so severe that she was not permitted to undertake any nursing for three full months. She was repatriated to Australia and never saw service in France. The consulting doctor recorded that her condition was not caused by war service but was *...aggravated by the sub-tropical climate.* The power of the medical diagnosis had far-reaching consequences for nurses and soldiers who had to find work again on her return if their medical condition was not due to war service. Ione arrived in Australia on January 1919 and was discharged from the AIF the following May.[19] Ione Nowland did keep working and she had a remarkable career after the war.

The Human Cost of the Salonika Campaign

The appalling conditions at Salonika gave rise to a late attempt to modify the uniform but the inclusion of more practical footwear for the harsh terrain and netting for mosquito protection was of limited value. Approximately sixty-two Australian nurses were invalided home from Salonika, many suffering from malaria and dysentery.[20] One such casualty was Elizabeth Rothery, who had finished her service on troopships while awaiting a permanent placement and was sent to Salonika. Eventually, she returned to Australia for a well-deserved rest. [21] While visiting friends at Beechworth on 14 June she developed appendicitis and her condition quickly deteriorated; the next morning she died of peritonitis.[22] The loss of such a fine nurse from the profession was incalculable, but the loss of a daughter was a catastrophe for her family who were already mourning the death of their son Norman.

A Homecoming and Farewell: May Hennessy

A Victorian, May Hennessy was born in Castlemaine (Dja Dja Wurrung Country) and trained at Gippsland Hospital, Sale (Gunaikurnai Nation). At the time of her enlistment with the AANS she was living in Melbourne at the Royal Melbourne Trained Nurses' Home in St Kilda Road and her parents had relocated to Bendigo.[23] When Hennessy embarked on the *Mooltan* in Melbourne on 12 June 1917 she was young to be a qualified nurse (23 years) and was in the peak of health. The *Mooltan,* which had transferred hundreds of AANS personnel all over the world, arrived at Suez on 19 July 1917 and within a week it was struck by a torpedo in the Mediterranean Sea where it sank (26 July 1917). [24] A week after arriving in Egypt (25 July 1917), she boarded the *Chagres* destined for Salonika, where she worked tirelessly under the leadership of Jessie McHardy White for sixteen months.

She developed renal and liver failure after her first bout of malaria. The severity of her illness required a prolonged recovery so she was transferred to Cairo on 27 November 1918. Initially she was listed as 'seriously ill' but slowly improved to the point where she was ready to begin convalescence at the end of January 1919. Every effort was taken to keep her parents, Helen and James Hennessy, informed of any change in her condition. During December they were twice informed that she was on the 'seriously ill' list but they must have been relieved to receive formal notification that she was improving each week throughout January until she was finally classified as a 'convalescent'.

It was decided to return Hennessy to Australia as an invalid on the *Novgorod* on 22 February 1919 but her condition en route deteriorated dramatically. Just when her parents nearly had sight of their young daughter they received a telegram at the end of March from the *Novgorod,* describing her *...condition still most critical...* because the malaria was *...complicated by dysentery, jaundice and suppression of urine.*[25]

The ship's medical officer wanted her admitted to a military hospital in Melbourne without delay and requested the ship go directly to Melbourne as opposed to Geelong.[26] The request was denied because there was a fear the returning personnel would spread the influenza virus, at this time the pandemic quarantine arrangements were considered paramount to the safety of the public.

May was admitted to Nurse Mackenzie's 'Rivera' Private Hospital in Myers Street, Geelong, which was not too distant from her home town of Bendigo. She remained there until her death from malaria and acute nephritis on 9 April 1919—her mother, Helen, never left her side.[27] Although May Hennessy lived for just over a week when she finally reached Australia, she endured a prolonged and very painful death.

The young nurse's remains were transported by train from Geelong and arrived in Bendigo at 4.45 pm. She was met by an assembly of fifty returned soldiers and nurses at the station. The soldiers standing to attention as a mark of respect as her body was placed in the hearse. As the cortege moved away from the station they saluted.[28] Her coffin was taken 'home' to 38 McIvor Road and the details of her funeral were finalised.

The subsequent funeral of May Hennessy was conducted amidst the language of martyrdom. She became a lightning rod for the grief of local families who had lost a son they could not bury. Her funeral was detailed in local papers and expressions of grief were reported in heart-wrenching detail. A mother of a dead soldier asked permission to *...place a piece of worn khaki on the coffin ... a tribute to the memory of one who had tended wounded soldiers in the hospital wards.*[29] This was a time for homage and the Archdeacon offered in prayer the need to *...praise and magnify thy holy name for the nurses who have met the deaths of martyrs to their duty.*[30] On 12 April 1919 at 2.15 pm, returned soldiers in uniform and bandsmen assembled at the fountain in readiness to follow the remains of May Hennessy to the cemetery and *...at different points en route to the cemetery thousands of people assembled to view the mournful procession.*[31]

So many sons would not be returning – their bones decomposing in the dried and blood-soaked mud of Flanders or on a remote peninsula in Turkey. This day Sister May Hennessy was feted as a heroine because she represented those who were absent. A *...woman with tear rimmed eyes...* expressed a wish to see the coffin before the funeral because she had lost two sons. So many mothers did not have the opportunity to face the reality of their loss – it was so abstract – these dead children on the other side of the world.[32]

Over one hundred wreaths were carried by an accompanying cab as the funeral procession and mourning coaches moved through the streets of Bendigo. The largest muster of returned servicemen seen in Bendigo marked the occasion. Returned soldiers carried the coffin and forty returned soldiers raised their rifles and fired into the air. Brass bands played and finally the last post was sounded. After the funeral local newspapers were filled with correspondence about the need to raise funds for a memorial to Sister May Hennessy. The community wanted May's sacrifice to be immortalised, and for weeks the pros and cons of granite memorials versus community-spirited practical memorials were debated ad infinitum.[33]

The honours, the memorials and the public mourning may have assisted the collective grief of the community but the fact remained: May Hennessy, 25 years young, was dead and buried. Whether the nurses and soldiers were buried at sea or in lonely quarantine stations or in mass graves in other parts of the world, the results were the same for those at home. After the fanfare of the funeral, Helen and James Hennessy returned home without their firstborn child. May was a casualty of a little known conflict, amidst a much bigger one, where Australian nurses suffered and died.

28 India and Mesopotamia

Just a week after our arrival we received 300 released prisoners from Bagdad… More emaciated from disease and starvation, one would never see – Gertrude Davis

When Queen Victoria was proclaimed the Empress of India in 1877, she was well pleased with her Empire. During the First World War her grandson King George V ruled two-thirds of the sub-continent's 320 million people by way of a human network of 6,500 British officials and local bureaucrats.[1] One member of this human network was an Englishwoman, Gertrude Bell (1868-1926) an archaeologist and gifted linguist who, when war was declared, spent nearly two decades in Mesopotamia (present-day Iraq) and Persia (present-day Iran).

Bell, a student of Persian since 1892, was conscious and respectful of the religious and cultural history of the East. This knowledge was used to good effect during the war as *…she put on the map a line of wells hitherto unplaced or unknown …of which Colonel Lawrence* (Lawrence of Arabia) *made signal use in the Arab campaigns of 1917 and 1918.* During the war she was gainfully employed as an intelligence gatherer in Cairo, Basra and Baghdad and afterwards she remained in the region and established the Museum of Antiquities in Baghdad. Gertrude Bell was an exceptional woman who had a vast repertoire of life experiences and knowledge.[2] In contrast, Australian nurses had minimal cultural exposure to the customs of the East prior to the war.

How Australian nurses came to be in India during the First World War can be logically traced back to two historical happenings: firstly, the desire of Florence Nightingale to improve the sanitation level of the communities of India in 1857; and secondly, the expansionist military 'drift' of the British Army nearly sixty years later.[3] Florence Nightingale's report to the Royal Sanitary Commission, of which Sidney Herbert was Chair in 1857, initiated the dramatic changes to public health in India, especially for the British Army personnel stationed there.[4]

Since English trained nurses were part of the military nurse establishment of British military hospitals with more than one hundred beds, the QAIMNS had been based in India since 1888.[5] However, when the war spilled over to the Mesopotamian front a significant number of casualties put pressure on health resources and the demand for qualified nurses increased.

Mesopotamia

Once the Ottomans entered the war, Britain needed to protect its Abadan oil supply, which was located near the Persian Gulf not too distant from Turkish-controlled Basra.[6] To this end Britain increased its presence in the Persian Gulf and on 21 November 1914 Basra was captured. Enemy forces began to reinforce the area but were decisively repelled. Further expansion of the British foothold was needed to maintain an adequate defence in the region and British forces, who were met with little resistance, moved steadily towards Baghdad. In response, the enemy consolidated their defences and forced the British back to Kut-al-Amara where they were isolated until fresh reinforcements were able to reach the remote area, but in April 1916 Kut-al-Amara fell to the enemy.[7]

There were 97,579 Anglo-Indian casualties from this enthusiastic but ill-conceived push toward Baghdad. The Mesopotamian front was an open wound which desperately needed a tourniquet of allied soldiers.[8] In 1916 when the British army engaged the enemy in Mesopotamia the boundaries of the war expanded, so the Indian government called on Australia to provide nurses to care for the casualties of the campaign.

A rather bizarre twist to Army policy was that nurses who served in India were considered to be on 'home service' not 'active service'. If they had not served on any other front they were invisible to history. The rationale was that India, like Australia, was considered British.[9] The injustice of this is obvious as the following pages show. The nurses who served in India are included in the author's nominal roll which takes the number of Australian nurses who served overseas during the First World War to 2,470.[10]

Conditions for Australian Nurses in India

The pay and conditions of the AANS was inferior to their colleagues in both the Indian Nursing Service and the QAIMNS, but what proved to be more distressing was their lack of opportunity to serve in Mesopotamia. The rationale for this decision did not relate to the competency of the AANS nurses but the unfair financial arrangement agreed to by the Australian Government. Australian nurses became the de facto nursing workforce in India.[11] The number of Australian nurses serving in India steadily increased until there were 320 working in Indian hospitals. A staggering five hundred Australian nurses served in India between 1916-19.[12]

On arrival in India they expected to be kept together as one unit, just as they had been in Egypt, but they were soon informed they were to be sent to various locations throughout the subcontinent, sometimes alone.[13] The nurses were assigned to either one of the main hospitals in Bombay, Deolali or Poona. Alternatively they were sent to station hospitals at Lahore, Calcutta, Mooltan, Naoshera or Sialkot or smaller station hospitals like Quetta, Tank and Gharial.[14]

To India via Egypt: July 1916

When the Mesopotamian Front failed to be a *...moral counterpoise to their* [British] *other failures...* negotiations began in May 1916 and the Australian Government initially agreed to send fifty nurses from Egypt, led by Matron Emily Hoadley. This was for a six month period in the first instance with an option for further re-engagement in another six months or until the end of the war.[15] Amy O'Grady was new to military nursing but a very experienced civilian nurse while Kitty Power and Letitia Moreton were seasoned military nurses by this stage. They were among fifty nurses transported on HMHS *Neuralia* under the capable leadership of senior sister, and later matron, Emily Hoadley. They reached India in July 1916.[16]

Kitty Power and Amy O'Grady in India

Kitty Power was now a member of the AANS but she was more Irish than she was Australian. As her time in Egypt demonstrated she had a complicated social and nursing path which ultimately led her to the Taj Mahal Hospital, Bombay. In some ways she was like Amy O'Grady, especially during the course of their AANS service, but there were significant differences in their backgrounds. They were both Irish Catholics and both trained nurses who saw war service in many of the same hospitals and locations in Egypt and India. It was in their early life prior to the war where their paths differed significantly.

Kathleen (Kitty) Power: Biography

Kitty Power was born in Kilkenny, Ireland, in 1888, and although her birthplace is geographically distant from Australia the two countries had a number of cultural ties. Her father Michael resided in a rural area, Piltown, in the county of Kilkenny, while his young daughter travelled the world before and during the First World War. Kitty Power was part of the British nursing service until 24 August 1915 and was immediately eligible to join the AANS because all members needed to be a *...natural born British subject or naturalised British subject.*[17] Her previous experience with the QAIMNS was not taken into account when she joined the AANS, making her an extremely experienced civilian and military nurse when she was sent to India as a staff nurse in 1916.

Amy O'Grady: Biography

Similarly, Amy Veda O'Grady was a well-qualified civilian nurse when she enlisted. She was born in Castlemaine in 1876 about 25 years after the first gold discovery put the tiny Victorian town, located 120 kilometres north-west of Melbourne, on the map. Her mother Ellen died the year after her birth and her father, Daniel, in 1899. Amy had older sibling; a brother and six sisters. She was aged thirty-nine years and when she enlisted on 10 August 1915.[18] In the year of her enlistment her brother, James, became the first parish priest of Preston, Melbourne. At the same time he purchased a parcel of land, about 5-6 acres, and *...some houses...* in the immediate surrounds.[19]

Amy O'Grady completed three years of nurse training at the Melbourne Hospital (1905) and was a member of the RVTNA.[20] She, like Grace Wilson and Jane Bell, trained in midwifery at the Queen Charlotte Hospital, London, gaining her second nursing certificate.[21] By the time she enlisted with the AANS she had also completed a massage certificate, making her a triple certificate sister with thirteen years' experience *...in the execution of medical orders...* making her an extremely well qualified AANS staff nurse.[22]

Nurses from Egypt to India: July 1916

While the service record of Kitty Power records that she left Egypt on HMHS *Devanha* on 22 July 1916 it was the *Neuralia* which transported the nurses from Egypt to India. She had been temporarily attached to 15 GH, Alexandria, for a few weeks. Kitty Power and Amy O'Grady were part of the contingent of fifty Australian nurses from Egypt to serve in India. Once they arrived at Bombay the Australian nursing personnel were despatched to various hospitals throughout the sub-continent.

Cholera Epidemic: August 1916

Florence Nightingale was appalled when she read sanitary reports from India in 1862 because British *...stations contented themselves by declaring their water as "smells good" or "smells bad"*.[23] Her recommendations for a concerted improvement in public health strategies were politely ignored and the prevalence of cholera was still widespread sixty years later. Nurses were aware of the risks because service in India was renowned for its harsh climate and high risk of infection. A cholera epidemic struck suddenly on 12 August 1916 just a few weeks after the first Australian nurses arrived in India. Kitty and Amy were infected. The Taj Mahal Hospital was immediately closed and both nurses were transferred to the Colaba War Hospital, an isolation hospital, located about twenty minutes drive from Bombay.[24] The hospital was on a hill near the sea making it an ideal location for the management of infectious diseases but the close proximity to the sea did nothing to negate the humidity – making conditions for the nurses enervating.[25] Kitty Power was listed as *...dangerously ill...* and died on 13 August 1916, the day after Amy O'Grady.[26]

When Sister Eileen Burke was stationed at Colaba about four months later she found the ...bungalows were very dilapidated looking but proved to be quite comfortable either single room or perhaps two in a large room and a servant between four of us, who called us in the morning, prepared our bath (which was a small tin tub), brought us our tea when off duty etc.[27] The amenities or comforts offered by the hospital would have been of little consequence to the two nurses, who were sufficiently aware that they stood a very good chance of dying.

Anne Donnell was serving with 3AGH in Europe when on 16 August 1916 she recorded in a letter home that ...we have just had such sad news from India to say that at the Taj Mahar [sic], in Bombay, some of our officers and two sisters had died suddenly ... The Sisters were here with us for a while – such bonnie girls – and the news has given us quite a shock. What a history Australia will have to tell after the war is over.[28] May Tilton also served with Kitty Power and she recorded in her diary that a ...dear girl, Kitty Power, was a victim.[29]

Notification of deaths

News from the Somme was dominating the minds and hearts of Australians in 1916.[30] The Reverend James O'Grady was now the recipient of the sad news of Amy's death. How he and his four remaining sisters received the dismal news is unknown.[31] While there is no image of twenty-seven year old Kitty Power when she joined the AANS, it is known that she had a fair complexion with brown hair and she weighed 69 kg and was 160 cm tall. Ironically her only distinguishing marks were ...*vaccination marks distinct on left arm.*[32] Although the basic description of her physical appearance fails to bring the young woman to life, she was obviously well respected by her AANS colleagues and missed by her family in Ireland.

Resting Places

India is a predominantly Hindu country and the Hindu custom of cremation caused a considerable ...*glare of the cremation grounds...* at the 1,000 bed Gerrard Freeman Thomas Hospital between September and October 1918, during which time there were up to seven hundred deaths from influenza.[33] Despite the increasingly popular view that cremation is a more sanitary method of disposing of the dead than burial, there is no evidence that cremation was used by Europeans – even in cases of contagion.[34]

Kitty Power, an Irish Catholic, was buried at the Sewri Cemetery (plot 10, line "V", grave no. 16) Bombay, India.[35] Her name is included on the AWM Roll of Honour, Canberra. Michael Power outlived his daughter, Kitty, and had the unenviable duty of organising delivery of a memorial scroll in honour of her service and subsequent death. It must have seemed surreal for this man, in a distant rural area of Ireland, to receive information relating to his daughter about ...*Where the Australians Rest.*[36]

It is not possible to ascertain the last moments of Amy O'Grady's life but one would hope that there was sufficient time for the last rites to be administered – not by her brother but by a stranger. Although Amy O'Grady was laid to rest at Sewri Cemetery (plot 10, line 'T', grave no. 3), Bombay, in a culturally different country from her Australian home, at least there were Australian nursing colleagues close by caring for her. Amy O'Grady died on 12 August 1916, the first anniversary of her enlistment with the AANS.[37] There is little doubt that irrespective of their religion or place of birth or death, nurses like Amy O'Grady and Kitty Power fulfilled their commitment to their God and their profession.

PM Gertrude Davis and First Australian Contingent

At the same time it was agreed to send another fifty AANS nurses from Australia on RMS *Mooltan* under the leadership of Gertrude Davis. Gertrude Davis, who later became the PM for India, found the workload for the AANS staff when they first arrived at Bombay was ...*very heavy as this hospital was the nearest to the docks, which were less than 5 min. away so we got all the most serious cases. Just a week after our arrival we received 300 released prisoners from Bagdad. When Kut-el-Amara* [sic] *fell to the Turks, Gen. Townsend exchanged able bodied Turkish Prisoners of war for his sick and wounded British prisoners held by the Turks. More emaciated from disease and starvation, one would never see. It took them three months to come from Bagdad to Bombay and although the greater of them were serious cases of dysentery, beri-beri and old septic wounds, we only lost two men out of the 300. For months the daily ration of these men was five biscuits and they looked as if they were made of pollard. They were so hard it was impossible to eat them without soaking them in some fluid and as water was the only drink they received it was no wonder they nearly all had dysentery. Tea they had not tasted for months, sometimes they had a little ginger to put in the water and on very few occasions a syrup. We were so sorry for them that we gave them too much to both eat and drink, but we discovered that day that we would have to go very slowly with their diet.*[38]

Australian Contingent arrives in India: *Mooltan*: August 1916

Nurses from Egypt had been working in India since July 1916 and O'Grady and Power had already died when the first Indian contingent was boarding RMS *Mooltan* in Melbourne on 22 August 1916. The Australian contingent was led by PM Gertrude Davis and included Elizabeth Rothery and Gertrude Munro. Others boarded en route, including Jessie Gibson who embarked in Fremantle.[39] They arrived at Bombay on 12 September 1916 and were sent to meet the QAIMNS matron at the Taj Mahal Hospital the next day. They found ...*suppressed excitement became apparent in the hotel. Cholera was then rampant, several medical men and sisters having succumbed, including two Australians from Egypt, Misses O'Grady and Power. It now became known that another case had occurred at the hotel, and the place was at once evacuated.*[40]

Gertrude Davis was faced with an unprecedented medical and nursing emergency when the ...First Contingent of Australian sisters arrived in India from Egypt per H.S Neuralia with Miss Emily Hoadley, Late Senior Sister No. 3 A.G.H., Abbassia, in charge. At the time of their arrival cholera was rampant and unfortunately two of our sisters, Sister A.B. O'Grady and K. Power, succumbed to its ravages.[41]

Despite arriving a month after their deaths, PM Davis found the administrative aspects of their burials had not been dealt with for want of clear delineation of responsibility for the Australian nurses. In March 1917, PM Davis wrote to the Army authorities in a state of agitation when it was brought to her attention that the burials of Amy O'Grady and Kitty Power had not been paid for: She addressed the matter in her usual efficient manner.[42]

Letitia Moreton: Life in remote India

On 13 July 1916 Letitia Moreton was struck off strength of 4 AAH in Egypt and set sail for Bombay on the *Neuralia,* disembarking on 23 July 1916 with Kitty Power and Amy O'Grady.[43] She was more than likely unaware that her two colleagues had died of cholera in mid-August, because Letitia spent just over a week at a hospital in Bombay. She was instructed to join another Australian nursing sister and they boarded a train together but her colleague alighted early. Letitia was destined for Quetta. The distance from Bombay, India to Quetta in modern day Pakistan is 1,400 kilometres. Letitia wrote *...unfortunately I happened to be chosen for Quetta and had to leave my mate.* The young woman travelled with her colleague for one day before their destinations diverged and she spent *...four days and three nights in the train alone.*[44]

Australian nurses at this time tended not to disclose emotions, especially fear, in their letters home. They were well aware the reader was worried about their safety and well-being. Even today such a journey might evoke a sense of trepidation for an Australian woman but it must be remembered that Letitia Moreton was an Australian nurse, a Christian, brought up on the propaganda of the White Australia policy.[45] Furthermore, it was unheard of for a respectable woman to travel unchaperoned. This was AANS policy which was reiterated by Matron-in-Chief Evelyn Conyers, who pointed out in a correspondence to Matron Creal *...it must be clearly understood that no Sister stays away for a night, unless she has been sent to a Rest Home or is on leave.*[46] Miss Conyers needed to add the proviso — unless she has been sent 1400 km across the subcontinent, alone, as part of the Indian Military Service. Letitia Moreton was reassured by her Australian colleagues before leaving Bombay that she was *...going to the best place in India, one of the nicest cities...* but the adverse climatic conditions and the long train journey were only made tolerable by the electric fans in the first class carriage.[47]

When Florence Nightingale reviewed the mortality levels of the British Army stations in India in 1862 she was outraged to find the death rate was 69 per 1,000. At the time she claimed a *...company out of every regiment has been sacrificed every 20 months...* but her advice to implement sound sanitation measures throughout India was not heeded.[48] However, the introduction of the Indian Army Service in 1888 ensured there were some improvements and Letitia Moreton was pleased to find a comfortable permanent army station hospital staffed by surgeons, five professional

QAIMNS sisters and well-trained orderlies who were available to do much of the heavy work.

Nonetheless, Letitia was not so pleased to find she was considered to be on 'home service' as opposed to 'active service' which was the reason for enlisting with the AANS.[49] Despite this distinction made by the Army, it is near impossible to consider Letitia Moreton's working conditions at Quetta to be akin to 'home service' when the next Australian soldier or nurse was a few days' train journey away.

Furthermore, any promotion attained during Indian service was null and void once the nurses embarked for duty to another front. For example, Christina Morrison (AANS) served from 1917-19 in the main war hospitals in Bombay, including Victoria and Cumballa, before nursing at Belguam Hill station, and she attained the rank of head sister. As soon as she embarked for England she reverted to the rank of SN because her service in India was considered to be of no military consequence.[50]

Unfortunately, no amount of nursing care could combat the onslaught of *salmonella typhi,* which infected Letitia Moreton's intestinal tract just three months after her arrival.[51] The earliest symptoms experienced are usually a headache and perhaps a sore throat, so not terribly alarming for a nurse in a tropical location during the war. However, before confirmation of the disease could be made the early symptoms of diarrhoea and a fever would have attracted the attention of Letitia's medical colleagues. As her condition worsened she would have been nursed in isolation by her English nursing colleagues, who would apply ice packs and give Letitia sponge baths to reduce her temperature. Fluids would be strongly encouraged because dehydration, especially in the tropics, was a serious risk.[52]

Her nurses would have closely observed Letitia for any signs of intestinal bleeding which would indicate a real risk of perforation of her intestine. Unfortunately this occurred and on 1 November 1916 her father was sent a telegram which read in full *...Regret reported daughter nurse LG Moreton dangerously ill enteric haemorrhage at Quetta India will furnish progress report when received.*[53] During the next two weeks her condition worsened and the bleeding bowel most likely perforated causing *...intense abdominal pain and tenderness, frequent vomiting, a rapid pulse, and a sunken and anxious* *face*.[54] It is not difficult to imagine the anxious face of Letitia Moreton, who no doubt knew she would soon die without seeing her mother, sister and father again.

On 14 November a second telegram was sent to her father from 'base records' which read in part *...condition causing gravest anxiety profound toxaemia...* but in fact Letitia had been three days dead by this time.[55] At the end of her life she most likely lapsed into delirium and periods of staring blindly into space, and although she was just twenty-six years old her death would have ended weeks of pain and distressing symptoms.[56]

On 11 November 1916 Letitia Moreton died from typhoid after suffering from enteric haemorrhage and toxaemia.[57] She was one of the few Presbyterians buried at Quetta Government Cemetery (2092) and her name can be found at the Delhi Memorial, India (43).[58] Sadly, it was a requirement that twenty-six year old AANS nurses left a will during the years 1914-1918. Many years later another Australian nurse was required to write her will before she left for service in the Vietnam War and she found it difficult because she questioned what she had to leave. Such a sad question given that it was directed to her mother.[59] Apart from her jewellery, clothes and books she left to her sister Doris, Letitia bequeathed all her worldly goods, including a life insurance policy, to her mother. A bequest most mothers would receive with absolute dismay.[60]

On the second anniversary of her death — 11 November 1918 — the fighting would finally cease when the Armistice was declared. It can only be hoped the little compliant donkey, the Anzac mascot she found lying so still in the soldier's bed on Anzac Day, just six months earlier, survived the war.

Jessie Gibson: Quetta: 1917-1919

Nearly a year after Letitia Moreton died another 1916 *Mooltan* recruit, Jessie Gibson, was sent to Quetta where she worked for two years. She had extensive experience in India by this stage in a number of hill hospitals. Jessie remained at Quetta until October 1919 at which time she was given leave in England and her military service was recognised with the award RRC (2nd Class). She returned to Australia aboard the SS *Megantic* but was admitted to the ship's hospital, diagnosed with *...general* *debility.* Her condition did not improve when she arrived home.[61] Nonetheless, when she was discharged in April 1920 she claimed to be fit and healthy.

Jessie was born in Victoria, 1889, but she trained at Perth Public Hospital and was discharged in Western Australia. Two years after her discharge she died there, in the repatriation section, aged 32 years of age.[62]

Jessie Gibson, Sister AANS, ARRC, endured four years of military service in one of the most isolated and medically complex areas of the war. Her entire service was in India and she died outside the timelines for inclusion on the AWM Roll of Honour. Reference to her service with the AWM is scant but her Service Record provides an outline of military nursing career in India. As is often the case her community remembered her by etching her name on a memorial in Kings Park, Perth.[63] Lest we forget those who came home debilitated from war service.

The Perils of Transport Duty

The nurses on transport duty near India and the Mesopotamian Front endured the worst of the tropical heat and storm activity. The severely wounded and ill soldiers from the front were at increased risk of dehydration, so it was imperative they were transported to hospital as soon as possible.[64] The following table (*table 4*) includes the name and rank of the AANS nurses who are known to have worked on transport duty while serving in India.[65] It provides a snapshot of the voyages undertaken by Australian nurses like Alma Bennett.

The following table illustrates the vast distances covered by the nurses while they were, ostensibly, serving in India. The journey of Sister Lillian Fletcher, who travelled on HMHS *Madras,* from tropical India to be confronted by the winter in Canada and Russia while caring for war casualties, tested her resilience.[66]

Table 4: Australian nurses who served on transport duty, India (1916-19).

AANS staff and rank	Transports	Voyage
Sister Minnie Walshe	Vareela	
Matron Annie Roberts	Ellora	
Sister EG Browne	Vita	
Sister Elizabeth Horne	Vita Sicilia Delta	To Basra Return from Mesopotamia to Suez & German East Africa
Sister Alma Bennett (in-charge)	Herefordshire	Bombay-Mesopotamia
Sister Gertrude Moberley	Herefordshire	Basra-Bombay
Sister Annie Low	Herefordshire	
Sister Lillian Ella Fletcher	Sicilia, Madras, Dilwarra-Madras	To Hong Kong – Vancouver, Vladivostok
Sister Gladys Larkan	Takada	From Basra
Sister Mary Lenton		
Sister Scanlan		Persian Gulf
Sister Blanche McKane	Devanha	Persian Gulf
Sister Muriel Robertson	Devanha Sicilia	

The value of victory (medal) - Muriel Robertson

Gertrude (Muriel) Norton Robertson was a Victorian qualified nurse in her thirties when she joined the AANS. She was sent to India and after a number of years' service she became seriously ill in June 1918. Her symptoms were complex and a number of medical officers provisionally diagnosed malaria, then sand fly fever, then meningitis. A final diagnosis of neuritis and debility due to service in India was finally decided upon. The relatively young woman who returned to Australia was described as ...*frail*... and from September 1918 until May 1921 she remained a patient at 11 AGH, Melbourne.[67]

Following her discharge from the AIF as ...*medically unfit*... she sought her Victory Medal, but to qualify as a recipient it was necessary to actually serve...*on the establishment of a unit in a theatre of war*.[68] India was not considered to be a theatre of war so her years of service under trying and enervating conditions were discounted. Muriel Robertson did work on HMHS *Devanha* (13 August - 3 September 1917) and *Sicilia* (7 April - 8 June 1918) but her service record was incomplete and there was no surviving evidence of this service.

Fortunately, Principal Matron Gertrude Davis kept detailed records and she confirmed the exact dates that Muriel Robertson had served on the hospital transports and the medal was issued.[69] The medal was physical evidence that she had been part of the war and that, just maybe, her contribution had mattered.

Florence (Narrelle) Jessie Hobbes: QAIMNSR: Biography

Narrelle Hobbes was determined to serve in the First World War. She travelled, at her own expense, to London in the company of fellow Australian nurses Rose Kirkcaldie, Elsie Welman, Kathleen Fitzpatrick and Sylvia Bell.[70] Narrelle was the daughter of English migrants John Hobbes and his second wife Margaret, who married on 11 March 1863 at Kiama Presbyterian church. Narrelle was born at Tilba Tilba on the south coast of NSW in 1878 and grew up as the second youngest child in a blended family of twelve living children. [71]

Nursing Experience

It was not uncommon for nurses who trained in small hospitals to complete a five-year certificate in one or more facilities. Hobbes trained at St Kilda Private Hospital in the Sydney suburb of Woolloomooloo (April 1903 - February 1905).[72] It had previously been under the matronship of Nellie Gould for a short period (1889-91) before she took up the position of Matron at SHSEH.[73] Hobbes then had a break before completing her training at Cobar District Hospital in western NSW (Ngiyampaa Wangaaypuwan Country) from March 1907 to May 1910. She was ATNA qualified on 5 August 1910.[74] However, she was immediately appointed Head Nurse at Cobar for ten months before accepting a position as matron of the Brewarrina Hospital (April 1911 - May 1912). While this area of NSW has a reputation for hot, dry summers, it did little to prepare her for the heat and dust of her overseas service in Malta, Mesopotamia and India.[75]

Narrelle Hobbes: QAIMNSR Military Service

Narrelle wrote many long and detailed letters to her friends and family giving her mother Margaret some reassurance, her father having already died.[76] While residing at 38 Guildford Street, Russell Square in London, Hobbes successfully joined the QAIMNSR in 1915 and sailed to Malta with Rose Kirkcaldie and Elsie Welman.[77] They nursed allied causalities during the Dardanelles Campaign but rarely cared for Australian soldiers who were routinely sent to the AGHs in Egypt or Lemnos.[78] March 1916 saw Sister Hobbes serving in Palermo, Sicily. She was in-charge of St David's Tent Hospital, Malta before being transferred to Mesopotamia in 1916.
The hospital in Mesopotamia was not ready by the time she reached India so she served at the Victoria War Hospital in the interim. In late August 1916 Narrelle was sent to Basra for duty, where she remained until October when she was sent further north to 32 BGH, Amara. It soon became evident that after two years active service Narrelle was not well. She was returned to Bombay for a detailed examination with the hope of a diagnosis.

Coincidences on Sea Transport: *Herefordshire* and *Mongolia*: 23 June 1917

Narrelle sailed on the *Mongolia* from England to Malta when she was first accepted for service with the QAIMNSR in 1915. She boarded SS *Erinpura* and was later transferred to HMHS *Herefordshire* bound for Bombay in June 1917; she was, coincidently, not too distant from the *Mongolia* which was also approaching Bombay. It was 23 June 1917 and three other Australian nurses, Evelyn Vickers Foote, CL Despard and Beatrice Mawson who had been loaned to the QAIMNSR and were required to return to Australia before they were enabled to re-enlist with the AANS, were on the *Mongolia.* The indomitable Evelyn Vickers Foote recorded what happened when ...*We got nearly as far as Bombay (nearly 45 miles off) and we were mined. It was exciting all right. Noon. Sank in less than 15 minutes. Out of sight in that time! The getting off was fine. There was a big list on one side. We had had good training beforehand. It was just like a rehearsal – no confusion. The Ship's officers were splendid, amazing. The fact that only 30 drowned speaks for itself – 15 minutes and a monsoon blowing. It was awful in the small boats in the big sea. We could not save a thing ... It was difficult to land. One boat capsized. There were rocks on the shore and it was pretty dark.*

Two got drowned landing. We had some biscuits and water ... we camped in our life belts in tropical rain, smashed up a couple of boats and made a fire.[79]

Narrelle Hobbes: Diagnosis

Fortunately, Hobbes made it safely to the sick sisters' quarters of the Colaba War Hospital, where Kitty Power and Amy O'Grady had died from cholera the previous August. A friend was relieved to see Narrelle in better health, because she had been *...horrified when she got back to Bombay from her holiday to hear I had been so ill on the way down ...that I had died and was buried at sea. Pathetic wasn't it, however, she says that if this is my ghost , it's a jolly healthy ghost – so I'm afraid they cannot get rid of me quite so quickly just yet.*[80]

A definitive diagnosis was not made while Narrelle was at Colaba War Hospital, but after two weeks of rest she recovered to the point where she was instructed to have one month's leave in a cooler hill station; she left in July 1917 and returned in February the following year. Unfortunately, her predilection for sight-seeing may have impaired her judgement, as she decided to make a sixteen hundred kilometre journey by train, car and dandi from Bombay to Binsar, located at the base of the Himalayas, despite still suffering severe abdominal pain.[81] At this time the correlation between cigarette smoking and cancer was not widely appreciated and a number of nurses, including Hobbes, smoked. Her father's early death from stomach cancer is suggestive of a familial predisposition to the disease.[82]

Hepatic Cancer

Hobbes developed a non-war related disease, hepatic carcinoma (cancer of the liver). This is a particularly painful condition due to the size and function of the liver, which is both a large gland (secretes chemicals for use by other parts of the body) and an organ (produces important chemicals), located in the upper right section of the abdomen. It has many complex functions including metabolism, detoxification of harmful substances and the breakdown of red blood cells. The liver produces bile – a clear orange or yellow fluid – which is then stored in the gallbladder and used as needed during digestion.[83] The jaundice or yellow pigmentation of Hobbes' eyes and skin was due to a failure in this function and the build-up of bile pigment in the blood. Her distance from appropriate medical and nursing care, combined with the lack of a diagnosis, caused additional hardship while she was supposedly recuperating.

Present-day nurses can easily access the most up-to-date information about the cancer-suppressing gene P59 or the complex surgical concepts regarding liver transplants, but in 1918, when Hobbes was diagnosed with advanced cancer, the level of knowledge was basic.[84] After a number of months in Binsar and then the long journey back, she arrived at Colaba War Hospital where she underwent an exploratory laparotomy on 19 February 1918. There is no question of the surgery being successful or not because on discovery of the cancer the surgeon would have had no option but to close the wound. Surgery for someone in an advanced stage of cancer is painful and traumatic and was likely to have accelerated her death.

Narrelle Hobbes longed to see her family and Australia again, but despite the best efforts of her colleagues and family she died aboard HMAHS *Kanowna* at ten o'clock on 10 May 1918, only approximately four days from Fremantle, WA. Her burial was a simple affair. A Church of England chaplain, her sister Elsie, who had travelled to India, and a ship full of soldiers and nurses witnessed her body, wrapped in linen, deposited into the water.[85] Her mother and family had her letters as a remembrance. The letter written to her 'darling people' dated 25 September 1916 recounting how she had reportedly died and been buried at sea must have seemed sadly prescient.

29 Controversy at 34 Welsh General Hospital, Deolali, India, 1917-1918

What a history Australia will have to tell after the war is over– Anne Donnell

Another outpost in India was 34 Welsh General Hospital (34 WGH) located 280km from Bombay. Nurses caught the train for approximately four hours, arriving at a major military depot for troops and a 2,000 bed hospital. The hospital spanned approximately three by one kilometres and consisted of old barracks, galvanised huts and stone bungalows. No air conditioning in these buildings was a major problem as the hot season in March-June had an average temperature of 35°C while the coldest month of January had a range of 13-31°C. The photographs show a desolate area with no trees or gardens to reduce the heat or lighten the senses. This was a harsh placement for AANS nurses but fortunately they were led by two remarkable women: Acting Matron Alma Bennett and Principal Matron Gertrude Davis.[1]

Acting Matron Alma Bennett: Biography

Biographical information about Alma Louise Bennett is thin on the ground. She was born in Beechworth, Victoria in 1877 and recorded her age as 38 years when she enlisted. She had trained at a Melbourne hospital. Given her age it can be assumed she was a competent civilian nurse with many years' experience when she was accepted for Indian Service in August 1916. Sister Bennett sailed on RMS *Mooltan* that same month with PM Gertrude Davis in-charge. There are no photographs of Alma but in 1916 she had a fair complexion with blue eyes and brown hair. Her build was slight as she weighed 66 kg with a height of 170cm. On arrival she served at a number of hospitals in Bombay but in May 1917 she was promoted to Acting Matron, 34 WGH, when her leadership skills came to the fore.[2]

34 WGH, Deolali, India: May to December 1917

Fortunately, Alma left a detailed account of her experience at 34 WGH immediately after the war. This account is, in the main, accurate. It was after less than one year of service in India, she *...was then informed that I had been appointed as matron in charge of the 34th Welsh General Hospital, Deolali containing 3000 beds, 4 hours train journey from Bombay and staffed by Imperial Sisters, who had recd. urgent orders for Mesopotamia.* She found it difficult to ensure her nurses were given adequate rest especially as the climate was particularly enervating and the risk of disease ever present. She records that *...each week we recd. convoys and September found us with 2188 patients. My staff had been increased 59 Australian Sisters & 15 Indian Temporary Nurses – 74 in all including myself, my assistant H[ead] Sister & Home Sister, Mess Sister & massage Sister leaving 68 for duty, both day and night. No more staff was available and I was at a loss how to relieve the pressure of work, for everyone was going at high tension, if not with actual acute cases, dealing with numbers.*

Smallpox

Given the workload the last thing she needed was a series of epidemics. She describes the complexity of dealing with the situation by writing ... *at that time also, an outbreak of small pox occurred in one of the wards, followed in three weeks time by an outbreak of plague in another wd. Thus began a strenuous and anxious time – all the Sisters, medical officers and orderlies having to be vaccinated against small pox & inoculated against plague, also all the patient contacts. The vaccinations against small pox were in most cases unsuccessful and it was fortunate that all the attacks were all of a mild nature. The patients were immediately taken to a marquee & isolated, the Sisters nursing them sharing the same fate. No deaths occurred. We were not so successful with the plague. Deaths occurred within 48 hours and we rec. orders to evacuate the whole of the nursing division 1600 patients. The convalescent division and Officers hospital of 40 beds remained as they were, being quite apart from the nursing division.*[3]

Smallpox, also known as Variola, is an extremely contagious viral disease which often proves fatal to those who come into contact with it. The virus is transmitted by droplets from the nose, throat and the fluid which forms blisters on the skin. Obviously nurses were particularly vulnerable and the most effective management was quarantine.

Bubonic Plague

Once the smallpox outbreak was under control, Alma Bennett and her staff faced another medical emergency. Bubonic plague is transmitted by fleas which are often carried by rats, or by droplet infection between humans in the case of pneumonic plague. The bacillus *Pasteurella pestis* is now treated with streptomycin but isolation of infected patients and the management of their symptoms was the only treatment option in 1914–18. The contagious nature of the disease often resulted in entire populations being wiped out, so a prompt response at the early stages of the outbreak was essential.

Once the patients were isolated their symptoms, including acute, painful swellings of the lymph nodes, chills, fever, vomiting, thirst, headache and generalised pain were managed.[4] Alma Bennett directed her nurses to ensure … *all the bed cases were to be accommodated in the new building then in the course of erection for the 44th BGH one mile distant, "up cases" to be accommodated in tents and marquees to no.6 camp about ¼ of a mile further on. I was nominally appointed o/c while they were there, with orders to detail any staff as they were required. There were several patients who could not be moved so they were left with us. The evacuation took place November 1st and everything went off quite smoothly and quickly. The Sisters were conveyed daily to the 44th in ambulances, dining in our own mess and occupying their own quarters. The duty hours were as usual, 2 hours off in the morning of their long day & every other ½ day – whole day a month. The CO of the 44th BGH was already there, also the medical officers having come down from Rawalpindi 4 days journey a few weeks previously, awaiting completion of their new hospital. They carried on the treatment of the patients, our own medical officers attending to the camp cases, Couval [illegible] Div & Officers Hospital. In the meantime our wards were thoroughly cleaned & the walls limed. At the end of three weeks all was ready to receive patients again.*

Acting Matron Bennett was diligent about providing sufficient detail in her narrative because the evacuation of a hospital due to an outbreak of plague was an atypical event in the career of an Australian nurse in 1917. The practical aspects of the management of such a situation warranted a comprehensive description. Shortly after the outbreaks of smallpox and plague were controlled, …*Christmas was then near & the hospital quiet, large numbers in but nothing particularly worrying. We gave up the whole day to make it a memorable one for the patients and I feel sure they enjoyed the whole day and greatly appreciated all that had been done for them. We had our Christmas dinner 8.30pm, 85 Sisters, including myself sitting down to our plentiful meal and I felt a glow of pride as I looked round on all those bright eager faces. They had proved so staunch & loyal in many busy, anxious days & night.*[5]

Background to Events: October 1917 to April 1918.

The early stage of 1918 was a turning point as these staunch and loyal nurses endured a series of accusations made against five of their number. The Australian nurses found to their detriment that a failure to understand the cultural and religious paradigms of those they were nursing created serious problems. In 1918 accusations of immoral behaviour were made by an English, male medico who was the officer-in-charge of 34 WGH, against five Australian nurses.[6]

The former officer-in-charge AW Sheen had earned the respect of Acting Matron Bennett and her staff but his replacement, Colonel Seddon only earned their contempt. Christmas was over and 1918 ushered in a New Year full of activity including a Vice-Regal visit.

Acting Matron Bennett recalls that …*Jan 2nd 1918 was to be a busy and interesting day. The Viceroy of India and staff (Lord Chelmsford) was paying a visit to the hospital. The visit has been promised and arranged when our former O.C. Col. A.W. Sheen was in command, so altho he had given up the command, he paid many visits to the hospital in his present capacity consulting surgeon, still as keenly interested as ever in the hospital he so splendidly organised in 1916 and carried on successfully until Oct. 1917. Both Mrs Sheen and himself were present to welcome the Viceroy and party, also our present O.C. Col. A.W.Maturin RAMC and Mrs Maturin.*

This narrative clearly establishes another officer-in-charge, Colonel Maturin, was in place when the plague and smallpox epidemic occurred and Colonel Seddon had not yet taken charge of the hospital. After the Viceroy visit in January, Alma Bennett goes on to describe her rationale for enabling her staff leave. She claims *...I allowed none of the Sisters leave during these months but as soon as good weather set in I arranged their leave. In early March we were inundated with Officers coming in suffering from Scarlet Fever, coming from the officers' convalescent hospital ... (of 60 beds) 7 miles away. We had to move all our patients into the corrugated iron & wood bungalows which I might state we do not use during the hot months, March to Nov. unless compelled. However, there was nothing else to be done.*

In some ways it is unfortunate that Acting Matron Bennett decided in ... *March and April I took my leave, the first time I had taken any leave whilst at the 34th ... The weather by this time was unbearably hot and I was really glad to leave the heat for 30 days, having waited over 12 months for leave, the Senior Sister carrying on my work in my absence.* Therefore it was during Acting Matron Bennett's absence that the new Officer-in-Charge, Colonel Seddon, gathered evidence that would be used against the nurses.

The Accusations: 7 May 1918

Acting Matron Bennett ... found the hospital very quiet on my return, but many changes amongst the personnel. Some of the medical officers had gone on to Mesopotamia to relieve others who had been there 2 years without relief.[7] On Tuesday evening, 7 May 1918, Acting Matron Alma Bennett was sent for by the Camp Commandant, Colonel Seddon. Colonel Seddon gave her a slip of paper with the names of five Australian nurses and an accusation that they were implicated in immoral conduct. Commander Seddon's quiet word to Acting Matron Bennett about the conduct of the nurses backfired dramatically. Not only did she not believe him, she sent a cable to PM Gertrude Davis, who made an immediate overnight train journey to the 34 WGH from Bombay. After interviewing the accused nurses, who refuted the allegations, the two nurse leaders demanded an inquiry to clear their reputations.[8]

Colonel Seddon believed the evidence of a Turkish interpreter, Signor Martirossi, who claimed the nurses behaved immorally with soldiers. One nurse was charged with intimate relationship with a Turkish prisoner-of-war, an orderly and a lower caste Indian. This interpreter for the hospital's Turkish prisoners was the main witness against the nurses. The charge against one nurse was that *...she was in familiar relations with the English patients in this Ward. Later on I was told by the same Turkish prisoners (by 2 of them) that one night they saw her in an empty tent in the arms of a "Mehtar". I could not believe this charge.*[9] It was a shame he did not believe it.

Implications of the Accusations

To place the situation in a religious, social and cultural paradigm: A female, Christian nurse was accused by three Islamic males who were the enemy during a world war of behaving in a promiscuous manner with a Hindi lower caste Indian male. The evidence was accepted and the charges were pursued with a vengeance by a male British Medico who found the Australian laxness about respecting the status of officers difficult to accept.[10]

To put the seriousness of the charges in perspective for the Australian nurses, it is necessary to consider appropriate behaviour for AANS nurses at the time. For example, the AANS Matron-in-Chief, Evelyn Conyers, heard reports that nurses from 14 AGH in Egypt had been behaving in an untoward manner by keeping late hours, taking wine in public places and smoking on the verandah while on duty. In response to Miss Conyers' claims, Matron Rose Creal promptly replied that there was no substance to the rumours: Leave passes ceased at 11 pm and nurses only took wine with their meals in restaurants and hotels, not public places.[11] She was quick to point out that no Sisters would dare smoke in a public place as they were aware that the consequences would be a return trip to Australia immediately.[12] It is not difficult to imagine the distress that charges of behaving in a sexually promiscuous manner would have caused these unmarried women in 1918.

The Court Case

Colonel Seddon's original note contained the names of four AANS nurses and one temporary nurse, Miss Alston, from the St John's Ambulance Service. However, on arrival in court after travelling for *...50 hrs thro' the most appalling heat ...*Sister McClean was excused as she was not the Sister the main witness had identified.[13] Daphne and Claudine Cadwallader were sisters and when the main witness informed the court that neither Daphne nor Claudine were implicated, they requested a written apology. They were both excused and it is unclear if they ever received their apology.[14] Therefore, the three remaining AANS nurses, McAleer, Kellaway and Bell plus Miss Alston had to attend court and face the charge levelled against them.

The transcripts of the court case make distressing reading but the findings of Colonel Fetherston, Director-General of the Australian Army Medical Service, who conducted an investigation into the charges and subsequent court case about six months later, provides an excellent summary. In part, he found when *...about to sail from Colombo I received from Defence, Melbourne, copies of papers which had been sent to Australia by the Viceroy of India without having been seen by the nurses concerned or by the Principal Matron ... In fact they had asked for copies and had been refused; therefore they could not forward any statement to you. I had previously gone into this matter very fully, interviewed all the nurses concerned, all those who could furnish any information on the subject, and had also seen the Officer in Charge Deolali Hospital ... I also saw the Chaplain of Deolali Hospital who had taken a great interest in the cases and was one of the very few who gave any help or assistance to the nurses who were falsely charged ... The papers showed that every nurse was completely cleared of any imputation, but the treatment they received from the authorities in Bombay and Deolali Brigade, as the district is known, was, in my opinion, scandalous. General Knight, the general officer commanding the district, allowed these vile accusations to be made the subject of inquiry without taking the least trouble to verify them or to find out what evidence and what class of evidence was to be produced ... When seen by Principal Matron Davis, he tried to excuse himself and stated that the whole trouble was caused by the nurses demanding a inquiry. The court ... consisted of four members and not one word of help was given except from one member, a combatant officer. In fact everyone seems to have taken the whole matter as settled and proved without trial.*

Insinuations at the inquiry were made and not allowed to be contradicted at the court. Hearsay evidence was admitted. No one was allowed to be with the nurses in court, and Sister McAleer had to sit alone for hours in the presence of several officers and hear the vile charges made against her without anyone as a companion.
One insinuation was made by Colonel Seddon that nurses had visited immoral houses. Two nurses, Sisters, (not those included in the charges) had one occasion gone to afternoon tea with the widow of a non-commissioned officer … Whilst at this house a Sergeant Clerk came. They were only there a short time on one afternoon and knew nothing of anything wrong at the place and still believe it was and is a perfectly reputable home. This seems to have been the real origin of the attack on our nurses. Speaking to a non-commissioned officer, which in the eyes of many imperial officers is an unpardonable sin, and not being able to prove anything against these two nurses, the Camp Commandant started a foreign spy to work, who, to show his zeal and acumen trumped up some cases and told lies…In justice to the Australian nurses, I consider that further action should be taken to ensure their protection or else they should be withdrawn from India…Not one word of sympathy was spoken to any of the nurses and not a word written by those in authority…This matter was brought under the notice of these officials by me and one and all expressed regret and tried to excuse their neglect for various reasons, but when their action was explained to General Sir G C Monro, Commander-in-Chief, he was also indignant and at once volunteered to write and did write a letter of sympathy to the nurse.[15]

Cultural Conflict

While General Fetherston may be correct in his analysis of why a British officer treated the Australian nurses with such disrespect because they failed to heed the policy of not speaking to an NCO, the reason why the Turkish prisoners-of-war (POW) turned against the Australian nurses may relate to an earlier misunderstanding. The AANS nurses treated the POWs very well and had endeavoured to accommodate their cultural and religious beliefs under trying circumstances. However, when Principal Matron Davis accepted the POWs from the Red Crescent ship the *Firefly* (which had previously been captured from the British) there was a great deal of interest by the Turkish officers about the nurses' badges of rank. Principal Matron Davis writes the … *T.O.s* [Turkish Officers] *were amused at our* *badges of rank and the conclusion they came to was: - That I was the wife of a captain; the sisters wives of 1st Lieuts. and the s/nurses wives of 2nd Lieuts. We did not bother to disillusion them.* Therefore, all the Turkish POWs believed the Australian nurses were married women.

Language Difficulties and Miscommunication

The reason why the Indian 'spy' may have been so persistent in undermining the respectability of the Australian nurses may relate to an earlier misunderstanding about the caste system that is part of the Hindu religion and culture. When Principal Matron Davis arrived at Victoria War Hospital in Bombay with her AANS nurses *...there was no matron to give any information as when I took over she was ill ... the ward work was performed by native servants of different castes and the main difficulties with them was to know what their duties were. There were ward boys who did the dusting, washing of lockers and dishes. Bhestis, who carried water to and from the patients. Sweepers, who swept floors and attended the latrines. Many were the mistakes made at first and as none of these servants could speak English and the sisters did not know Hindustani so all communication had to be made by sign and gesture.*

In retrospect it is surprising that more problems were not caused by the lack of preparation of the Australian nurses. They were expected to manage an 800 bed hospital during wartime when the staff did not speak the same language; they were required to understand the intricacies of the Hindu culture through sign and gesture; they provided personal body care to male Islamic POWs who believed they were married Christian women. These incidents occurred earlier than the Deolali accusations but Principal Matron Davis makes a quick but important point *...we never had less than 500 T.P. of W. ...the 34th WGH Deolali, which I shall mention later took most of them.*[16]

The above observations are mentioned as a possible explanation for the events at Deolali and are not intended to excuse or blame any party. General Fetherston's reference to the need for an apology to one particular nurse was justified. The charges against her, which she had to sit in court alone and listen to, included that she had sexual relations with a number of soldiers, orderlies, POWs and a lower caste Indian who was a sweeper. The charges were so damaging to her reputation that when asked in court if she had any statement to make she replied that... *"I am not guilty of any of the accusations made and I have nothing further to state except that I consider that I have completely vindicated myself by my consent to be examined by a Medical Board."* This nurse, a member of the AANS, signed a consent form on 14 May 1918 which gave permission for a Medical Board, consisting of three male doctors, to examine her at the Sisters Quarters of 34 WGH. The result of the medical examination is recorded as ...*The Board having assembled pursuant to order, proceed to examine the above named nurse and found that she is "virgo intacta"*. All charges of immoral behaviour against her were dismissed.[17] The nurse was not given the opportunity to charge her accusers with unethical behaviour.

The Cover-Up

The injustice of the accusations was matched by the ability of the Army to keep the entire incident quiet. Historian, Jan Bassett, claimed ...*The matrons' discretion was such that neither Miss Davis nor Miss Bennett even mentioned the inquiry at Deolali in their later accounts of their wartime experiences written for the official medical historian.*[18] However, the evidence that Principal Matron Davis and Acting Matron Bennett were ordered to withhold information about the incident is overwhelming. This was achieved through censorship because the Viceroy of India considered it desirable to avoid scandal and publicity.[19]

Despite all of the charges against the Australian nurses being dropped due to lack of evidence and mistaken identity, the three nurse leaders —Acting Matron Bennett, Matron-in-Chief Conyers and Principal Matron Davis —do not mention the incident in their narratives and the medical historian, Colonel Butler also omits the inquiry from the Official History.[20]

Even after this trauma the nurses did not receive apologies or an opportunity to vent their anger. Sister McClean who was mistakenly identified as one of the accused nurses makes a vague reference to her time at Deolali as being unpleasant.[21] Claudine Cadwallader claimed that during her time at the 34 Welsh General ... *Matron & Nursing Staff were Australians and the male personnel RAMC, but it worked extremely well'*.[22] This claim is incongruous with the court proceedings that indicate she and her sister, Daphne, requested a written apology for being falsely accused. Furthermore, Daphne Cadwallader makes mention of the incident in a letter to her parents at the time of the inquiry. She writes there … *has been a Great Scandal (that all ended in smoke) in Deolali; Avenal will send you the letters telling you all about it. It was an amazing thing – like a cheap novelette, & the Australian Sisters you – may bet your life – are going to have full reparations to say nothing of Sweet Revenge. Everyone is regarding us as perfect heroines, but we'd much rather they hadn't had the chance.*[23]

Tragically there were neither reparations nor sweet revenge. Just silence.

Consequences

There was no personnel reference to Colonels Seddon, Sheen or Maturin or Acting Matron Alma Bennett by the official medical historian. Principal Matron Gertrude Davis had a distinguished career and she is mentioned a number of times but there is no reference to the Deolali incident.[24] However, the decision to censor the incident does not mean the Army did not take the situation seriously and a fair assessment would be that it was a political decision, not a military one.

General Fetherston was instructed by the Secretary of the AIF to make a full inquiry into the matter by visiting India on his way back to Australia after a tour of inspection in Egypt.[25] General Fetherston did this with his usual vigour and his sense of outrage was ignited whenever members of the AANS were treated unjustly. In many ways General Fetherston was a true advocate for the AANS nurses.[26] He has been criticised for implementing policies such as making nurses wear symbols of rank and thereby inadvertently preventing them from having social contact with non-commissioned officers. However, there is little evidence that this was his intention.[27] His reports are littered with expressions of frustration at the lack of consideration given to the nurses in places like Lemnos, Salonika, India and at the frozen CCS's in France. They are also full of praise for the good sense and straight thinking that many of the AANS nurses displayed when faced with such adversity.[28]

Nevertheless, the Deolali incident was different because these nurses were not enduring hardships because they were caring for soldiers who needed them. They were being victimised and it was not in the nature of the AANS nurse to relinquish the role of advocate and adopt that of a victim. The request to General Fetherston was sent some three months after the inquiry and there is evidence that the nurses at 34 WGH had begun to express their outrage by sending their account of the situation to civilians in Australia. An extract of a letter dated 6 June 1918 was obviously written by a nurse at 34 WGH but the name, signature or any other identifying marks have been removed.[29] This letter was attached to correspondence from a Melbourne solicitor to the Acting Prime Minister, WA Watt, and reads in part that the *...lady who has written the enclosed to me is known to me as an exceedingly conscientious and capable woman. She struggled hard to become qualified as a Nurse so that she might give her services to her country in this war. You will see from the enclosed how disgracefully these women have been treated.*[30] Those in authority were outraged but the result was the same — silence. The matter had already been brought to the attention of the Deputy Chief Censor in May 1918 by the Viceroy of India who believed it was *...desirable avoid scandal or publicity and trust measures will be taken in Australia with conformity this end.*[31]

Rumours of the matter did reach Australia.[32] The *Sydney Bulletin* published a small article on 1 August 1918 outlining the snobbishness of civilians in India to the private soldier and how negative rumours about the conduct of Australian nursing sisters had begun to circulate. The article makes no reference to the Deolali incident but was noted by the AIF and a copy of the article was included in the archival file relating to the accusations.[33]

Influenza Pandemic: 34 WGH: 1918

Acting Matron Alma Bennett continues her narrative in August 1918 recalling that*...everything went on quietly until August when the Spanish Influenza made its appearance in the station. We were getting in all the local admission cases, as the 44th BGH had been converted into an isolation hospital the previous month. There were thousands of troops in the station, so we began to be busy again. In September it was at its worst. Continuing until Oct. and Nov. Until that time the health of my staff had been excellent but early in Oct. they were attacked with influenza having been then nursing the cases some* *weeks they were tired and soon fell victims, 18 being off duty at one time. To my intense regret one of my staff nurses died Oct. 17th from pneumonia following influenza, only five days ill. Another on the D.I. [dangerously ill] list for 5 weeks had a tremendous fight for her life and ultimately made a good recovery. I had a sick Sisters hospital attached to the hospital and it was a veritable haven of rest to those poor tired Sisters after the distressing time they had had.*[34]

Emily Clare Biography: 1890- 1918

The deterioration in the quality of media reporting during the twentieth century can be appreciated when the *Stawell News* (Victoria, Djab Wurrang Country) was quoting John Locke's treatise on education when reporting the dancing accomplishments of the local children on 17 November 1900. One such child was Emily Clare who had turned ten years old the previous September and on the night in question not only *...danced an Irish jig which brought down the house...* but managed to compose herself later in the evening when she performed a *...graceful skirt dance.* The reporter claimed that, according to the philosopher John Locke (1632-1704), the effect of dance on children like young Emily was *...not confined to the body, and that it gives to children not mere outward gracefulness of motion, but many thoughts, and a becoming confidence.*[35] It is difficult to fully appreciate if Miss Bates' dancing lessons were solely responsible for Emily's confidence but she needed a degree of self-confidence in 1917 when she left Australia to serve with the AANS in India.

Emily had two older brothers and one younger as well as four older sisters, making her the youngest daughter and giving her a special place in this large Catholic family. Her mother Mary and father Peter were married in Albury (NSW, Wiradjuri Country) in 1874 but most of the children were born in Victoria. Emily was born at Footscray (Victroia, Kulin Nation) on 11 September 1890 and baptized in 1904.[36] She attended Footscray State School until she enrolled at the Stawell State School in July 1899 where she remained until mid-1902. She left just prior to her twelfth birthday to go and live with her maternal uncle, Henry Edhouse, who owned a brewery and was a local councillor. Given that her father was deceased when she enlisted with the AANS it is possible that she was sent to live with her uncle to reduce the financial pressure on her widowed mother. Emily remained with the family until she was old enough to commence her nurse training at the Stawell Hospital.[37] On completion of her three-year nurse training she worked at the Caulfield Military Hospital and was finally accepted to join the AIF on 7 November 1917. Irene McPhail and Emily Clare boarded HMT *Canberra* in Sydney on 16 November 1917 as reinforcements for 14 AGH. En route Kathleen McAleer boarded in Fremantle. However, when the *Canberra* arrived in India the nurses were both dispatched for duty to different locations.[38]

Emily Clare had been at 34 WGH when her colleagues, including Kathleen McAleer, had been unjustly charged. She worked throughout the inquiry and nursed soldiers and POWs suffering from cholera, smallpox, bubonic plague and finally influenza, which compounded with exhaustion, caused her own death. Her family received word that she was dangerously ill, but by the time the telegram reached them she had died at the family hospital which was attached to 34 WGH. Emily was buried in the Roman Catholic section of the Camp Cemetery of the Deolali Government Cemetery (M.2.22) on 17 October 1918 – she was twenty-eight years old.[39]

Her family and community mourned her passing, as did her nursing colleagues. Her name appears on many honour boards in Stawell and on the Roll of Honour at the Australian War Memorial. Her uncle (who loved her like a daughter) ensured she would not be forgotten, by having her name included on the tombstone of her maternal grandmother. The inscription reads …*Nurse Emily Clare – died on active service in India 17th October 1918, aged 28 years – Deeply regretted. She made the supreme sacrifice.*[40]

Irene McPhail

On completion of her training Irene McPhail enlisted with the AANS (3 MD) in South Yarra (Bunurong Boon Wurrung Country & Wurundjeri Woi-wurrung Country) and travelled overland to join her unit's ship, HMT *Canberra,* which departed from Sydney on 16 November 1917.[41] Irene designated her paternal aunt, Josephine MacNeece from Rhode Island (who was married with two children and living in Australia), as her next-of-kin. Despite the expense of life in India she allocated forty per cent of her net salary to her aunt while on overseas service, seemingly conscious of the ongoing financial burden endured by those at home.[42] After four-and-a-half months service in India, Irene McPhail developed a persistent cough and became languid, easily tired. Her voice was weaker from laryngitis and she was losing weight rapidly. While at Poona, phthisis (pulmonary tuberculosis) was diagnosed so she was transferred to Egypt, as a patient aboard HMHS *Devanha,* and had a medical board assessment at 14 AGH, Port Said, on 1 June 1918.[43] A decision was made to transfer her back to Australia aboard the HMAHS *Kanowna* on 22 July because her condition was considered so serious that ...*the medical officers had grave doubts that she will live to reach Australia.*[44] On her return to Australia she was admitted to 11 AGH, Caulfield, where she had worked before enlisting and received excellent nursing care and had worked before overseas service.[45]

Leaving India: November 1918

Some of these poor, tired nurses were given the opportunity to leave India and they took it. Acting Matron Bennett recounts that ...*Nov. 18th I recd. orders for 16 of my staff to report to Head Quarters Bombay in 24 hours for embarkation to UK. The excitement was intense – after waiting so long it had at last come. I forgot to mention that 13 Sisters were transferred to Egypt in Sept. and not replaced so you can see I was very short of staff during the epidemic. Nov. 24th again urgent orders for 8 more Sisters to report Head qrs. for embarkation to UK including myself if I wished to go. Needless to say I reported to head qrs. With the Sisters already mentioned. 20 Sisters having reported to me for duty a few days previously just arrived from Australia. Miss A. Scott of the AANS having come aboard in 1914 & returned to Australia taking* the *position rendered vacant by my transfer to UK so ended my Indian Service, also my rank as Matron. I reverted to my former rank of Sister on choosing to leave India, having received my promotion in India for Indian service only.*[46]

It is difficult to imagine a nurse leader who better deserved to retain her promotion. While the AWM refers to her as achieving the rank of ...*Matron...* there is no evidence of this in her Service Record. If every Sister of the AANS had the capacity to lead her staff under such trying conditions as Alma Bennett, it is little wonder that the reputation of the AANS was one of excellence.[47] Alma Bennet had the good sense and kindness to choose Kathleen McAleer to accompany her to England in November 1918.

Kathleen McAleer Biography: 1892-1977

Unlike many of her colleagues Kathleen McAleer lived a long life. Born in Broken Hill (NSW, Wilyakali Country) in 1892 her family had moved to Western Australia, where she commenced her training at Perth Public Hospital. ATNA qualified and having attained the position of Charge Nurse before she enlisted in August 1917 Kathleen was ready for military service when she embarked on HMT *Canberra* at Fremantle on 23 November 1917. Aged just 26 years Kathleen had a dark complexion including brown hair and eyes. She was of medium build being 165 cm tall and weighing 58 kg. She nursed in Bombay for a few months and was sent to 34 WGH in January 1918. As previously noted, this was a time of change. After enduring the ordeal of being unjustly accused of immoral behaviour, this young Catholic woman continued her work with no time off or special leave. She just got on with it.

Fortunately, she was enabled to leave for the UK with Acting Matron Alma Bennett on 18 November 1918, a month after the funeral of Emily Clare. A short stop-over in Egypt saw the Indian contingent board SS *Kaiser-i-Hind* for the UK arriving on 12 January 1919 at which time Kathleen was despatched to 3AAH, Dartford. A few months later she was accepted as a midwifery student at the Rotunda Hospital in Dublin where she underwent her training from 24 April to 24 October 1919. On her return to England she was granted leave before RTA aboard HMT *Matatua* arriving in Perth on 28 January 1920. It would appear that Katheen McAleer was an extremely healthy woman who did not suffer any ill-effects, physically or psychologically from her military service.

It is known that she was nursing at the Prince of Wales Hospital in Randwick, a suburb of Sydney, in the 1930s. A military hospital during the war, it was later a repatriation hospital and many military nurses elected to continue caring for returned soldiers. It would appear that Kathleen was such a nurse. She did eventually return to Perth where she resided until her death in 1977 aged 86 years. She is buried at the Karrakatta Cemetery in the RC section.[48]

Conclusion

The Commonwealth War Graves Commission refers to the Kirkee Memorial, located at Poona near Mumbai, which ...commemorates more than 1,800 servicemen who died in India during the First World War, who are buried in civil and cantonment cemeteries in India and Pakistan where their graves can no longer be properly maintained.[49] Kitty Power, Alma O'Grady, Emily Clare and Letitia Moreton fall within this category of ...servicemen.

Australian nurses in India were not confronted by the horror of nursing soldiers with severe battle wounds, shell-shock or the effects of gas. However, the AANS nurses went to one of the more incapacitating climates to care for soldiers from all religious and ethnic persuasions. Furthermore, nurses who endured unjust treatment, like those who served at Deolali, deserve to have their experiences validated. At a military level, service in India may not have captured the imagination of the Australian psyche in the same way as *Anzac*, *Beersheba* or *Pozieres* but from a nursing perspective the adverse conditions endured by our number deserves a place in our history.

30 War is Over but Peace is Elusive

... Horror it is and carnage, yet are both
Part of the price of peace- Cpl. Comus, *The Anzac Book*

Despite the carnage of Gallipoli, the fledgling Australian nation embraced the experience as evidence of collective courage. The Gallipoli Campaign was a failure from the Allied perspective, but ironically it was on a ...*British dreadnought in Mudros on the Aegean island of Lemnos*... where the Turks surrendered unconditionally to the British at the end of October 1918.[1] The armistice was formally accepted as 11 November 1918 but 1918 was a year of turmoil for the global population.

By promoting veracity in intellectual discourse within society, free thinkers were enabled to contribute to improvements in health, economics, science, technology and a number of other disciplines. The war promoted dramatic advances in medicine, nursing and allied health areas such as physiotherapy and psychology. Claims that war provides the impetus for improvements in health cannot be judiciously dismissed, but if the same rationale is applied to all areas of discourse it could be claimed, for instance, that global economic depressions are useful in improving the financial knowledge base. There must be better ways to learn such lessons.

St Paul's Cathedral, London, was chosen to hold a Roll of Honour which included the names of 350 nurses from all parts of the Commonwealth. Beside their names was written their cause of death. Simple words – 'drowned', 'died of wounds', 'accidentally killed' and next to the name 'Edith Cavell' the word 'executed'.[2] The price of peace was endured throughout the lifetimes of partners, children, parents, siblings, friends.

Treaty of Versailles

The administration of the peace was a complex process and at a global level it was not particularly well done. After the war a frustrated John Maynard Keynes left negotiations at Versailles and wrote *'The Economic Consequences of the Peace'*. He foreshadowed the impact that Article 231 — that related to German war guilt and reparations included in the Treaty of Versailles — would have on Germany. Professor Sir Hew Strachan claims *...there was no inevitable link between it* [the Treaty] *and the outbreak of a second war twenty years later.*[1542] However, it can be argued that the failure of the victors to restore a level of self-sufficiency within Germany did expose the German people to the competing political agendas of Fascists and Communists in the 1920s.[4]

Administrating the Peace

Four years after their dinner in Egypt, Alice Kitchen and Evelyn Conyers had endured very different wars: Conyers as Matron-in-Chief of the AANS stationed in London (16 January 1916 - 6 March 1920), and Kitchen as a front-line nurse in France. The responsibilities of Conyers included *...postings, promotion, pay, discipline, leave, invaliding, reinforcements and other concerns of AANS members in Egypt, England and Europe (not including Salonika).*[5] Despite her heavy workload, AANS nurses who arrived in London for duty were required to pay their respects and report to the Matron-in-Chief.[6]

Evelyn Conyers was not a distant administrator but a nurse leader. She was often in France with Maud McCarthy reviewing the conditions being endured by her nurses. Neither she nor McCarthy recoiled from the danger of the front-line.[7] This did not stop nurses perceiving her job to be cushy and merely *...watching other people work.*[8] By the time the war was at an end even her dinner companion in Egypt, Alice Kitchen, grew *...increasingly bitter towards Australians and Australian hospital administration.*[9] Nurses who served under a variety of services such as British, Canadian or French became more judgmental of their own leaders. The war gave them an opportunity to make comparisons and to learn from other mentors. Tragically, not all mentors survived.

'I am her mother': The Death of Nellie Miles Walker

Apart from the identity of those who died in the war there was occasionally confusion about the next-of-kin. Every member of the AIF had to make a will before they left for overseas service. They had to also clearly state their next-of-kin, but just as circumstances changed during a war for those who were sent overseas, so too did family situations at home. This was a time when patriarchy reigned and a father was the assumed next-of-kin ahead of the mother.

In October 1918 Matron Miles Walker was in London nursing the ever-growing numbers of influenza victims when she became ill and died. Her death was keenly felt and Anne Donnell, who had experienced her kindnesss, recorded that we *...have just lost one of our Matrons from this terrible influenza – Miss Myles-Walker* [sic]. *She was such a fine woman, and all we Nursing Sisters abroad have indeed lost a friend. Matron and I have just returned from her funeral at Sutton Veny. It was a military funeral and very representative. The coffin was draped with the Union Jack, but when I saw her red cape and white cap lying on top of the beautiful wreath of flowers it fairly broke me up.*[10]

Her Anglican burial at the Sutton Veny churchyard was well attended by her colleagues and when the Armistice was declared Anne Donnell could not shake a heavy heart.[11] She confided to her matron that she would give anything to feel happy and the matron empathetically replied that she understood because *...we must not forget in our joy to think of others in their sorrow.*[12] Nellie Miles Walker was the most senior AANS nurse to die and the tragedy of her death after four years of continuous service, within a fortnight of the Armistice, was apparent to her heart-broken mother.

Louisa Walker was unable to claim her daughter's personal possessions without first proving her relationship because her son, Albert, was the designated next-of-kin. The correspondence on this subject between the Army and Louisa Walker is both extensive and heart-wrenching. A particularly poignant remark displays the level of distress experienced by the grieving mother who *...was in close correspondence all those four years with my beloved daughter. Cheering and helping her and now to think there should be a doubt about me being her "Mother" ... the very smallest trifle belonging to my child is most precious to me, and I wish no other hand to touch it first. This may sound sentimental but if you have ever loved anyone deeply you will understand it.*[13]

The letters of Louisa Walker bring the grief felt by those who waited at home for more than four long years into sharp historical focus. To be robbed of the much anticipated reunion at the last moment reminds us that the millions of dead soldiers, nurses and civilians left behind a world filled with soul destroying grief.

Missing Presumed Dead

The scale of death during the war, combined with the slow process of family notification, often created an atmosphere of hope that a mistake had been made even when the dreaded knock on the door came. The only positive confirmation of death came from a nurse or a comrade who was present at the time of death. Nurses spent much of their spare time writing to the relatives of soldiers who had died. Matrons were particularly conscientious when it came to reassuring relatives that their charges had been well cared for up to the time of their death.[14] When a nurse died they were even more diligent because they felt responsible for the health and welfare of their nurses.

It was a natural hope that when the war was over the missing son or daughter would just walk through the door. The brother of Edith Jackson (AANS), who served in Salonika, went missing during a battle. His father wrote to the Defence Department in 1920 seeking any possessions belonging to his missing son. He was informed that a ...*Court of Inquiry...* had judged his son, Private HC Jackson (37 Battalion), to have been ...*Killed in Action.*[15] Such an unverified judgement was not easy to accept.

The words 'presumed drowned' also left scope for doubt about whether the nurse or soldier was actually on the ship when it sank. Transport nursing was difficult and hazardous because of the U-boat risk and sea mines which littered the waterways like confetti. The following summary of ships which were sunk during the war provides a snapshot of the risk of sea travel for wounded soldiers and non-combatant nurses.

Salta

While stationed at 26 General Hospital in France, Sister Trantar (AANS) recorded in her diary on 28 June 1917 that we ...*had to attend the funeral this morning of Sister*

Dawson. Her body was washed up near our camp. She was on a hospital ship that was torpedoed in the Channel. There were about one hundred Sisters and VADs present. The service was at the mortuary, then we all walked to the grave headed by three kilties playing the bagpipes. The coffin was covered in the Union Jack and flowers. After it was lowered 'Last Post' was sounded by two Jocks and two Tommies. This cemetery is beautiful, kept flowers on each grave, name, number, regiment and date of death of the soldiers on a plain wooden cross at the head.[16]

The person was most likely Matron Eveline M Dawson (QAIMNSR) who died, aged 49, on 10 April 1917. This was the same day that a number of QAs, who were serving on the *Salta,* were lost at sea.[17] The Chief Officer, who had shot himself when the *Salta* ran aground the previous year, was at least spared this tragedy which resulted in loss of life.[18]

Asturias

Similarly, on the night of 20-21 March 1917 the British hospital ship *Asturias* was torpedoed. British Staff Nurse J J Phillips drowned along with twelve RAMC orderlies; in total forty-one people perished at sea.[19] Initially she had been identified as an Australian nurse but she has since been acknowledged as a British sister and her name is recorded with two hundred QAIMNS colleagues who died during the First World War.[20]

Britannic

The *Britannic* was the sister ship of the *Titanic* and was refitted as a hospital ship transferring the wounded from the Dardanelles.[21] After finally being given the all clear for typhoid, Sarah Furnifull served on the *Britannic.* On arrival she was not required to immediately re-embark, but she was grieved when on the *...trip to Naples the* Britannic *was sunk, and two of my nursing friends were lost.*[22]

On Tuesday 21 November 1916 the *Britannic* sank in shallow water in the Kea Channel off the Aegean Sea at 9.07am. The shallow water caused the bow to hit the bottom before the rest of the ship. Unfortunately two lifeboats were launched far too early, causing them to be sucked into the still-turning propellers and resulting in the only deaths.[23] Of the 1,100 people on board only thirty died.[24] It is more likely Sarah's nursing colleagues were British as there is no record of Australian nurses perishing on the ship. However, they may have been unidentified Australian nurses who served with the QAs.

Glenart Castle

The *Glenart Castle* was where the youngest member of the AIF, Private James Martin, died of typhoid off the coast of Gallipoli on 25 October 1915.[25] Edith Blake, aged 32 and a trainee of the Coast Hospital (1908-12), was one of eight nurses and 162 people who presumably died when the ship was sunk on 26 February 1918.[26] It was a Union Castle ship (previously named *Galicia*) and was sunk by UC-56 near Lundy Island in the Bristol Channel during a voyage from South Wales to France.[27]

Edith's parents, Catherine and Charles (Chas) Blake, were from Sans Souci (NSW, Dharawal Country) and may have had a sense of security about her safety because their son, William, was residing in London during the war. Edith travelled to England and joined the QAIMNSR. There is no uncertainty about Edith Blake's death from a legal viewpoint due to the volume of correspondence from her mother and solicitor to the Army. There is little ambiguity about Edith Blake being one of the four Australian nurses who died while serving with the QAIMNSR.[28]

She suffered a traumatic death while doing her duty as a service nurse and although her physical remains are forever lost her name can be found at the Hollybrook Memorial, Southampton, and on the AWM Commemorative Roll.[29] The Coast Hospital history recorded that ...*Sister Enid* [sic] *Blake (1908-12) was reported missing probably drowned on 26th February 1917* [sic] *while on transport duty on the hospital ship 'Glenart Castle' which was torpedoed and sunk.*[30]

The last word

All too often the nurses had to relay to the parents of soldiers how their sons had died.[31] Olive Haynes (AANS) recorded that we ...*always write to their mothers if they die. I have had some of the sweetest letters from the poor mothers. I just love the Scotch people. They are fine. Some of the baby Jocks (as we call them) are only 16 or 17 – it is so sad to see them die. They are plucky little boys. You'd give anything or do anything to save them.*[32] Despite the sadness suffered by those who received news of the death of a daughter or a son during the war, it was harder for those who were illiterate to get news. The education level of nurses enabled them to read letters to, and write letters on behalf of, their soldier patients.[33]

The accuracy of the letters is debatable. When Vera Brittain's brother was killed she sought information about how and where he died, but when told by an Army official that he was shot through the head by an Austro-Hungarian sniper at the end stage of the war, she did not believe what she was hearing. She *...realised only too well from the agitated efforts of Army Sisters to mitigate truth with compassion in letters describing the last moments of men who had died in hospital – the colonels and company commanders on the various fronts were so weary of writing gruesome details to sorrowing relatives, that the number of officers who were instantaneously and painlessly shot through the head or the heart passed far beyond the grounds of probability.* However, when this version of events was confirmed by other independent sources she felt more confident about the veracity of the official account.[34]

Occasionally new friendships, founded upon the battlefield, ended abruptly when a wounded soldier left the regiment. The remaining men would reflect that they *...have had no letter ... but hardly expected one as he never wrote to anyone.*[35] Given the emphasis upon the mail it is surprising that a soldier would not write either to his family or to his mates if he had the literacy skills to do so. Soldiers and nurses on overseas service were desperate for news about family members and the events occurring in Australia. News from home was essential to the morale of troops, but during the First World War news was communicated through the written word. It was a cruel situation for those at home not to be able to write to a loved one in a war zone. It was tragic for those who could not read the telegram reporting their loved ones recovery or impending homecoming. They were unable to read of the injury or death which, in turn, rendered them powerless to dispute the accuracy of the words or be comforted by the written words of a nurse who witnessed the death.

Logistics of Marriage

When the war was over, the logistics of transferring AIF personnel home was complicated by the marriages of soldiers and an influx of children being born. Initially the soldiers had to pay the fare for any dependants, but when it became obvious that families were being separated because of the financial inability of soldiers to pay, the government relented and offered free passage if the marriage took place prior to 1 September 1919. The government expected to transport 6,000 dependents but the number swelled to 15,000.

Once aboard, men and women were berthed separately and each ship included a *...women's general hospital...* but *...nurses with midwifery training were scarce.*[36] Many AANS nurses did have a midwifery certificate but their recent nursing experience was in military surgery and infectious diseases - not midwifery. Experienced military nurses resented being assigned to family ships instead of military transports.[37] Nonetheless, nursing on the family ships was not easy. For instance, nurses were used to seeing dead soldiers and even their own colleagues draped in the Union Jack before being lowered into the water, but the sight of a three-month-old baby who had died of diphtheria being *...lowered into the stormy and raging sea...* was a whole new heart-breaking experience.[38]

Mary Harford and Catherine Adaway: Physical and Mental Health of Nurses

Nurses who remained in the UK awaiting transport duty continued to undertake non-military employment (NME) courses, or travel if they were due leave but were primarily nursing soldiers in auxiliary hospitals. Nurses who continued working were affected by the strain of the war. For instance, Matron Bessie Pocock was in-charge of 3 AAH, Dartford, when Mary Rosa Harford joined the staff. Mary was born in 1881, in Penrith (NSW, Mulgoa and Darug Country) and took up nursing on leaving school. On 8 October 1915, she enlisted with the AANS and was assigned to the Quarterly General Reinforcements, 2 AGH as a SN with Catherine Adaway. They left Sydney on HMAT *Orsova* the same month, served in Egypt at 2 AGH (Ghezireh) and left Alexandria on 26 March 1916, arriving at Marseilles on 4 April 1916. On arrival at Etaples, they served at 23 BGH and later at 2 AGH (Wimereux).

Mary was given leave in keeping with the new policy by DMS Howse in January and again in August 1917. During her second term of leave she was declared medically unfit for further service. This suggests she was adversely affected by service on the front line, because from August 1917 to April 1918 she nursed at 2 AAH (Southall) and then 3 AAH, Dartford. Significantly, 3 AAH was in Kent, where air-raids occurred. In April 1918, Matron Bessie Pocock recorded an incident in which Mary Harford refused to do night duty because she basically hated it. It is not difficult to conclude Mary suffered from PTSD and she was frightened to admit she had any form of mental health problems. She was a competent and experienced military nurse who was unwell. Following disciplinary interviews with Matron Pocock, the Commanding Officer and eventually DMS Howse, and Matron-in-Chief Conyers, she continued to refuse to perform night duty. She was placed under virtual arrest at Dartford and was not allowed to leave the hospital for more than one hour at any one time while she awaited transport back to Australia.[39] She returned to Australia in April 1918 and was discharged from the AIF in June of the same year.[40] The reason for such unusual behaviour was not forthcoming, but the claim by Matron Pocock that it was due to laziness lacks credence when Harford's war and post-war activities are considered.[41]

Mary Harford and Catherine Adaway (both RC) travelled extensively after the war, including in …*America, where as Australians, they were welcomed and promptly engaged to Nurse in various hospitals.* They nursed returned servicemen in a military hospital in Vancouver, Canada and then travelled to the USA including Seattle, Portland, Chicago, New York and San Francisco.[42] The extensive overseas trekking of Catherine Adaway was surprising given she served in Egypt and France where, following a paratyphoid inoculation in May 1917, she became very ill. She developed pleurisy and was five weeks in bed as her condition worsened due to anaemia, debility and strain. Eventually she was RTA and was nursed at 4 AGH, Randwick where it was decided to send her to Cavell House, then located at Prospect Road, Summer Hill, for further convalescence. When she was 28 years old she was discharged with a pension of £2.7.9 per fortnight in 1918.[43] Although she managed to continue to nurse throughout the USA and was still in San Francisco in 1920, the following year a letter dated 15 November 1921 appears in her service record requesting information about her will. Nurses continued to work but it does not mean they were physically or mentally well.

Going home or suicide

Some soldiers chose not to come home. There is no record of any nurses committing suicide, but such statistics were unlikely to be recorded. Records of soldiers committing suicide are often disguised. The rationale for disguise is usually to protect or hide.[44] The practice of keeping soldiers suffering from shell-shock isolated on the return voyage proved unwise, as a number committed suicide before they reached Australia.[45] It is not easy to read the accounts of soldiers and nurses who served in various fronts of the war without understanding why *...some men shot themselves, others went mad.*[46] Vera Brittain waged an exhaustive battle against a nervous breakdown for more than 18 months after the war and she *...drifted to the borderland of craziness.* She was overwhelmed with her mirror image which reflected a woman who was either growing a beard or turning into a witch. This period of time demonstrated to her the *...thinness of the barrier between normality and insanity.*[47] Fortuitously, she eventually managed to survive the transition from war to peace.

George Merrick Long and the Merrick Scheme

George Merrick Long (1874-1930) was an extraordinary educator and one of the earliest Australian born Anglican bishops. He enlisted in 1917 and while in France came under the notice of Major General Brudenell White who appointed him Director of Education. Teaching the divisions was difficult but once the Armistice was declared he negotiated with educational institutions and industry organisations throughout the UK so that soldiers and nurses could undergo education or training while awaiting transportation home. It was an innovative idea which proved remarkably successfully for the 12,880 soldiers and nurses who underwent non-military employment (NME) under the *'Merrick Scheme'*.[48] George Merrick Long was awarded honorary LLD degrees from both Cambridge and Manchester Universities and appointed CBE in 1919 for his services.[49]

Merric Boyd and the Merrick Scheme

Merric Boyd was a gentle man who loved Doris Gough and the year that war was declared he created her in sculpture. Dr Guy Springthorpe, who achieved an insight into the psychological ramifications of war, was a close friend and neighbour of Merric Boyd, who suffered the torment of epilepsy. Springthorpe's close association with the family was fortunate because epileptics were often doomed to reside in *...madhouses...* and were treated with disdain socially. Merric's younger brother, Penleigh, returned to Australia suffering from the effects of poison gas on the Western Front in October 1917. That same month, Merric Boyd left Doris to join the Australian Flying Corps and served in Britain as a transport driver. It is difficult to imagine a man so unfitted to the business of war.

After the Armistice, under the NME program, Merric Boyd used the opportunity to study art and pottery at the Central School of Science and Technology in Stoke-on-Trent, which he completed with a commendation. Once he completed the theoretical training he worked at the Wedgwood Factory *...under the tutelage of Thomas Mellor.* On his return journey to Australia, Merric Boyd gave soldiers pottery lessons as a form of rehabilitation. Nine months after he returned to Doris, their first son was born. Merric Boyd became *...Australia's first and most original art potter...* and his son, Arthur, become one of Australia's greatest artists and philanthropists.[50]

AANS Nurses and the Merrick Scheme

Readapting to the peace was not easy for many men and women whose recent past had been war-centred. The scheme was more than a diversion because these experienced soldiers had to readjust to different employment opportunities on their return to Australia. After the war, 14 AGH was disbanded and Rose Creal and her staff were transferred to England. Rose Creal used the opportunity to undertake elocution lessons under the Merrick Scheme and was granted ten weeks' paid leave to tour British hospitals and learn as much as possible before returning to the SHSEH, where she resumed the matronship in April 1920.[51] One of the nurses, Jessie Tomlins, did not realise she would be waiting nearly eighteen months for a return to Australia and regretted not enrolling in a midwifery course while she continued military nursing at 3 AAH, Dartford. However, many nurses chose courses unrelated to nursing in a bid to find alternative employment on their return to Australia because they felt it was time to ...*take a saner hold on life.*[52] The employment choices available to nurses had to comply with the limited socially acceptable paid employment opportunities for women. One occupation which did not appear to be available for returning nurses was farming, because they had difficulty accessing the Soldiers' Settlement Scheme.

The Soldiers' Settlement Scheme

On her voyage home Anne Donnell witnessed a great gathering of soldiers as ...*Mr Agnew gave an address to the troops on the Imperial League*... (a precursor to the RSL). Donnell and the ...*Sisters sat on deck chairs, sewed and listened. It was very interesting and we enjoyed the last tit-bit when he advised all the boys to buy a little farm and invite someone to share it with them.*[53] The Soldiers' Settlement Scheme aimed to establish returned soldiers in rural areas and included the provision of a loan which did not exceed £625 per settler.[54]

Although 36,000 farms were established under the scheme, few succeeded because of the allocation of unsuitable land and a lack of farming expertise by the soldier.[55] Some soldiers, especially Light Horsemen, were able to combine their land allocation with that of their family. They were in the enviable position of returning to an extended family and supportive community in an area well known to them.[56] Land management of the small, government-allotted blocks was near impossible for men who had no history with the land and no cumulative knowledge of the rural landscape in which they were expected to operate a business.[57] The consequences were dire for many returned soldiers and their families, especially during the economic decline of the 1930s.[58] Poor land management also had a negative impact on the health of the soil and during the Second World War governments were eager not to repeat past mistakes.[59]

Nonetheless, soldiers were more fortunate than returned nurses who were ineligible for one of the 100,000 houses made available by the Repatriation Minister in 1919. The houses were ...*built at a maximum cost of £700 each to be repaid over thirty-seven years with interest at 5 per cent.*[60] When Canadian nurses returned home they were dissuaded from applying for settlements because …*Nursing sisters, though technically eligible, were urged to look elsewhere for re-establishment*. Apparently it was believed that they could not cope with …*the rough and strenuous duties of settlers…* so in 1920 an amendment formally excluded nurses from even applying.[61] The Canadian nurses who served in Salonika and in CCSs of France were certainly capable of strenuous duties. Apparently, demonstrations of strength by women during wartime were tolerable but during peacetime it was actively discouraged. There is conflicting evidence regarding the eligibility of Australian nurses for land under the Soldiers' Settlement Scheme.

Nurses as farmers: Elizabeth Helene Draper and Evelyn Percy Wright

Elizabeth Draper (b. circa 1879) was born not too distant from Sydney in Strathfield (NSW, Wangal Country), but her family were living in the Forbes district during the war. She served in Egypt at the 4 Auxiliary Convalescent Depot and later in Salonika.[62] Elizabeth attained the position of acting matron and in 1919 she was awarded the ARRC and the Greek Medal of Military Merit.

She returned to Australia on 16 June 1919 and made an application for land under the Soldier Settlement Scheme 1919-20 in NSW. If a nurse married or had male relatives who would work on the land, she had some chance of receiving an allocation. Being from a rural area and knowing the business of agriculture and animal husbandry made little difference if the applicant was a single woman. Nonetheless, Elizabeth Draper was a successful grazier and she remained Miss Draper until her death in 1974, aged 95 years.[63]

Evelyn Percy Wright enlisted with the AANS in May 1915 and later saw service in France. In 1919 she enrolled in a NME scheme and attended the British College of Cookery for three months.[64] On her return home she nursed for a short period in Tamworth (NSW, Kamilaroi Country) and then turned her attention to animal husbandry. There is no evidence of an application or receipt for a settlement block and it is more likely that she was given the opportunity to manage cattle by her father, who was operating a property near Walcha (NSW, Dhanggati Country) at the time of Evelyn's return from the war.[65]

Evelyn Percy Wright and her sister, Irene, operated a successful Hereford beef cattle property east of Walcha in the 1920s and were respected members of the grazing industry for a number of years.[66] Evelyn Wright was not the archetypical cattle woman as she was small in stature (153 cm tall and 51 kg when she enlisted) with grey eyes, fair complexion and golden brown hair. She lived a long and full life on the land, dying aged 103 years in 1985.[67]

The changing face of 'home'

Just as soldiers and nurses had changed during four years of war, so too had many homes. There was no respite from illness and death for the civilian population, which is illustrated by the personal experience of one American soldier. He confided to his Australian nurse, May Tilton, that *...there were only three of us: two elder brothers and me ... my two brothers were killed in the same stunt I was in. Then a cable from home announced the death of both mother and father.* The 19-year-old soldier spent the war doing all he could to *...get knocked and follow them...* but he survived the war without any physical injuries or illness. His nurse could not speak for crying so she *...stooped and kissed him. He broke down and sobbed.* He felt desperately alone with no home, and despite promising to write to May Tilton she never heard if he found a new family and a new life after the war.[68]

The changing face of 'home' for Sarah Furnifull

In 1917 Sarah Furnifull was in London enjoying a well-earned break when two significant events occurred. She was awarded a MID and she met *...the love of her life...* but preferred to keep his name to herself. After an eventful furlough she returned to France.

Confusion in France during the German offensive was commonplace and Sarah was sent to a hospital which had been taken over by the Germans. Fortunately she narrowly missed proceeding too far over the ever-changing front line, but her family was notified that she was missing, causing them great angst. Sarah finally made it to the Champagne district of Epernay where she and her group nursed many casualties in a hotel which was bombed each night, so they sought nocturnal sanctuary in the wine cellars. Villers-Bretonneux was the next location where she nursed many men, allied and enemy, in a mental institution.

After long and grueling days of work during the 'Big Push,' Sarah was offered a mug full of cherry brandy which she drank quickly and fell asleep for three days. While she slept her unit moved many miles but made sure Sarah remained with them. They crossed the Hindenburg Line and continued to nurse many casualties until they were only a few miles from where the Armistice was signed.

She *...vividly remembers the silence on the 11th hour of the 11th day. All the guns stopped firing. We were hysterical, laughing and crying. But it was quite peculiar, we didn't feel much like celebrating. Only crying. That night in my tent 18 men died of pneumonic flu.*

The war was over for this ordinary Australian nurse whose wartime experiences read like an adventure novel. The Armistice was signed and she had survived.

They moved to Cologne and she requested immediate leave to go home as her mother was ill. The three-month trip home was not easy. Sarah Furnifull had endured hazardous war service and her large and loving family was within reach in NSW. She deserved great happiness after all she had endured. Eleven thousand Australians died during the influenza pandemic and the day before Sarah arrived back in Australia her beloved mother became one of them.[1536] Sarah was made aware of the fact when she landed. At the same time she received word that *...the love of her life...* had been killed in action just prior to the Armistice.

Like most returned nurses Sarah Furnifull regrouped. Decades after the war she recorded her history for her training hospital ending with *...A few weeks after my return I accepted the position of Matron at Muswellbrook Hospital. It was strange coming back to a civilian hospital but I soon settled down to the routine. It was a good hospital with 50 to 60 beds, and we had three trained nurses and five probationers. I was there for seven happy years. I had a little T-model Ford and sometimes went out into the country with the nurses. There I met my last love, got married, and lived happily ever after.*[69]

Elsie Grant and May Tilton: RTA 1918

The transportation of Australian nurses was variable but there is one constant –

they worked. Elsie Grant and May Tilton were physical wrecks and in need of convalescence. In January 1918 Elsie returned to 3 AGH at Abbeville, France, where the frozen conditions affected the staff and patients adversely. By February it was obvious to the Medical Officer that both nurses needed to be returned to Australia because they were at risk of a complete breakdown. It was believed that Elsie was suffering from a nervous condition resulting in a painful swelling of her face so she was transferred to 2 AAH, Southall where Pearl Goodman was also a patient.[70]
Despite their physical and psychological exhaustion they did not receive a free trip home but returned to Australia on transport duty. They boarded RMS *Kenilworth Castle* which took them as far as Cape Town, South Africa where they enjoyed two days leave and then another nine days in Durban. Both nurses had been fortunate to have had twenty days of touring and sight-seeing in England and Wales before they were transferred to the hell of France, and they enjoyed leave in South Africa before enduring a nightmare trip on the SS *Field Marshall.*

The voyage of the damned – the *Field Marshall*

The *Field Marshall* was originally a German ship. She had spent seven months under water after being sunk by the British during the early stages of the war. She was refitted but on the first day at sea the Commanding Officer deemed her to be unseaworthy. Unfortunately, there were no other vessels available, so the CO had to accept makeshift alterations. The voyage to Australia was traumatic for all concerned due to the high seas; only one engine operating effectively; tropical temperatures; insufficient food and space for the troops. When the *Field Marshall* finally arrived in Fremantle, there was much rejoicing by those who were able to disembark in one piece. An inquiry into the seaworthiness of the ship was held and when it finally concluded, May Tilton *...received notice to report to military barracks. I was told the* Field Marshall, *under another name, had been refitted and made more comfortable to return, and as sisters must be sent on her, I was asked not to talk about our experiences on the ship.* In response Tilton *...promised not to unless I was requested to by anyone who was sailing on her; and to avoid doing that, I would make myself scarce.*[71]The refitted name of the ship and the fate of its passengers remained a mystery to Tilton.

Once in Fremantle many of the soldiers and three AANS nurses, who were returning as invalids, were transferred to the eastern states aboard HMAHS *Kanowna*. Although Elsie Grant's service record claims she RTA on the *Kanowna*, she remained with her soldier patients and her friend, May Tilton, on the *Field Marshall* for the final leg of the trip.[72] On their arrival in Melbourne the nurses were transported by rail to their original MDs and finally home.

Quarantining the flu

Anne Donnell was one of ten nurses who returned to Australia on a troopship with 600 soldiers, mainly orthopaedic cases. Apart from a few days of seasickness aboard the recently commissioned HMHS *Marhga* she found the trip ...*divine*.[1516] It was not uncommon for ships expecting to land at Fremantle to be diverted to Adelaide for fear of infection by a 'dirty ship' - one containing the influenza virus. The *Margha* was deemed to be a clean ship after the Medical Officer inspected the soldiers and nurses' hands but the situation in Fremantle was dire and permission to land was withheld. Despite the obvious disappointment of soldiers, nurses and their waiting families it was a wise decision because Perth and Fremantle were inundated with sufferers of influenza.

Anne Donnell was bitterly disappointed, as were families who had travelled overland to welcome their loved ones home from war. Instead, off the coast of Fremantle, Anne watched, disgusted, as ...*an ugly old tug comes along and off go our WA boys with cheers from their shipmates. Can it really be true. Can one realize that not a smile is given; not a sign of welcome; not a flag even, except the one with the yellow dash on it.*[73] The welcome home was different for every ship and every person.

Families were relieved to finally embrace their daughters. Many like Anne Donnell had been away for three-and-a-half years. Her disappointment at being prevented from landing at Perth and embracing her family was acute. However, it must have made the meeting in Adelaide even more memorable. Nonetheless, Australia and its health system was heaving under the weight of the influenza pandemic and nurses were once again in the battle.

31 The Human Tragedy of Influenza

Thompson buried today. They would not let us go to her funeral- Susie Cone

There was an Armistice on a number of fronts of the First World War in October and November 1918 but the question of victory is moot. The human toll can only be estimated: Ten million soldiers dead; twenty million soldiers scarred; incalculable numbers of civilians who died from …*starvation and disease rather than bullets and shells*… and in the aftermath of war there were twenty million dead from the influenza pandemic.[1]

There were two main cohorts during the influenza pandemic: the victims who died and the survivors who mourned. Rarely did a family, a community or a profession escape the touch of the virus or the war. Surely, one disaster would have been enough but the back-to-back tragedy of 1918-20 is difficult to reconcile. The euphoria of the peace was permanently marred by the virulence of the virus because the global population was in a physically and psychologically depleted state.[2] Ultimately, these small surface proteins (H1N1) joined forces and killed more people than the arsenals of the great nations. The pain and grief of the Australian nurses and their families was one small and penetrating splinter from an avalanche of falling trees.

Influenza had been with the Australian nurses and soldiers throughout the war. On 29 August 1917 an indigenous Australian soldier, William Punch, who survived the massacre of his family during the Colonial Wars died of influenza at Bournemouth Town Hall, which had been converted to Mont Dore Hospital. He was under the care of Australian nurse Constance O'Shea (QAIMNSR) and his burial ground was not on country but in the English countryside of Dorset.[3]

Unfortunately the influenza pandemic did not allow the returning nurses an opportunity to build upon their experience and transfer it to the civilian setting in a timely and constructive manner. The response to the cessation of hostilities was mixed as some felt relief while others felt great sadness as they remembered those who had died or were wounded. After the Armistice, influenza became as mobile as the troops who were eager to return home. Quarantine was strict but it was impossible to contain the spread of the disease as soldiers wanted to get home and communities wanted to embrace their heroes. Many men and a number of nurses died after the peace.

Coping with the Influenza Pandemic in Australia: Victoria

Clinical facts and the social consequences of the influenza pandemic provide a snapshot of life for Australians during the immediate aftermath of a world war. Civilian and military nursing merged once again as civilian nurses were caught up in the unprecedented devastation of a pandemic. Despite years of war, religious sectarianism also continued. When the influenza pandemic was raging in Melbourne in 1918 the Exhibition Building took on a life as an emergency hospital and Archbishop Mannix offered the services of the nursing nuns in the East Melbourne district.

Initially the offer was gratefully accepted by the government of the day but confusion about the role of the secular matron, the indomitable Jane Bell, and the Mother Rectress of St Vincent's Hospital resulted in the arousal of public suspicion.[4] Suspicion soon deepened and became evident during hostile church meetings where it was asserted by a leader of the Wesleyan Church, the Reverend H Worrall, that the *…garb worn by the nuns and brothers, the ceremonies they observe, and the customs they follow are not things which should be introduced into a public hospital.*[5] The competence of nursing nuns is beyond rational debate as they preceded the establishment of secular nursing by centuries.[6] Nonetheless, exhausted Australian nurses returned from four years of war only to, once again, roll up their sleeves to combat one of the worst pandemics of the twentieth century. They had witnessed too much and had little energy left to deal with religious bigotry. As usual, they just got on with it.

Coping with the Influenza Pandemic in Australia: South Australia

Margaret Graham had a relatively uneventful war after she left Egypt. Apart from transport duty back to Australia on one occasion, she returned to England where she served at 3 AAH, Dartford, from July 1917 until January 1918. She was appointed matron of St Albans Convalescent Home for Nurses during the latter part of the war.[7] After being stationed at St Albans she was posted to AIF Headquarters in London and was finally discharged as medically unfit on 28 August 1918. She was 58 years old and recognised for her contribution with the RRC and MID (1916).[8] However, she had little time to recover from the war when she returned to Australia and resumed her role as matron of the Adelaide Hospital.

In May 1919 she was assigned to supervise the management of the pneumonic influenza patients in the Adelaide Exhibition Building.[9] Margaret Graham dealt with the situation in her usual no-nonsense way but was also asked to provide nursing reinforcements for the overworked nurses at Woodman's Point Quarantine Station (WA, Whadjuk Noongar Country). She sent four nurses, including Doris Ridgway, Blanche Morrison and ...[Harriet] *Jackson's sister'*.[10] Margaret Graham was well aware of the risks associated with nursing infectious patients because she suffered from typhoid fever during her nurse training, which necessitated having three months off duty.[11]

AANS Home Service Nurses

Blanche Morrison joined the AANS in 1917 and worked at 15 AGH. In December 1918 she volunteered to nurse influenza victims in 5MD and left on 21 December 1918.[12] This appears to be common for home service nurses as Florence Watts, who trained at Adelaide Hospital, volunteered to nurse influenza victims in Victoria in January 1918.[13] Lily Nugent (b. 1893) was also an AANS home service nurse, who died in Sydney on 21 February 1918. Although she was born, trained at St Vincents Hospital and died in Sydney she had a great deal of experience in the Riverina district of NSW, particularly at Wagga Wagga District Hospital (NSW, Wiradjuri Country).[14]

Coping with the Influenza Pandemic in Australia: Western Australia

Originally named the *Melbourne* and commissioned in 1912 by the German-Australian Steamship Company she was renamed HMAT *Boonah* and refitted as a transport ship when war broke out. There were twenty-seven enemy ships in Australian waters when hostilities began. The *Boonah* spent four years of war transporting troops and horses. At the time of the Armistice she was transporting Australian servicemen overseas, so she was forced to wait in Durban Harbour for further orders. While waiting, a number of local workers boarded the ship to trade and coal the furnaces. It soon became apparent the locals were infected by the influenza virus and the men on the *Boonah* quickly became casualties.[15] It was decided to land the soldiers at Woodman's Point Quarantine Station to avoid any risk to the civilian population of nearby Perth.[16]

The *Wyreema*

The granddaughter of Thaddeus O'Kane, Rosa, trained at the Townsville Hospital and was appointed matron of Winton Hospital (Queensland, Koa Country) before enlisting with the AANS (1 MD) on 17 November 1917.[17] She served in a military hospital in Brisbane and was eventually called up for overseas duty on 7 October 1918 when a contingent of nurses was required to serve as reinforcements in Salonika.[18] She departed on HMAT *Wyreema* from Sydney on 14 October 1918 in the company of a number of AANS personnel. En route to Salonika the nurses put on a play to entertain the troops and Rosa played *...the part of Bluebeard splendidly.*[1564] Rosa and her colleagues never reached Salonika because the Armistice was declared, so the *Wyreema* was recalled to Australia. During the return journey the *Boonah* radioed the Officer-in-Charge stating Australian servicemen were dying from the Spanish flu.

On landing at Fremantle the matron of the *Wyreema* called for twenty nurses to volunteer for duty at the Woodman's Point Quarantine Station, located on the outskirts of the town. Only twenty nurses were required but despite being aware of the risks, 26 of the 45 nurses aboard the *Wyreema* volunteered, so the nurses *...drew lots for places.* Rosa O'Kane and Ada Thompson were successful.[19] A similar situation arose in the Second World War when the Matron of 2/5 AGH, Kathleen Best (aged 29 years), needed forty volunteers from her staff of 75 nursing sisters and 9 masseuses to remain at Elaki (near Athens) during a German advance in 1941. She devised a system whereby the nurses would write 'go' or 'stay' on a piece of paper and she promised she would be the only one to know of their decision. Despite being informed that there was every chance the volunteers would be captured, the system was shown to be flawed when every nurse wrote 'stay'. Eventually, the twenty nurses, including Matron Best who was the granddaughter of a pioneering nurse, were safely evacuated.[20]

Woodman's Point Quarantine Station: Fremantle, WA

The provision of adequate staff, drugs, dressing or even food and water had never been a feature of service for the war nurses. The conditions under which the nurses from the *Wyreema* found themselves were graphically recorded by Staff Nurse Cone. Susie Cone recorded that the nurses *...started to get things ready for the boys coming off the* Boonah. *Wilkinson, Hamilton, Bradshaw and I were in W3, a hut holding 8 beds and 10 tents. No conveniences of any kind. About 10 am the boys began to come up from the jetty. Our tents and hut were soon full. Poor lads were in a terrible plight. Filth and dirt all over them terribly sick, we had no drugs, no clean shirts or pyjamas to put on them. All we could do is to wash them and get them as comfortable as possible. Three died the first day.*[21]

Woodman's Point is an isolated location even by contemporary standards and the Australian summer heat was an additional hardship. Susie Cone had known Rosa O'Kane during the voyage and she along with the other '*Wyreemians*' were shocked and saddened by her death at 1.45 pm on 21 December 1918 from *...pneumonic influenza.*[1573] Her nursing colleagues mourned her passing and recorded *...Poor old O'Kane died early this morning, one can hardly realise that she is gone, everyone very depressed about it. We gave her a military funeral to-day at 4pm. It's sad to see we old Wyreemians have decreased. Only nine of us on duty now.*[22] Poor old O'Kane was 28 years old.

Burial of Rosa O'Kane

Rosa O'Kane had a *...most impressive...* burial with *...full military honours...* and the *...cortege was made up of staff nurses in uniform and the medical officers. A guard of forty soldiers followed the coffin and fired a volley over the grave and the ceremony concluded with the playing of the 'Last Post'.*[23] Her death was keenly felt by the nurses and there was a subsequent reduction in morale at the quarantine station. Unfortunately this had an impact on the management of subsequent burials. On the other side of the country Rosa's mother had recently received a letter dated 9 December, 1918 (before volunteers were requested) from her only daughter saying that she hoped to be in Fremantle the next day and home by Christmas.[24] It is difficult to know whether her grandfather would have been proud or angry but Thadeus would have most likely felt something akin to grief tied in with anger at the waste of potential through the loss of a young life.

Crisis Management

Initially the AANS volunteers were told they would be led by a competent nurse who had four years' war experience, Matron Brown, and they anticipated working under adverse conditions but with strong and effective administrative support. Unfortunately a civilian matron, Miss Prosser, was appointed 'in-charge'. She was so appalled at the lack of basic nursing necessities for seriously ill patients that she left on the first day, but was persuaded to return two days later. Matron Prosser succumbed to the disease just prior to Christmas but fortunately recovered.[25]

The rate of illness amongst the nurses was indicative of the highly contagious nature of the disease. Others who became ill included Ridgway, Thompson, Wilkinson, Manning, Hamilton, Walker, Newby, Kymer and German. Susie Cone, the diarist and record keeper, became ill herself on 12 January 1919 and another six unidentified nurses succumbed on 17 December 1918.[26] Sisters Kymer and Williams and Matron Prosser were civilian nurses who contracted the disease, bringing the total to seventeen.[27] This correlates roughly with information contained in a letter to the press from the military sisters who claimed *...the sisters numbered about forty...* and by 21 December sixteen had contracted the disease.[28]

There was confusion about the delineation between the roles of Miss Brown and Miss Prosser and this, combined with a lack of a sympathetic response to the physical needs of the over-worked nurses from the senior medical officers, contributed to a period of serious discontent. On 21 December a letter appeared in the *West Australian* which was signed *...Military Sisters, Quarantine Station, Woodman Point...* and among other matters they wanted to set the record straight because they disputed the statement previously made by the civilian matron and Chief Medical Officer claiming the sisters were *...happy and contented.*

The Reality of Nursing in a Quarantine Station

Apart from the administrative anxieties caused by a lack of nurse leadership from a non-military matron, they outlined the day-to-day conditions endured by soldiers and nurses. They wrote in part that *...when the boys arrived from the* SS Boonah *some of them were in a dying condition. The only thing ready for them was a clean bed. Nothing in the way of nourishment was ready for them. An hour after their arrival a lemon drink was procured instead of the nourishing drinks which the boys so badly needed. Later in the day cocoa made from condensed milk was obtained for them. Fresh milk for the boys arrived only two days ago ... Now for a word about the sleeping accommodation provided for the sisters who numbered about forty. Less than five yards from the sisters' sleeping quarters were pitched tents in which were many of the worst cases. Is it any wonder sixteen sisters have already contracted this terrible pneumonic influenza?*[29] The letter ended with the plea *...trusting you will help us by publishing this letter...* but its publication caused a great deal of controversy among the civilian population. Initially the WA community rallied when news of the plight of the *Boonah* became known. School children raised funds for foodstuffs while the local Red Cross continued its excellent *...war work...* at home. A number of local charitable organisations such as the YMCA made donations and the local council endeavoured to *...provide Christmas cheer.*[30]

Susie Cone described the situation just before Christmas and after the letter was published. She recorded that a *...letter from the Perth military sisters here appeared in the daily paper and caused quite a stir. Meetings etc being held about it. We are forbidden to talk to the officers and men except while on duty and all Xmas festivities have been knocked on the* *head. Xmas eve and the unhappiness*[sic] *I have ever spent … News that we have to move from our present quarters down to tents about half a mile down a dusty track. How we are going to walk that distance every day goodness only knows or cares.*

The good people of WA would have been further outraged if they had been made aware of the consequence of their concern. However, a quarantine station is by definition isolated and the exhausted, sick and dying nurses felt that isolation keenly. Susie Cone described her first Christmas since the Armistice when she had

…my first day off. Spent it moving to our new camping ground. What a day, hot and dusty as possible to be. Xmas dinner was a scream. Our tent was the only one fixed up. So when the others came off duty and found their beds strewn all over the paddock and their luggage and bedding God only knows where, they all went up to the main building to attack that little beast Dr Park. He, as is typical of him, did nothing for us so we all went back again. The convalescent boys offering to put up our beds and cart luggage etc for the girls it was midnight before things were finally fixed up. Did not sleep much tents don't agree with me.[31]

A second nurse dies: Ada Thompson

Ada Thompson became ill at the peak of the Australian summer and took twelve days to die. She had sailed on the *Wyreema* and had left Sydney on 14 October 1918, but Susie Cone noted that *…Thompson very ill…* and on New Years Eve *…Thompson of NSW very ill still.* This was in conflict with the official announcement published the same day in the *West Australian* claiming that *…Sister Ada Thompson … has also shown sufficient improvement to warrant her transfer to the seriously ill list.* Ada died of pneumonic influenza at 5 pm on New Year's Day 1919. The year which ushered in the peace.[32]

Susie Cone recorded an interesting deviation from the normal practice of a full military funeral for any member of the AIF who died on active service. She noted in her diary on 2 January 1919 *…Thompson buried today. They would not let us go to her funeral.*[33] The rationale for not allowing the nurses to attend the funeral of their colleague was prompted by the reduction in morale that followed Rosa O'Kane's funeral. The negative press reports about the mismanagement at the quarantine station were having an adverse impact on the decision-making of those in charge.

Civilian Nurses Volunteer and Die

William and Louisa Williams had made a comfortable life in Claremont but the grief of losing their only son, Arthur, was still acute. Their daughter Alice was overseas serving with the QAs in 1918 when their other daughter, Hilda, volunteered to nurse the men from the *Boonah* at nearby Fremantle.[34] Hilda Williams, born on 20 August 1892, followed her older sister's example and completed her nurse training at the Perth Children's Hospital in December 1913.[35]

Susie Cone first mentions that Hilda Williams became ill on 30 December 1918 and was sick for a number of days before becoming *...very ill...* on 4 January 1919 and finally dying late that night. A nephew of Hilda Williams, Bruce Wright, recounted that the *...hospitals were asked to send volunteer nurses, and Hilda Williams offered. My mother (Edna) told me that Hilda wrote a quick note to her mother and posted it before she left. Ten days later her mother had a telegram to say that she was dead. Along with her brother Arthur who was killed in France, Hilda was the second casualty in the family in* WW1.[36] She was buried the next day on 5 January 1919. Hilda Williams was twenty-five years old and her parents were not allowed to visit her while she was dying. Unlike wartime deaths when distance prevented a parent from being at the bedside, the situation for all family members was cruel. Furthermore, her parents were not permitted to attend Hilda's funeral.[37] These precautions were due to the stringent isolation requirements and the absolute panic of the general population. While necessary, they were brutal.[38]

A new recruit to the AANS: Doris Ridgway from South Australia

Ada and John Ridgway were anxious about the health and welfare of their two soldier sons, Hugh and Victor, as they mourned the death of Eric. Meanwhile Doris completed her training, immediately enlisted in the AANS (21 December 1917) and gained post-training experience as a charge nurse for three months. She was accepted into the AIF on 24 August 1918 and served at 7 AGH, South Australia. Doris Ridgway was an attractive and intelligent woman and although petite, weighing less than 49 kg and just 153 cm tall, she was obviously robust because she never had a day off during her training. Doris was also an outstanding student who received four first-class passes and *...was a gold medalist.*[39]

Like families around Australia her parents welcomed the news of the Armistice and anxiously awaited the return of their two sons. Ten days after the Armistice was declared, Doris volunteered to reinforce the nurses at Woodman's Point Quarantine Station. She and four AANS colleagues, including Blanche May Morrison, travelled from Adelaide to Perth on the East-West train. This was not an easy or quick journey in the Australian summer heat.[40] The conditions at Woodman's Point were dire on their arrival and within four days she had taken ill and died.[41]

On 6 January 1919 Susie Cone recorded that *...Ridgway died this evening. Such a dear little girl.*[42] A Protestant service was most likely performed when she was buried the next day in consecrated ground near the bodies of Rosa O'Kane, Ada Thompson and Hilda Williams.[43] Staff Nurse Ridgway had just turned 27 years old when she became the fourth Australian nurse to die at Woodman's Point Quarantine Station.[44] Her parents, a large and loving family, colleagues and her community were bereft.

Futility of inoculation

Doris Ridgway's medical record at the time of her appointment to the AIF on 21 December 1918 indicates she was a healthy young woman. The general population was encouraged to be inoculated against influenza but it was a requirement for the staff of the Woodman's Point Quarantine Station to receive a course of two doses of the influenza inoculation A and B. Influenza A contained 25 million organisms per cubic centimetre and the body was given time to adjust to the presence of the organism before the second dose containing 125 million organisms per cubic centimetre was administered seven days later. Doris Ridgway and the other three nurses who died had all been inoculated, as had the other nurses who contracted the disease and recovered. Resistance and survival was a lottery.[45]

In retrospect

While there is some truth in Kingston's claim that *...World War One and the subsequent influenza epidemic were probably blessings in disguise for both the hospitals and the nursing profession...* it was not an ideal way to progress the profession or the health system.[46] Reactive policies rarely become institutionalised and tend to create professional insecurity. Furthermore, a number of Australian nurses, unrecorded, died in civilian settings as they cared for family members, neighbours and patients. The loss to the profession was incalculable. The circumstances surrounding the death of the four nurses at Woodman's Point Quarantine Station gives a fleeting glimpse of the working lives of nurses. The actions of their families provide insight into how their deaths were felt by those they loved.

Woodman's Point is now a recreational area and an access road to the public launch ramp has been named in honour of Rosa O'Kane.[47] She was a nurse devoted to her profession but she was also the only daughter of a long-widowed mother, Jeannie, and sister to Frank and John. Her brothers rallied the people of Charters Towers who raised sufficient funds to place a large memorial marking the place where Rosa was buried.[48] It has been claimed that over a three-day period in June 1958 all the military graves except for Rosa O'Kane's were *...disinterred and transferred to the Perth War Cemetery at Karrakatta.*[49] Rosa O'Kane's family and community wanted her impressive memorial transferred as well but this was not possible under the guidelines of the War Graves Commission, as each grave must be uniform.

It is not clear if the father of Ada Thompson, William G Thompson, had pre-deceased her but he is absent from any official correspondence.[50] Although her mother was her designated next-of-kin, her sister, Miss H C Thompson, managed her financial affairs after her death and another sister, Miss Ethel Thompson, was the sole beneficiary of her will.[51] Normally any personal belongings would be transferred to the next-of-kin after the death of a service nurse, but in the case of the four nurses who died in quarantine the *...Deputy Assistant Adjutant General, Defence Department, Perth has been requested to have the effects of those members of the AIF who died in quarantine at Fremantle, fumigated and forwarded to this Branch for disposal.*[52] Given the protracted correspondence between Ada's family and the Army this process was very slow.[53]

There is a plaque to the memory of Ada Thompson at the Perth War Cemetery Garden of Remembrance (Wall 5, Row I).[54] However, for reasons which are unclear, Ada Thompson was disinterred from Woodman's Point and transferred to the public cemetery at Fremantle (Anglican, A 806). She is one of 120 war dead buried there from the 1914-18 conflict.[55] Once you know of her sacrifice, her headstone looks out of place amongst the burial plots in the cemetery. Surprisingly, the small town of Pallamallawa has no obvious memorial to one of their own who died while nursing the soldiers at Woodman's Point but her name can be found at the First World War memorial in Kings Park, Perth, and on the Roll of Honour, AWM, Canberra.[56]

Doris Ridgway received a number of honours befitting her sacrifice. In 1925 her name was forwarded to the Commandant of 4MD in connection with the York Minster 'Five Sisters' Window Memorial and her name is listed on the honour roll of the now Royal Adelaide Hospital.[57] Her body was disinterred from Woodman's Point Quarantine Station in 1958 and she now rests at the Perth War Cemetery amongst the graves of sixteen soldiers who were also re-interred.[1626] Her name, along with that of Ada Thompson, can be found on a brass plaque in the Garden of Remembrance in the same cemetery at Karrakatta, WA. The names of three of the four Woodman's Point nurses (O'Kane, Thompson, Ridgway) are recorded in brass on the Roll of Honour, AWM, Canberra.

However, it is a less grand monument which gives the true impact of their story. Cooke's Plains is a small locality in South Australia with an old Soldiers' Memorial Hall *...erected in memory of Cooke's Plains Heroes...* and from the door hangs a list of seven names including Nurse D. A. Ridgway and her brother, E. B. Ridgway.[58] Their parents, Ada and John, mourned the loss of their children into their old age.[59]

A family snapshot of the Williams children prior to 1913 indicates their parents had every right to be hopeful. Furthermore, an image of Hilda shows a young woman ready to embark on life with the confidence that emanates from a strong and loving family. The family did not talk about the sadness of the war years. What is there to say when their only son, Arthur, is dead in France since 1916 and the peace brought with it the death of Hilda? Their grief was compounded in 1924 when Edith, mother of two little boys, died. Hilda's father died in 1937 *...because he was worn out...* and her mother died ten years later.

Hilda Grace Williams was a civilian nurse, consequently her grave remains unchanged from the day she was buried on 5 January 1919. A small white cross marks her final resting place with the words written in coarse black writing 'Nurse H Williams RIP'.[60] Eighty-six years after her death, her nephew made the salient point ...*She gave her life just the same as her brother had.*[61]

Coping with the Influenza Pandemic in Australia: New South Wales

Elizabeth McGregor had a busy war serving with the Red Cross. Her sparse record of service with the British Red Cross basically consists of two entries: Serbian relief in Serbia and Corfu from October 1914 until April 1916 followed by service in Salonika from May 1916 until June 1917.[62] The locations and conditions in those war zones are well known but Elizabeth was still invisible to the Australian war authorities. She managed to return to Australia with a view to signing an AANS enlistment form so she could be sent overseas for further service. She nursed the servicemen at 4AGH, Randwick but never managed to be part of the AANS. Elizabeth volunteered for service at North Head Quarantine Station near Manly (NSW, Gayemagal Country) when a dirty ship arrived.[63]

There was a call to arms from the Italian Government for Italian reservists to return to their country of origin and replenish the dwindling number of soldiers. HMAT *Medic* left Sydney in October 1918 with a large number of Italian reservists and AIF soldiers intended for service in Europe. It was soon apparent the Armistice would be declared, so the ship was recalled to Australia but had to first refuel in Wellington, New Zealand. It was at this port of call that the influenza virus was transferred on to the ship.

Elizabeth McGregor: North Head Quarantine Station, Sydney

When the *Medic* arrived in Sydney on 21 November, over a third (335) of the total crew and soldiers (989) were infected and the ship was quarantined. Elizabeth McGregor volunteered and within a week of the ship docking she became a victim. She died of 'pneumonic influenza' six days later at 7.15am on 5 December 1918 and was buried at the third burial ground. Although Elizabeth McGregor did not achieve her goal of joining the AANS, she was buried with full military honours by soldiers of the AIF. Australian soldiers collected local wildflowers and placed them on her grave. She died close to home and her war experiences included nursing the people of the war-torn Balkans, which confirmed the rigour of her training as an Australian nurse.

Today her resting place has sweeping views of one of the most beautiful harbours in the world. Even in November 1919, a Scottish war-bride claimed that her ship was *...led slowly inside the world's most famous harbour, Sydney. It really is beautiful, with all the little islands and beautiful bays.*[64] Nonetheless, the absence of the Sydney Harbour Bridge isolated the quarantine station and the summer heat made the terrain most inhospitable.[65]

Given the absence of evidence that Elizabeth McGregor sailed on the *Medic* from Sydney in October 1918, it is more likely she volunteered when infected soldiers returned to Australia. In a number of ways her experience was similar to that of Doris Ridgway and Hilda Williams except she had spent three years on active service in the middle of Europe.[66] However, unlike Doris Ridgway there is no evidence that Elizabeth McGregor was *...a member of the Army Medical Corps Nursing Service who was accepted or appointed by the Director-General of Medical Services for service outside Australia...* thereby disallowing her from inclusion on the AWM Roll of Honour or Commemorative Roll.[67] Her story and sacrifice was unrecorded and unacknowledged.

Catherine McGregor was still on overseas service with the Military Masseuse Corps at the time of her sister's death. Ten years later, in 1928, she attended an Anzac Day commemorative service at Sydney University when the university's War Memorial Carillon was officially opened. Bell number 23 is inscribed with the name 'Elizabeth McGregor'. May her contribution finally resonate throughout the pages of history.[68]

Annie Egan

During the influenza pandemic, hospital administrators made public pleas for assistance from *...Certified nurses, untrained nurses and wardsmen.*[69] Annie Egan was an untrained nurse who had commenced her training at RPAH on 7 July 1914 but left the following year on 1 May 1915.[70] There is no evidence that she was ATNA qualified which indicates she did not complete a course of nurse training at any other recognised hospital. However, it was not uncommon for unqualified nurses to gain extensive experience in community settings and there is little doubt that her practical expertise was valuable during the pandemic. Tragically, her service at North Head Quarantine Station ended with her death, aged 27 years old, on 3 December 1918.[71]

Kate Porter: Matron 4 AGH Randwick, NSW

In the middle of April 1919 Sister Kate Porter was assigned to transport duty and she arrived home after more than four years away on 1 June. Her homecoming was a special civic occasion with a public meeting to celebrate the return of their *...District Heroine...* who locals referred to as the *...Milton Angel.* Her respite from military service was brief because she accepted the position of matron of one of the larger military repatriation hospitals, 4 AGH, Randwick. The Milton community was proud of Kate Porter's war service and her appointment to the Military Hospital was recognised as an extremely prestigious position.[72]

On 16 July 1919, just three weeks after commencing her appointment, Kate contracted pneumonic influenza and died. She was buried with full military honours at Waverley Cemetery (NSW, Gadigal Country) and was attended by a number of AANS nursing colleagues. Her contribution during the war was acknowledged when she was awarded the ARRC just prior to her death.[73] The loss of Kate Porter to her family, her community and her profession is inestimable. This 33-year-old woman had the potential to make a marked contribution to the progress of nursing on account of her experience and expertise. The war was responsible for the premature deaths of many returned nurses, thereby depleting the Australian nursing profession of great leaders.

A personal postscript to her life was a letter dated 1922 from a soldier who sought the address of Sister Kate Porter who served at 25 BGH in France during 1918. A story left untold.

Margaret Graham

Finally, the pandemic subsided and Margaret Graham returned to the Adelaide Hospital in 1920. She was sixty years old and retired in December of the same year. She returned to England where she died 22 years later in her birthplace, Carlisle. While her body rests in England, it is in Australia where she is remembered as an outstanding nurse leader. An innovative woman who furthered the development of secular nursing in Australia, she cared for allied soldiers and the citizens of Adelaide by being a positive influence on the professional development of more than 3,000 probationary nurses.[74] Her influence left an indelible mark on the Australian nursing profession The Margaret Graham Building which forms part of the present-day Royal Adelaide Hospital complex is a fitting tribute to an outstanding nurse and a remarkable woman.[75] The war brought to the public's attention the new role and responsibilities of professional nurses and the influenza pandemic sealed their respect and affection for nurses.

32 Nursing and Medical Legacies

... surgeon is not so likely to have cast in his way that bug-a-boo of the internist – the "chronic".
– Crandon & Ehrenfred

When Australia said goodbye to its soldiers in November 1914 the expectation was a quick victorious return. Instead a generation endured conditions and torment previously unimaginable during the next four long years. The impact on the individual soldier was witnessed by health professionals as well as community members who joined volunteer organisations. A groundswell of interest in the sick and disabled soldier was created.

Triage in Battle: Gallipoli 1915

During the landing at Gallipoli many soldiers were wounded. Diagnosis was undertaken by over-worked and over-wrought medical officers so it was not uncommon for seriously ill and wounded soldiers to be admitted to auxiliary hospitals and convalescent depots while some of the less serious cases were sent to the main AGHs.[1] The term *...less serious...* is used rather subjectively because the level of disability and illness was relative during the war.

A *...travelling medical board...* reselected the boarded cases to determine which were best suited for the available transports but an experienced officer noted that *...there appeared to be few guiding principles as to the class of man who should be invalided, and these were liable at any moment to entire revision.* The so-called *...six months policy...* was initially a three months policy that caused difficulties for military medical officers who had little guidance about what constituted an invalid as opposed to a convalescent. The ability of a doctor to discern, at the time of injury or illness, whether a soldier was likely to completely recover was a near impossible task.[2]

Return to Australia

The lack of a coherent procedure for the classification of casualties had a bearing on the diverse range of conditions of the soldiers who were *...returned to Australia...* in 1915. When a sufficient number of soldiers were in need of repatriation to Australia the matron would assign nurses to transport duty in the same way they were rostered for theatre duty. While at 1 AAH (Luna Park, Cairo), May Tilton recounted that the nurses *...principal duty was keeping order among our eleven hundred men waiting there for transport to Australia, wounded men from Gallipoli who ... wait until transport was available to take them home.*[3]

HMHS Kyarra: Melbourne: July 1915

The civilian population came face-to-face with the human consequences of the failing Dardanelles Campaign on 17 July 1915 when the sick and wounded soldiers began to return. The hospital transport *Kyarra* arrived in Melbourne carrying the first wounded soldiers from Gallipoli. There were 56 wounded soldiers but 242 were sick and 103 suffered from venereal disease aboard. Unfortunately*...the first reception of wounded was not an unqualified success.*[4]

Ballarat: Sydney: August 1915

By August 1915 the situation improved and when HMAT *Ballarat* arrived in Sydney the 116 soldiers, who were transferred through the streets to 4 AGH, Randwick (a suburb of Sydney), were accompanied by *...vast demonstrative crowds.* Muriel Knox Doherty was one of four VAD nurses sent to assist the soldiers as they made their way to the hospital and she was overwhelmed by the *...cheer upon cheer burst forth from the thousands in the Domain.* She was only young but felt embarrassed when *...on the corner of College and Oxford streets the reception was deafening...* and the VADs *...blushingly acknowledged the shouts of* "God bless our brave sisters". She need not have blushed because her future was one of distinction. After a number of years she was asked by the matron of RPAH, where she had trained and worked as a VAD, to undertake her nurse training which she commenced in 1921.[5] She served with distinction in the next world war and was matron of the Bergen-Belsen concentration camp following its liberation from the Germans in 1945.

Repatriation Military Nursing

Just as the crowds in the Domain had difficulty differentiating between a VAD and an AANS sister, the medical and nursing personnel in Australia had no appreciation of what the soldiers had endured or, in many cases, how to treat them appropriately.[6] Gradually, the AAMC and AANS personnel returned to civilian and military hospitals during and after the war. This enabled the sharing of knowledge with staff who had not experienced war service which, in turn, improved the chances of the soldiers receiving appropriate care. It is impossible to effectively nurse a patient if one is unaware of their history.

The reality of wartime nursing started to permeate the letters of nurses writing to other nurses. At the end of July 1915, while serving at a military hospital in Valletta, Malta, Narrelle Hobbes wrote to a nursing colleague in Australia with this advice …*I don't owe you a letter but I want to get some things off my chest and as you are a nurse, you would understand things a bit better than a non-nurse … stay where you are my dears, stay right there, and if you must look after the men we are sending and for gods sake make up to them for all they have gone through over this side … I could howl over the patheticness of some of the cases up in this division.*[7]

This explains, to some extent, why many Australian nurses returned to work in repatriation hospitals after the war and why many others married returned servicemen.[8] There was no need to discuss the horror of what had happened because the nurses had witnessed their sufferings, creating an unspoken understanding.[9] Returned nurses expected their colleagues and communities to ensure the suffering of the soldier to be alleviated when reached home, but those at home could not comprehend the reality of war.

A dual health system

The overriding response to the rehabilitation needs of soldiers, at a policy level, was one of fluidity. Reverence toward the wounded and sick soldiers was matched by a community desire to offer practical support and ensure they received the best treatment possible. In effect, the Defence Department implemented a health system which functioned separately from the civilian health system, although there were examples of overlap such as tuberculosis sanatoriums. This decision was not always the most advantageous to the soldier because those who had been disabled from wounds or debilitated from illness were placed in general repatriation facilities instead of specialist civilian hospitals, without particular emphasis on their condition.

Detail camps: Australia: 1916

The rapidity of changes to military policies relating to the management of injured and sick soldiers was unprecedented. For instance, in 1916 there was a significant change to facilitate the transition of military convalescents away from the authority of medical officers and back to military command. Initially, soldiers who were ill or wounded were treated in hospital and, when deemed fit returned to their unit for duty, or otherwise were discharged from the AIF. While in Australia, it became apparent that a period of adjustment after hospitalisation and before redeployment was needed.

In each MD a detail camp was established which, unlike the hospital system, was under the command of combatant officers. A range of qualified medical staff and a small hospital was available where massage and minor treatment was performed if necessary. Initially, soldiers were treated in the hospital portion of the camp and then introduced to barrack living where they started 'light duties'. Gradually these duties were increased until they were certified fit for duty. Medical officers would examine the soldiers every week or fortnight and once satisfied that a soldier was fully fit he was transferred back to a military camp.[10]

Private Bequests: Graythwaite

Individuals also donated homes for the convalescence of returned servicemen. Men like Sir Thomas Dibbs who donated Graythwaite, a beautiful estate including a large home located on 2.6 hectares of land on the north shore of Sydney, in 1915. It provided much needed respite to returned servicemen for decades but despite it being bequeathed to the state in perpetuity a court case in 2008 saw it being placed on the open market for sale. The court valued the property at $16.8 million and the Federal Government was prepared to pay $20 million to keep it in public hands. The neighbouring Private School, Shore, paid $35 million for the property. During and immediately after the war there was no need for iron-clad legal bequests, as the emotional climate of the nation was one of generosity fuelled by grief.[11]

Role of the Red Cross

Even after hospitalization it was apparent that not all soldiers would be restored to full health or independence. An Australian Branch of the British Red Cross Society, co-operating with the Defence Department, was initiated to develop a scheme of VADs to work in …*Red Cross auxiliary convalescent hospitals.*[12] Policy changes were frequent as the government attempted to come to terms with the logistics of caring for an army of returning wounded and ill soldiers. Federation was in its infancy and state-federal responsibilities for the health and welfare of soldiers was unclear. Local communities often supported families who were the main carers of ex-servicemen.[13] Red Cross services were created as needed throughout communities and often initiated by war widows or families of returned servicemen.

Convalescent Homes or Asylums

To understand the concept of a 'convalescent home' it is necessary to differentiate it from the then commonly used term 'asylum'. Pressure on acute hospital beds was augmented by the provision of additional beds in the asylums for chronic cases of illness such as rheumatism, heart disease and paralysis.[14] In 1913 the Department of Public Health in NSW collected £12,187 from the Commonwealth Government for maintenance of old-age pensioners cared for in state asylums for the infirm. These asylums were provided by the state for the use of old people in the community who were without means or friends willing to provide for them. The term 'home' described an establishment requiring less acute care for a specific cohort of individuals. For example, the 'Cottage Homes for Aged Couples, Parramatta' provided safe and secure accommodation for elderly couples who were without financial resources.[15]

The Red Cross dominated fundraising events and harnessed public support for Red Cross auxiliary hospitals and Red Cross convalescent homes. These facilities were complementary to the official hospitals. For example, the military hospitals in 1915 in NSW were 4 AGH, three auxiliary hospitals and six Red Cross homes, which provided 950 beds in total.[16] Ultimately, the Red Cross convalescent homes dealt with a wide range of inmates (as they were then referred to) recovering from an acute episode like pneumonia, and others with severe spinal injuries who had no chance of restoration to full physical function. Some soldiers, who had no expectation of leaving, were admitted and died in these facilities. Admission was not necessarily determined by their disease, injury or even the likelihood of a full recovery but it was a place where soldiers, who had endured the shared experience of war, could just be.

Psychology

A diagnosis of shell-shock included a variety of physiological symptoms which varied in intensity and consistency. This enabled the psychological impact of war to be defined within a construct of the acute medical model. A model which doctors who at the time, were more familiar and therefore more comfortable with but which did little to help the soldiers. The physical manifestations of shell-shock included delirium, delusions, transient blindness, hallucinations, stupor, acute dementia, aphonia (stuttering), anarthria (inability to speak due to impairment of speech organs), mutism and other symptoms of affected speech.

As previously outlined, the Gallipoli *...campaign belongs to a stage of the war when the idea of a psychiatric problem had simply not entered into the minds of the medical service.*[17]

While the term 'shell-shock' was used to describe a diverse range of symptoms, it was not the only psychiatric condition suffered by soldiers. Evidence of alcoholism and depression are scattered throughout the diaries and letters of soldiers, nurses and doctors but they were, in the main, undiagnosed and consequently remained untreated; cases of suicide were also recorded.[18]

One English nurse recounted an event where suicide was used to obfuscate dishonour. Sister Harries had served with 3 AGH but was on transport duty aboard HMHS *Salta* from August 1916 as the ship moved casualties from Le Havre to Dublin. On 29 September the ship struck rocks at Culver Cliff near the Isle of Wight. The 800 patients on board behaved well and the low tide and calm sea prevented the ship from breaking up but the …*Chief Officer shot himself and died about 11am.*[19] There were no other deaths from this incident.

There is some evidence that there were attempts to introduce a basic level of psychological rehabilitation during the Gallipoli Campaign. Although there were only twenty beds in the 'military mental hospital' established for the accommodation of Australian soldiers who had served at Gallipoli, there was a system of rehabilitation in place.[20] Usually the soldiers were given a short stay in hospital where they received nourishment, rest and massage and resumed wearing civilian dress. However, if their condition was considered chronic they were returned to Australia.

Shell-shock was a grey diagnostic area and depended upon the sympathetic diagnosis of the attending doctor. However, as the war continued and the number of shell-shock casualties increased, the Army came to the conclusion that medical officers were too soft-hearted and lacked military discipline.[21] Although there was a lack of consensus by medical and military personnel initially, it soon became apparent that when …*men admitted for "nervous breakdown" had won as large a proportion of "honours and rewards" as the general body of soldiers…*, military authorities began to review their position.[22]

As an act of kindness to those soldiers who would otherwise be inflicted with …*the stigma so cruelly associated with mental disease – a relic of the days not long distant when "possession" by the devil was a theory of pathology…*, special military hospitals were commissioned in Australia.[23] Therefore, the AIF admitted shell-shock casualties to military hospitals in Australia to avoid the indignity of their being certified insane.[24] Five designated Red Cross …*nerve homes…* were commissioned in NSW throughout the war because it was found that general convalescent homes were unsuitable for …*those suffering from nerves* [who] *are still our most disturbing problem.* It was noted two years later that …*the Nerve and Shell-shock Home has been a great help to the Red*

Cross, affording a suitable rest for these cases, who are not bad enough for No 13 AAH, and yet not suitable for an ordinary Convalescent Home.[25]

Foreign Wars bring Foreign Health Problems

The morbidity and mortality statistics of the 1914-18 conflict are confronting. An estimated ten million soldiers, young men from around the globe, were dead. Add to this picture twenty million soldiers rendered invalids due to limb amputations, facial disfigurements, blindness, deafness, speech and breathing difficulties due to the effect of gas and the residual effects of diseases such as depression, cholera, malaria and tuberculosis combined with years of chronic undernourishment.[26] The treatment of injuries caused by gas, shrapnel, bombs, bayonets and the extremes of temperature in the deserts of Palestine or the muddied trenches of Europe emerged as the war progressed. It soon became apparent the acute medical model of treatment was limited and slowly a multi-disciplinary approach to rehabilitation was introduced, albeit in an ad hoc manner.

Rehabilitation

The type of wounds sustained by soldiers at Gallipoli was a shock to nursing and medical personnel. They provided care on the beach, on transport ships and in the hospitals located in Egypt, but by the time soldiers returned to Australia the extent of their disabilities was apparent. During the First World War, nurses observed how soldiers responded to certain therapies and they progressively introduced the concept of rehabilitation within their nursing plans.[1300] This was done without specific reference to medical officers who had less time to take an interest in the recovery of a chronic patient during the war.[27] Therefore rehabilitation occurred more often by chance than design and the implementation of programs was not universal.

Elizabeth Kenny: a non-ATNA qualified AANS Nurse

There are examples of the medical model being overtly challenged by nurses. For example, Elizabeth Kenny who served in the AANS but was not ATNA qualified spent four years nursing the First World War soldiers.[28] Despite determined effort from the AANS leaders to see evidence of her ATNA qualification she managed to evade confirmation. She is the only AANS nurse to have feigned her ATNA qualification and when later asked about being known as 'Sister Kenny' she claimed it was an honorific earned as a bush nurse and military nurse. Nonetheless she returned to Australia where she formulated new rehabilitation therapies for sufferers of poliomyelitis. After the war her rehabilitative techniques were widely adopted despite being constantly ridiculed by the Australian medical profession. She became a household name in many parts of the world, particularly the USA, where her controversial and revolutionary treatment for poliomyelitis was embraced.[29]

During the war the personal and interactive nature of rehabilitation and convalescence fell more easily within the range of the duties of a nurse. Allied health professions such as social work, occupational therapy and physiotherapy were evolving but the underlying principle of modern-day rehabilitation was just beginning. While the medical establishment dominated the health portfolio at a political level, the nursing profession had undergone a drastic change in knowledge and confidence during the interval between the South African War and the First World War.

Convalescence

Definitions of the terms 'convalescent' and 'invalid' were fluid during the First World War. These terms, as commonly used and understood by laypersons and civilian trained medical/nursing personnel prior to the war, began to take on different meanings when applied to soldiers. Until this time the medical establishment had not considered rehabilitation of particular interest because progress of the chronically ill was often time-consuming and a cure was unlikely. For example, in 1914 surgical convalescence was deemed to be *...comparatively brief, and the surgeon is not so likely to have cast in his way that bug-a-boo of the internist – the "chronic"*.[30] The average length of stay in a suburban public hospital in 1926 was just over eighteen days and the mixture of acute and convalescent patients in one ward was still the norm at this time.[31]

In 1939 an edited text was published of 23 *British Medical Journal* articles and the topics covered *...a wide range of war-time casualties, whether falling within the surgical, psychological, or chemical domains.* Unsurprisingly the index makes no reference to the words 'rehabilitation', 'convalescence' or 'invalidism' because the medical model is based on a cure not management.[32] During the war these concepts melded to such an extent that it rendered any attempt to define them as arbitrary.

Electricity and Massage: Modern Physiotherapy

Today it is widely recognised that physiotherapy is an integral part of rehabilitation but prior to the war the discipline was in its infancy. During the First World War, 'electricity' and 'massage' were used to relieve pain, improve circulation and relax muscle spasm.[33] The aim of massage was *...the restoration of function.* It worked in two ways, '*reflexly*' and '*mechanically*'. The reflex effect was used to treat patients suffering from nervous conditions such as insomnia or neurasthenia. This is a term commonly applied to shell-shock during the First World War. It is disputable that the severe pain which accompanies a *...comminuted fracture of the neck of the humerus...* which is a severe break in the upper arm, would gradually disappear following *...very gentle massage.* Nonetheless, the mechanical effect of massage benefited lymphatic drainage, improved circulation and reduced contractures.[34]

One example of electrical treatment involved the application of rounded electrodes covered by saline-soaked pads or blankets applied to the skin. The pads and blankets were constructed of flat coils, kept separate by embedding them in a top and bottom layer of asbestos which acts as an insulator, and the *...electrical current passes through the resistance wire and becomes heated.* The current spreads evenly in the salt solution and the heat permeates the skin, reducing pain, releasing muscle tension, increasing circulation thereby bringing leukocytes to the area in a bid to destroy bacteria. Electric immersion baths were also used but electric treatment was not without side-effects, shock being the most significant. The observation that *...with a minor shock the patient may be frightened and possibly hysterical...* while a *...severe shock may cause loss of consciousness and cessation of respiration...* indicates that physiotherapy was by no means a pedestrian therapy at this time.[35]

Only two physiotherapists trained at the Melbourne Hospital in 1907 and SHSEH introduced training for their nurses in 'electricity and massage' in 1902.[36] One of the Melbourne Hospital-trained physiotherapists, Edith Pratt, served on the Masseurs' Registration Board.[37] An eminent physician, Dr Springthorpe, who played an important role in the development of a scientific approach to war neuroses in the First World War, was instrumental in the formation of the Australasian Massage Association in Melbourne.[38] Medical and nursing personnel developed an awareness of the important role massage played in surgical convalescence as well as general rehabilitative benefits.[39]

Almeric Paget Massage Corps: England: 1914

Initially, qualified nurses who had some training in massage were recruited with a view to training orderlies to perform some of the basic massage treatments.[40] In 1914 Almeric Hugh Paget, 1st Baron Queenborough, and his first wife, American socialite Pauline Payne Whitney, recruited fifty privately funded masseuses and instigated the *Almeric Paget Massage Corps* which was given permission to operate within Territorial Force General Hospitals. The success and importance of the service within military hospitals, command depots and convalescent hospitals was confirmed in May 1917 when the War Office took over financial responsibility and changed the name to *Almeric Paget Military Massage Corps*. During the war 3,388 masseuses and masseurs joined the service and when the Armistice was signed 2,000 were at work.[41]

Physiotherapists in the Australian Massage Reserve: 1915

In August 1915 the first twelve physiotherapists left Australia for service in Egypt and England; men held the rank of sergeant and women that of SN. Their brief, as members of the Army Massage Reserve, was to *...prevent muscular atrophy after nerve injury, promote nutrition in the tissue of amputated stumps, and prevent atrophy in stiff limbs and contractures of muscle and tendon after bullet wounds*. In addition to the initial twelve, a physiotherapist was assigned to each hospital ship and ten more were sent overseas in October 1915.[42] Given their comprehensive brief, the staff ratio was not generous, especially when Australia had 60,000 killed and 152,000 wounded soldiers.[43] Occasionally, the names of masseuses have been identified within the ranks of the AANS, while a number of AANS nurses had additional qualifications in 'massage' and worked predominantly in this specialty.

The chaos of the initial stages of the war meant that doctors, who had thousands of men waiting for treatment in CCSs, amputated limbs without considering the implications for future prosthesis. As the war progressed the rehabilitative value of a below-knee, compared to above-knee, amputation became common knowledge. The knee joint greatly assisted the fitting of prosthesis.[44]

Dietetics

Dietetics had not evolved into a specialised health-related discipline at the beginning of the war. Australian nurses were taught the importance of providing nutritious food to their patients because it was one of Florence Nightingale's first priorities in the Crimea.[45] Adequate food for the patients and nurses was a constant concern. The nurses initially lived on bully beef and biscuits but later the diet was changed to include rice topped with marmalade three times a day.[46] In France, Matron Phyllis Boissier was respected by her nurses because she *...has been marketing and striking bargains wholesale in the food line...* which gave each of her nurses *...a bonus of Fr 30 from the mess funds.*[47] Just as war created 'bands of brothers' on the battlefields, the adversities endured by nurses cemented professional and personal camaraderie within nursing units.[48]

Invalid cooking was a core component of the ATNA examinations, so AANS nurses were aware of the relationship between nourishment and rehabilitation. As previously mentioned, Blodwyn Williams (AANS) received soldiers from Ari Burnu who were *...skin and bone...* at 2 AGH (Mena House).[49] Nurses like Williams were aware that the lack of nourishing food compromised the recovery and eventual rehabilitation of many soldiers. There is also evidence that the dietary preferences of Muslim POWs were respected by Australian nurses who served in India.[50] The matron, who was responsible for procuring foodstuffs from local markets, quickly became aware that war created a scarcity of goods which benefited the seller and not the buyer. Australian soldiers had hearty appetites so local farms were scoured by nurses for fresh eggs and vegetables.[51]

On her return to the Melbourne Hospital, Jane Bell introduced a number of reforms including a diet kitchen and dietetic department. Furthermore, she emphasised the important role that diet played in a patient's convalescence and ensured her qualified nurses undertook six months' training in dietetics when the hospital's first dietician was employed in 1930. The dietician, Nesta Miller, was a qualified nurse who was sent to Toronto General Hospital in Canada to train in dietetics. She then visited Ann Arbor University Hospital and the Mayo Clinic in the USA as well as major hospitals in London and Edinburgh to gain practical insight into how a dietetics department should function. Comparative major hospitals in Australia, which were led by nurse leaders who had not served in the AANS, were less inclined to invest resources in dietetics.[52]

The procurement of eggs was also a priority in Australia. The Western Suburbs Cottage Hospital ran an egg appeal in 1916 during which time 1,080 dozen eggs were donated, mainly from the chicken runs in most backyards. An annual allocation for patients was set aside and the remainder was sold with the funds being used to improve the hospital. Due to the success of 'egg days' they became a regular hospital fundraising event.[53]

Diversional therapies

Nurses spent prolonged periods with their patients and they observed rehabilitation required time. Due to the varied nature of the wounds endured by the soldiers, the subsequent disability and expectation of recovery was not usually known. Nurses began to involve patients in diversional activities because *...as the patients become convalescent, they also become restless.*[54] These activities ranged from assisting the nurses with their ward work to organising sports days, musical evenings, special meals and reading rooms.[55] While serving in France, Emma Cuthbert (AANS) noted in her diary that *...the fields around us are during the season full of beautiful large poppies and yellow daisies, and we don't have any trouble in gathering great arms full for our wards, and on these little excursions any convalescent patients just about ready to return to the line,* *love to be asked to accompany us and help bring back their share of the flowers.*[56]

AANS nurses considered diversional activities to be the domain of the unskilled worker or VAD but not the professional nurse. Matron Mary Finlay served at 2 AAH, Southhall, England, where a large number of limbless soldiers were nursed and she claimed *...here is very little scope for skilled nursing, and the work could have been done equally well with fewer trained nurses, which would have released more qualified women for general war nursing.*[57] This was a common attitude amongst the AANS nurses.[58] During the war, Red Cross convalescent homes incorporated diversional activities and encouraged the *...inmate...* to participate in *...Activities of Daily Living.*[59]

Nursing staff shortages in Australia

Matron Finlay found the employment of qualified and experienced military nurses a waste in convalescent wards and this was compounded by the shortage of qualified nurses in civilian hospitals back in Australia. Community and political acceptance of nursing was heightened during the First World War. Previously the profession sought respectability but nurses were the only group, other than soldiers, who were in uniform and overseas, sometimes close to the front-line. Despite the demotion to a 'staff nurse' position, which was irksome to the more senior nurses from civilian hospitals, the consolation of overseas service was worth the indignity. Military nurses enjoyed a special kudos but civilian nurses, at home, also benefited.

During the war, recently qualified nurses in Australia were required to undertake varied responsibilities due to staff shortages. For instance, Ivy Little had not long completed her training when she was sent to the operating theatre where the surgeon, not recognising his new assistant, asked who she was and she succinctly replied *...Senior Nurse, Acting Sister, doing Matron's theatre work.* There is evidence that nurses, including Ivy Little and her colleague Amy Bembrick, were *...deemed to have completed their training ... six months before the expected date...* to cope with the additional demand for military and civilian nurses.[60]

Some nurses saw the shortage of nurses at home and their added responsibility as an opportunity to negotiate individual workplace agreements, such as Agnes Annie

Bindley. She had completed four years of training at Armidale and New England Hospital (NSW, Anaiwan Country) and passed the ATNA examination in September 1915. The ATNA examinations were brought forward to increase the available pool of qualified nurses.[61] Six months after passing her ATNA examination Nurse Brindley approached the hospital board for a pay increase. She sought £90 per annum but was offered, and accepted, £80 per annum.[62] Her salary, when compared to nurses who worked in a comparable public hospital like Ballarat for £60 per annum, was generous.[63] Despite securing this substantial pay increase she was not promoted to head nurse for another six months until 30 September 1916. Nonetheless, pay rises could not compete with the lure of overseas war service and she resigned on 30 March 1917 to enlist.[64]

AANS leadership reforms

The reforms to the AANS leadership following the Jane Bell incident were dramatic. Nurses in diverse parts of the world, nursing men their own age or younger, needed to feel confident in their professional leaders. They were civilian nurses who respected leaders who guided them through their training and were known to be competent nurses themselves. It was difficult for an incompetent or uncaring clinical nurse to gain the respect of her cohorts.

The administration of hospitals in Egypt during the initial stages of the war was sufficient to meet the needs of the Gallipoli casualties, but it would have been easier for the nurses if the question of leadership had been addressed earlier. The delineation of roles between doctors and nurses has been a source of consternation since the inception of the Nightingale reforms. Nightingale's first order of business on arriving at Scutari related to medico-nursing politics but she out-waited the doctors who in the end asked for the assistance of her nurses. Bell operated within the framework of the Nightingale system when she refused to accept the decision of Ramsay Smith just because he was a doctor. She had no qualms about accepting direction from those with bona fide authority over her such as the Surgeon-General, Egypt.

The complex relationship of doctors and nurses during the war is best exemplified by a nurse who claimed the only personnel who swore in front of nurses were not soldiers, but doctors. Soldiers were more likely to relate to the nurses as women, mother-figures and even angels because they saw them as special, even heroic. Doctors who recognised the importance of nurses to the recovery of their patients viewed them as colleagues. There are many examples of collegial relationships during the war founded on mutual respect and trust when doctors viewed nursing as an autonomous profession which complemented medicine. Doctors were also aware of the personal cost endured by many nurses and were solicitous of their welfare. Unfortunately, there were also examples of doctors who treated nurses with disdain and disrespect, as if the exposure of women to the degradation of mankind, which is war, in some way, degraded the women themselves.

However, the group which created the greatest tension and animosity were doctors like Ramsay Smith, who behaved in a paternal, patronising manner suggesting that the nursing profession was designed for the benefit of doctors and not for the welfare of patients. This situation was intolerable for nurses, especially those like Jane Bell who had endured many personal and professional difficulties to achieve a leadership position. Her example, no matter how controversial, demonstrated to those who came after her that civilian nursing achievements were not to be relinquished because a nurse wore an AANS uniform. War could demand a great deal from a nurse but never that. The result was the *...authority of the ward sister ... the head matron in relations with the medical officers, were not only recognised in fact but were laid down in military regulations.*[65]

Nurse leaders like Nellie Miles Walker, Rose Creal, Ethel Davidson, Jessie McHardy White, Evelyn Conyers and Maud Kellett created a new era of leadership which started in the civilian sector but was confirmed by their war service, creating a period of extraordinary potency for Australian nursing.

Rose Creal, Matron, SHSEH

Despite all the advances in medicine and nursing, the post-war period was a dangerous time, especially for worn out nurses. It was more than a year after the Armistice when Rose Creal disembarked from HMAT *Aeneas* on 12 January 1920.

She was discharged from the AIF at the end of May. At the time of her discharge Creal had developed a *...post influenza cervical adenitis with pressure on left brachial plexus causing neuritis in left arm*...but signed a medical report stating that *...I am not suffering from any disability due to or aggravated by war service and feel fit and well.*[66] Adenitis is defined as *...inflammation of a gland...* but she most likely had nerve compression in her cervical spine which caused pain in her shoulder, radiating down her arm.[67] Creal's decision to seek medical advice demonstrates that she was not opposed to approaching doctors for help when needed and her behaviour the following year was indeed out of character.

Rose Creal was immediately reinstated as matron of SHSEH and started the hard work of managing a major hospital during the influenza pandemic. In August 1921 one of her nurses remembered that her matron *...had acute abdominal pain and refused to see a surgeon. Dr Walker Perry was the Medical Superintendent at the time. Miss Creal absolutely refused to see a surgeon until the pain became unbearable, then it was too late. Miss Creal was taken from her bedroom straight to the operating theatre (ruptured appendix). But all the surgeon could do was incision and drainage tubes, after about a week, an embolism and her death in a few hours, (Sir Herbert Maitland the surgeon).'*[68]

Rose Creal's death certificate supports the nurse's account of the cause of death on 7 August 1921. It states... *appendicitis (one week) and pyelophlebitis (one week).*[69] Pyelophlebitis is defined as *...inflammation of the portal vein* [supplies the liver] *which gives rise to severe symptoms of septicaemia or pyaemia...* [toxins in the blood]. Basically, she had a ruptured appendix resulting in a severe infection throughout her body. The best course of treatment is antibiotics which were still twenty years from development.[70]

Early surgical intervention may have saved her life and the reason for such irrational behaviour from an otherwise rational person is difficult to discern. As already outlined earlier, she was noticed by a surgeon as having a natural aptitude in the operating theatre as a young woman.[71] Therefore, the operating theatre held no particular fear for her as a nurse and it is unlikely that she did not trust the surgeon. Sir Herbert Maitland was a renowned neck and head surgeon who mastered the skill of plastic surgery at a time when many soldiers were returning home disfigured.

Although he was a specialist surgeon there is little doubt he would be able to perform a simple appendectomy.

He had ...*lectured to Sydney Hospital nurses in 1900-09, and was an early medical member of the Australasian Trained Nurses' Association from 1899 and on its first board of examiners (1906-08). He was first lecturer in clinical surgery when Sydney Hospital became a clinical school of the university in 1909. Students and young doctors were attracted to the hospital for the sole reason that Maitland was there.* So Creal and Maitland were contemporaries. Ironically, two years after Creal died, Maitland felt a little unwell and went to his rooms where he died of coronary vascular disease. He, like her, was buried with Anglican rites at Waverley Cemetery.[72]

Three days after her death Rose Creal was given a full military funeral and St James Anglican Church was filled to capacity, with hundreds of mourners being turned away.[73] Media tributes were extensive and in one titled ...*Farewell Matron Creal – Mother Chief of Hospital – Friend of Broken Humanity*... she was described as a ...*woman with a deep religious belief.*[74] Rose Creal was known as a Protestant but her siblings remained Catholic — including her only remaining sister, Elisabeth, who was later interred with Rose in her Protestant grave.[75]

Given her humble beginnings Rose Creal's estate was extensive and included cash, shares in public companies, furniture, paintings, war bonds, property and interest earned from a number of mortgages to individuals. Her total assets were valued at £5,892 or ($577,000 in 2024) and her debts in the vicinity of £166 ($16,000 in 2024). She was a very competent businesswoman. Her last will and testament was signed on 18 August 1916, the day before she enlisted with the AIF; her sister and remaining two brothers were the only legatees.[76]

Following Rose Creal's death nurses contributed to a collection to provide academic nursing prizes in her memory and maintain her grave. The monies were invested and a cheque to the value of the interest (6% in 1925) was drawn each year by the Board of Directors; the amount was divided equally between the two nurses who gained the highest passes in the May and November fourth-year examinations. The Rose Creal Memorial Prize was highly valued by nurses of SHSEH but was discontinued in 1985 following the transfer of nurse education to the tertiary education sector.[77] On a visit to Rose's grave the author found it in a state of disrepair and attempted to find how these funds were now administered. They had apparently been absorbed into the new Area Health Service but were made available to the Sydney Hospital Graduate Nurses' Alumni, who ensured Rose Creal's grave was restored. Given her remarkable life and her contribution to the profession and her community, it is the very least she deserved.

33 Professional and Personal Legacies

Lady, fiancé killed, would gladly marry officer totally blinded or otherwise incapacitated by the War
– London Times

Australian nurses emerged from the war confident in their standing with their international peers. The nursing profession was depleted of remarkable leaders like Nellie Miles Walker and Rose Creal, but they were remembered by military nurses who transferred their example and knowledge into the civilian sphere.

Wives and mothers: Elsie Grant

After the war May Tilton wrote *The Grey Battalion* about her wartime experiences and dedicated it to her close friend, Elsie Grant. The book's foreword was written by Evelyn Conyers, who resumed private nursing after the war.[1] Elsie Grant and May Tilton had become firm friends by the time they said their heart-felt good-byes. Tragically, Elsie returned to find her dear mother had already died.[2] On her return to civilian life Elsie married Carl John Hock and they had four children, but her wartime experiences did not recede. When Elsie was 37 years old she committed suicide on 25 September 1927. One of her children, a daughter aged six at the time, remembers her as a *...kindly spoken gentle and loving person.*[3] The loss of a mother cannot be quantified but there is little doubt that the impact of war was ongoing. Those left to grieve included the children of nurses when mothers who died before their time.

There is no direct evidence Elsie Grant died because of her war service. However, a number of fit and healthy women, who were accepted for service with the AANS, died an early death.[4] At the time of the 1933 Census there were 1,844 returned army nurses *...who saw service in the Great War...* living in Australia, but the original count did not include those who served in India and later joined other units.[5]

Wives and Mothers: Alice Williams

The unique social dynamics which resulted in dramatic demographic changes caused by the war and the influenza pandemic are illustrated by the subsequent life of Alice Williams. The Williams family of Claremont (WA) lost a son, Arthur, and a daughter, Hilda, and were pleased to welcome home Alice, who had served with the British Red Cross in England. Nursing was a hazardous occupation during 1914-18 and they were no doubt pleased their second daughter, Edith Lillian (b. 1891) had elected to be a schoolteacher. She married Lionel Sargent, a chemist from York (WA) who joined the AAMC and served at Gallipoli and later on Lemnos *...where he had a tent with all his pharmaceuticals (not pills in those days but potions) ... He then moved to Egypt and then to Marseilles through France to Calais. Lionel Sargent went to 31 different depots in France. Then he went to England and had a lot to do with medical supplies at Horseferry Road (AIF HQ).*[6]

When Lionel returned home he married Edith and they had a son, John. Edith tragically died from septicaemia following the birth of their second son, Peter, in 1924. The risk of death during child-birth was ever-present and in Australia during the ten years after the war *...more women died in childbirth...* than soldiers died at Gallipoli.[7] Alice returned home and took responsibility for her sister's small children. She continued to care for Lionel and Edith's two sons and eventually married Lionel Sargent in 1926.[8] Alice Williams two sisters and brother were dead and her responsibilities to the living continued.

There were instances of nurses marrying returned soldiers, ex-patients, with whom they had a long history. Some women craved the opportunity to be linked with men who had endured the war, in the absence of a loved one returning. In the early stages of the war a bereaved woman placed an advertisement in the London *Times* which read *...Lady, fiancée killed, would gladly marry officer totally blinded or otherwise incapacitated by the War.*[9]

Nursing Sisters: Irene and Doris Ridgway

Ada and John Ridgway had lost Eric and Doris to the war and the influenza pandemic respectively. They were relieved when their sons Hugh and Victor returned to Australia on HMHS *Oxfordshire* in August 1919. They *...decided to move to another district possibly with the idea of keeping the remainder of the family together for a while longer.*[10] This was an understandable but vain hope. Their eldest child, Irene, known as Rene, remained at home with her parents throughout all their moves but after the war she decided to commence her nurse training at the Adelaide Hospital where Doris had trained.[11] Her motives for emulating her deceased younger sister are not known but it was not dissimilar to the action of Victor, Eric's younger brother, who had felt it was his duty to takes his dead brother's place in the AIF.[12]

On completion of her course in 1922 Irene Ridgway remained on the staff as a sister.[13] Like her sister, Doris, she contracted pneumonia and despite all efforts to save her, she died. While Irene was ill her mother, Ada, was recovering from surgery and she was, once again, unable to be at the deathbed of a beloved daughter. The tragedy of the situation is best related by one of Ada's sons who remembered *...Rene's death was a sad blow to her, more so as she was not able to see Rene in her last days ... in her grief requested that the hearse with the coffin be brought to the house front gate so that she could at least have a memory of her eldest child (a happening that was enough to make the angels weep).*[14]

The Uren Family Dynasty of Nurses

The entire contingent of AANS members whose surname began with 'U' were from one family, the three Uren sisters from South Australia.[15] They came through the First World War unscathed. Ethelda Uren, who served with distinction in Salonika, graduated from the Adelaide Hospital in 1895. She then travelled to Glasgow where she completed her obstetrics training and returned once again to South Australia, taking up leadership positions within civilian hospitals. In 1915 she was Principal Matron of 4 MD until she led the third contingent to Salonika from Melbourne in June 1917. Ethelda returned in August 1918 after more than two years and she received the RRC and Order of St John of Jerusalem for her service at 60 BGH, Hortiach, Salonika.[16]

Her younger twin sisters, Amelia and Catherine, also trained at the Adelaide Hospital, graduated in 1905 and served overseas from June 1915 until after the

Armistice, returning to Australia on 19 November 1918.[17] Two of Ethelda Uren's nieces, Honor and Elizabeth, also trained at the now Royal Adelaide Hospital and served in the AANS during the Second World War. Captain Elizabeth Uren (ARRC) left a descriptive and moving account of her service in England where *...the nightly blitz became a habit. Sisters were put into training for gas, fire squads and rapid casualty handling. Through all this, the English remained steady and hospitable.* She and her unit left Gourok, Scotland, for the Middle East, where a generation of nurses and her family before her had served. In 1941 they were in Alexandria and the hospital was filled with casualties from Greece, Crete and Tobruk. There were *...scenes of pathos and sacrifice that will ever live in our memories. How sad to see young boys of twenty-one, dying of wounds, and how glad we were to be there as women to soften the absence of their mothers.* Irrespective of the date, type and cause of wars the dynamics of being at the deathbed of boys changes very little.[18]

Margaret de Mestre: Manunda, 1942

Elizabeth Uren returned to Australia when the Japanese bombed Darwin (Northern Territory, Larrakia Country) in 1942. Margaret, the niece of Sarah de Mestre who had sailed on HMAS *Grantala* to Rabaul during the First World War, was on the hospital ship *Manunda* in Darwin Harbour when the bombing began. Margaret de Mestre died and another colleague, Lorraine Blow, received serious abdominal wounds but fortunately recovered.[19] Families of nurses continued to endure losses in war.

Nursing and marriage

In England, the ex-VAD Vera Brittain had lost her beloved fiancé and a brother to the war. When she finally decided to marry she considered that he was *...of the War generation, and that was all that really mattered. Had he been post-war I could not under any circumstances have married him, for within the range of my contemporaries a gulf wider than a decade divides those who experienced the War as adults from their juniors by only a year or two who grew up immediately afterwards.*[20] Brittain became a feminist, labour delegate and writer after the war. She provided a commentary on the experiences of a VAD in her book and also provided excellent insight into the social consequences of the war for nurses in England.

Public health and specialty nursing

One of the more dramatic changes after the war was the recognition of a number of specialities within nursing and medicine. Initially, the ATNA certificate was often referred to by nurses as a qualification which equipped them as 'Able To Nurse Anything'. However, changes in the nursing management of surgical cases and anaesthetics required the continual updating of knowledge. The influenza epidemic demonstrated the need for specialised nursing skills during a pandemic and the importance of public health nursing was recognised. Furthermore, the role of nurses was under scrutiny by emerging health professions as it became apparent that nurses could not be 'all knowledgeable' when it came to the health and welfare of their patients.

Management and administration of public hospitals

The collective experience of the First World War nurses created a milieu of problem-solving and a level of responsiveness to changing circumstances which brought with it special respect from their colleagues when they returned to a civilian setting. The names of matrons of public and private hospitals throughout Australia during the two decades following the First World War are often found in the list of AANS personnel or those who served overseas as part of other nursing units during the war. Those who served often became managers and leaders of public and private health facilities. They also undertook further education and introduced specialised courses to the nursing curriculum. It is not clear whether there was resentment toward returning Army nurses from those who remained at home and were by-passed for promotion. There is evidence that returning nurses, who wore a specially designed veil to differentiate themselves from those who had not served overseas, were held in high esteem by their colleagues. The contribution of the nurses continues to be acknowledged with a Roll of Honour in the foyer of most public hospitals throughout Australia.

Unfortunately, it did not take long for some members of the general community to articulate resentment toward returning soldiers who were being offered employment in the form of positive discrimination. However, nursing was a closed shop to some extent and just as nurses were proud of their matron and training hospital, so too were they proud of their senior nursing staff who had served in the war.

The Kellett Legacy

Maud Kellett returned to England in March 1919 and was appointed assistant collator of historical records until May 1919. She used the time to interview nurses who were awaiting transport home. The 'interviews' were a set of questions the nurses were required to respond to in written form. Given the position of authority exercised by Kellett, the responses appear to be stilted and even rehearsed when compared to the narratives elicited by A.G. Butler years after the war. Butler was a medical historian and he requested information about the nurses' experiences. Free flowing memories brought colour and detail to the narratives. Nonetheless, the interviews by Kellett are a valuable record of the nurses' experiences but as demonstrated by certain interviews, the lapse in time between the event and the interviews/narratives occasionally resulted in factual discrepancies.[21]

Maud Kellett returned to Australia on HMAHS *Kanowna* and disembarked in Sydney on 26 October 1919, after five years of service. After the death of Kate Porter she was appointed matron of 4AGH, Randwick. When Rose Creal died Maud Kellett became matron of her training hospital. She continued her association with the AANS and in 1924 was appointed Principal Matron of 2 MD and retired from that post on 31 August 1929. In 1920 she held the position of First President of Returned Army Nursing Sisters Association in NSW and she sponsored the first regular reunions of SHSEH nurses from 1923.[22] One of the most important aspects for professional nursing was the acceptance of the Australian Nursing Federation (ANF) as the national body to represent Australian nurses in the International Council of Nurses. The First World War nurses continued to dominate the profession, as the 1937 ATNA delegation list indicates. For instance, Jane Bell, from Victoria, was proxy for A Maud Kellett, President of the newly formed ANF.[23] Like Jane Bell,

Grace Wilson and many other military leaders, Maud Kellett supported improvements in nurse training and education. The preliminary training school at SHSEH bore the name of Kellett until absorbed into the Lucy Osburn School of Nursing in 1968.[24] As a memorial to AM Kellett, a fund was established for an Annual Memorial Prize for the highest marks in the written examination for general nurses.[25]

Maud Kellett was matron of SHSEH from 1921 until 1944, the year before her death. She died on 12 April 1945 at the War Memorial Hospital, Waverley, and was cremated after a service at St James' Anglican Church, Sydney. As befitted her military accomplishments, she was given a full military funeral one year before the cessation of hostilities in another world war. Maud Kellett's name is included on the Kellett family memorial at St Stephen's Anglican Church, Penrith and a memorial tablet can be found in the hospital chapel.

As Maud Kellett was being laid to rest, many RAANC nurses were being released from POW camps. Some of their colleagues had been raped and massacred by the enemy following the fall of Singapore. Their reality during World War Two is still in dispute to this day.[26]

Rehabilitation - Muriel Knox Doherty

While a number of nurses specialised in management and education, clinical nurses also furthered their knowledge-base after the war and sub-specialties of nursing began to appear. During the war, convalescence and rehabilitation increasingly became the domain of nurses. After the war Muriel Knox Doherty, who had served as a VAD nurse, trained at RPAH (1921-25).[27] She had an eminent career and co-authored one of the first definitive nursing textbooks, which became a recommended text of the Nurses' Registration Board of NSW. The book offers a working definition of rehabilitation which is described as an approach *...whereby a positive attitude is adopted, the individual's disability and ability is studied and bedfastness is reduced to a minimum. Stress is laid on restoration to maximum physical and mental capacity and independence.*[28] This definition has survived the test of time and underpins the main philosophy of rehabilitation.

When military nurses returned to Australia, many expected to work in repatriation hospitals and continue nursing their soldier patients. This was feasible in NSW and Victoria because of the relatively high population base, but less densely populated States like WA allocated wards within specified general hospitals for the management of returned soldiers. For example, Perth Public Hospital had three general wards allocated for the care of rehabilitation patients.[29] Minnie Lightbody (AANS) became one such patient. She served in France where, following an infection, she developed shortness-of-breath and persistent laryngitis. In 1917 she was deemed to be too ill to continue overseas service but well enough to be on transport duty during the return trip to Australia. In March 1922 she was admitted to her training hospital, Perth Public, with a diagnosis of endocarditis (inflammation of the inner lining of the heart), where she died.[30] Her name appears on the Kings Park Memorial, Perth.[31]

Convalescence and chronic care - Mary Stafford

On 26 August 1917 Mary Stafford returned to Australia on transport duty aboard HMAT *Benalla* and disembarked with her patients in Melbourne. She then proceeded overland to 4MD and worked at 15 AGH in Adelaide while she awaited an opportunity to re-embark for transport duty and further overseas service. The main convalescent hospital in Adelaide was 7AGH, but during the war it was necessary to commission additional auxiliary hospitals such as Torrens Park Military Hospital, near Adelaide, 15 AGH. A number of returned nurses found home nursing irksome because it no longer seemed real compared to the CCSs and the hospital ships.[32] However, Mary Stafford did not get an opportunity to return overseas but remained at 15 AGH caring for returned servicemen.

There is an unwritten law in civilian or military hospitals that when a nurse is ill and becomes a patient they are cared for like family. Mary Stafford had been working at 15 AGH for two years when she was diagnosed with acute lymphatic leukaemia in February 1919. Her workplace became her hospice during the four weeks leading to her death on 20 March 1919.[33] Her aunt was local but her sister was married and living in Perth.[34]

Mary Stafford was buried at the West Terrace AIF Oval in South Australia next to the returned servicemen she had nursed. Her name, along with that of Doris Ridgway, joined the York Minster 'Five Sisters' Window Memorial and is also included on the honour roll of the now Royal Adelaide Hospital.[35] Two exceptional nurses from the Adelaide Hospital who held such promise but tragically died when they were both twenty-seven years old. Of the 306 South Australian nurses who enlisted with the AANS, 235 served overseas and Staff Nurse Mary Stafford was the only one to die. One death too many for her aunt and sister.[36]

Repatriation

When sick or disabled returned nurses arrived home it became apparent they would have to rely on charity or their professional colleagues for support. The policy of Major General Sir Neville Howse to destroy the medical records of AIF personnel caused many returned servicemen and nurses problems accessing war pensions.[37] The situation was further compounded when doctors who had not served had no appreciation of what it meant, for instance, to suffer 'nervous debility' due to shell-shock or to experience recurring attacks of malarial fever. Howse had a prominent career in politics and was the Federal Minister for Health during the 1920s.[38]

Fortunately, the Australian nursing profession took care of many returned nurses from funds raised by public donations to the Edith Cavell Trust Fund.[39] Contingencies were made for returning nurses on a State-by-State basis. When the war was in progress and a number of nurses found themselves returning to WA sick or infirm, nurses like Eleanor Harvey were acutely aware that they had no place to live if they could not work. The benefit of nursing had been that it provided accommodation via the nurses' home as well as employment. When nurses were physically or psychologically unable to retain paid employment they were in effect destitute, unless they had private reserves or family who were in a position to help. Nurses did not have a pension system and Eleanor Harvey, who had remained in WA during the war, felt a keen sense of responsibility toward her returning colleagues. As a member of the ATNA Council she worked tirelessly to provide a scheme in which nurses did not have to rely on charity when they were no longer able to work. Some nurses had no alternative but to live out their lives in a womens' home. Through hard work and fundraising she developed a civilised and respectful place for aging nurses appropriately named the Eleanor Harvey Home.[40]

Many repatriation claims were made by nurses in their old age. Edith Dina Jackson, whose brother went missing and was later declared to have been killed in action, was seriously ill with broncho-pneumonia in Salonika. It was not until 1963 that she applied for a repatriation pension.[41] Staff Nurse Jackson married but it was often the unmarried nurses who endured the stigma of poverty. However, it was not unusual for the Edith Cavell Trust Fund to receive requests for financial assistance from married nurses who were caring for their husbands – often ill and disabled returned service men.[42]

Irene McPhail

Irene McPhail is a case in point. She had RTA suffering from pulmonary tuberculosis and remained amongst her family of colleagues at 11 AGH for another two years. She became increasingly emaciated and in March 1920 she weighed just 52 kilograms and had *...extensive tubercular invasion of both lungs with extension to larynx.* At the time Irene was still a young woman who was described as having a *...cheerful...*disposition with *...good...* habits.[43]

At the end of June 1936 the Repatriation Commission was responsible for the treatment of 206 ex-soldiers who were eligible for a service pension in repatriation hospitals or sanatoria and were suffering from pulmonary tuberculosis. An amending act was passed the same year to include provision for AANS personnel who had embarked on overseas duty.[44] Fortunately the spirit of the legislation was being implemented much earlier and a decision was made to discharge Irene McPhail from the AIF on 9 April 1920, with a recommendation that she remain in a sanatorium for a year. There is little doubt her death was expected and given the debilitating progress of the disease she herself may have welcomed it on 4 August 1920 at 11 AGH.[45] Irene McPhail had a difficult early life, which did not appear to impede her progress as a decent human being. The name 'Irene McPhail' represents the last AANS nurse who served overseas during the war and died within the timeframe for inclusion on the AWM Roll of Honour.

The Unionisation of the Nursing Profession

Prior to the First World War, ATNA was, in effect, a quasi-union/regulatory body.[46]It is interesting to note that Rose Creal recorded on her demobilisation form that she was not a member of a trade union, but under the question regarding her level of education she simply records 'ATNA'.[47] Unionism had distinctive political connotations at the beginning of the twentieth century. ATNA was often referred to as a credentialing association but there is no doubt that ATNA performed union-like services.[48]

In March 1912 Margaret Graham was asked to explain to the Board of the Adelaide Hospital her use of the phrase *...union is strength...* while addressing a group of nurses. She accepted the allegation but denied the words were used to incite the nurses to rebellion. The Board sought advice from the Chief Secretary with a view to dismissing Graham but was informed that any such action was most likely illegal.[49] Unionisation had specific social connotations but the middle-class position of nurses, coupled with a need for an extensive qualified female workforce after the First World War, created divisions within the post-war profession.

The Trained Nurses' Guild

When Drs Barrett and Ramsay Smith returned to Australia after the war they settled in Melbourne and naturally crossed paths with Jane Bell, matron of the Melbourne Hospital. James Barrett took a particular interest in the Bush Nursing Service and was the Honorary Secretary of the Victorian Bush Nursing Association for more than thirty years. He has been described as a champion of nursing interests and claimed that his bush nurses were better paid than those of any other branch in Australia. During the 1920s his involvement in the development of the Bush Nursing Service caused another rift with Jane Bell.

The concept of bush nursing services was innovative as it ensured that people who lived in rural and remote areas accessed quality and skilled nursing services. However, the program introduced by Barrett was not a free service. Furthermore the

Constitution of the Association specifically stated that the nursing of the sick patients was to be carried out under the direction of the medical practitioners except in cases of emergency.[50] A direct deviation from the Nightingale principles whereby nursing was carried out under the direction of nurses.

Jane Bell was intimately involved in the evolution of the RVTNA and its function was of paramount importance to the credibility of the profession until it was superseded by the introduction of the Nurses' Registration Act (1924). When Barrett founded the Victorian Bush Nursing Association he wanted the three-year nursing training course to include midwifery. Up until that stage this was an additional course and provided nurses with a second certificate. The importance of midwifery skills to bush nurses is apparent but there was no reason why the nurses could not undertake the additional six-month midwifery course after they completed their general training and then apply for bush nursing positions. This was the course of action advocated by the RVTNA.

Barrett opposed the Bill, which delayed the implementation of the Nurses' Registration Act. Confusion about the function of the Registration Board, which was designed to hold a register of qualified nurses who had passed a State Registration examination similar to the previous ATNA examination, resulted in a chasm within the Victorian profession. The Registration Board was never designed to act as a union or representative council. In 1921 about one hundred nurses formed the Trained Nurses' Guild further confusing the public about the role of the Registration Board. Jane Bell and a number of the First World War leaders who had nurtured the professional development of nursing focussed on educational standards and the power-base of nurses within the hospitals. Conversely, the guild viewed nursing as an industry with poor pay and working conditions. Advocacy was focussed on improvements in pay and conditions for nurses as opposed to the furtherance of the profession.[51] The collective energy of the profession was split and therefore power dissipated.

The privatisation of nursing

James Barrett regarded nursing as an industry and the individual nurses as units of labour. He wanted well-qualified units of labour and did not appear to see the hypocrisy of hiring nurses who were trained within public hospitals and paid during their training as public employees. His claims that the *...difference between working in hospital wards with Nightingale nurses – gentle women – on one hand and untrained male attendants and domestics on the other – is so great that to go back to the old system of so called 'nurses' in public hospitals caring for the sick would be repugnant for me...* suggests that Nightingale herself missed an opportunity to become a captain of private enterprise.[52] The trained Nightingale nurses were viewed by Barrett as a commodity.

Dr Barrett was a supporter of medical fees and he believed that hospitals were being abused by those who were anything but utterly destitute. He was also of the view that doctors were being subjugated by patients who could afford to pay for their services but were not required to. He wanted payments for medical services in public hospitals to be an integral part of the health system. This philosophy of 'user pays' for the Bush Nursing Service, in areas where many lived off the land and found it difficult to access cash even during good times, was mean spirited.

As previously mentioned, the British Medical Association expelled William Ramsay Smith for unethical behaviour in Adelaide. In contrast, (Sir) James Barrett had an illustrious albeit controversial career and was elected President of the British Medical Association in Melbourne in 1935.[53] His association with Melbourne University was long-standing and he was a Council member (1901-45); Vice Chancellor (1931) and Chancellor (1935-39).

NSW Nurses' Association

Two of Rose Creal's trainees, Ione Nowland and Jessie Tomlins, were great mates and pleased to catch up with each other in Egypt in 1917. Ione Nowland suffered from the effects of service in Salonika while Jessie remained with 14 AGH.[54] After the war Ione Nowland joined the Nurses' Registration Board and among other duties inspected training schools. She was appalled at the conditions under which nurses lived and trained during the Depression. When the Lang Labour government advocated compulsory union membership, Nowland, via a suggestion from Jessie Street, formed the NSW Nurses' Association and she was its first president in 1931. Ironically, the legalisation for improved conditions for nurses was resisted by ATNA which saw the establishment of a union as undermining its role.[55] Nonetheless, the NSW Nurses' Association grew to become one of the most powerful trade unions in Australia in the 1970s. Few student nurses would risk not having the protection of the union during their training and few registered nurses would forgo its powerful bargaining position with the government of the day.

Psychiatric nursing

In March 1931 the Australian press reported that a respected Australian officer of the First World War, Major General Harold Edward (Pompey) Elliott, had died of *...haemorrhage while undergoing treatment in a private hospital.* In fact, he was found by a nurse at 4.25 am with a razor blade *...embedded in a deep gash near his left elbow.*[56] Unfortunately his suicide and years of torment were not reported in the media, so thousands of men, who quite rightly admired and respected him, never knew their torments were shared.

The claim by Edmund Conklin, Professor of Psychology at the University of Oregon, in 1928 that the term 'insanity' was *...being rapidly dropped and some think that it will soon be obsolete...* was premature.[57] Nonetheless, steps were taken in Australia to introduce psychology as a discipline and in 1929 Henry Tasman Lovell, a scholar and philosopher, occupied the first full Chair of Psychology at the University of Sydney.[58] Advances such as this underscored an attitudinal shift and a better understanding of mental illness.

While the civilian medical, nursing and allied health professions learnt from the high number of traumatised soldiers, nurses and civilians from the 1914-18 conflict and transferred that knowledge to sound reforms, there is some evidence that the Army did not. First World War medical historian, AG Butler claimed that *...Mental "disease" can only be studied "scientifically" as a biological and physiological not a behaviouristic phenomenon.* However, he also noted that there were overlaps with the three types of ...*conduct disorders*... and doctors had to be diligent otherwise ...*the question whether a soldier should be "shot at dawn" as a military criminal, or be discharged possibly as a battle casualty with a "wound stripe" and war-pension*... may be answered incorrectly with dire and tragic consequences.[59] This volume of the Official History was published in 1943 at a time when soldiers were once again facing the horror of shell-shock in similar places against new enemies during the Second World War.[60]

The First World War did bring forth reforms in psychology and psychiatry because nurses and doctors were immediate observers of the impact of terror, fear, pain and shock on the human psyche. Ironically, the management of casualties after the Battle of Messines in 1917 was considered an unqualified medical success, but it was during this battle that Dr Roy Winn (AAMC) suffered an injury which resulted in the amputation of his right foot. Winn was a competent medical officer (MC, MID) during the war, but his decision to undertake further study in psychoanalysis was met with derision by his medical colleagues. After the war his enduring interest in the suffering of the mentally ill led him to become the first full-time private psychoanalyst in Australia.[61]

After the war Bessie Pocock specialised in psychiatric nursing and was matron of a psychiatric hospital in Newcastle (NSW, Awabakal and Worimi Country). She was later appointed Matron of Gladesville Psychiatric Centre, which enjoyed a reputation for the innovative management of diseases of the psyche. Like a number of the First World War nurses, including her nemesis Nellie Gould, she owned and operated a private hospital in Sydney with a war-related name. Pocock named her hospital '*Ismailia*' while Gould called hers '*Ermelo*' from her time in the South African War.[62]

Occupational Nursing: Enid Cherry

Enid Cherry trained at the Adelaide Hospital and sailed on the *Mooltan* as part of Ethelda Uren's Salonika contingent in 1916. She was invalided home with dysentery but recovered her strength and completed a certificate in midwifery. At a time when occupational nursing was a rarity, Enid Cherry joined the staff of the Myer Emporium and was responsible for the health and welfare of the staff for 23 years.[63]

The Grace Wilson Legacy

Grace Wilson was matron of Rosemount Military Hospital on her return home. Grace resumed civilian nursing as matron of the Children's Hospital in Melbourne in 1920.[64] This placement proved to be particularly difficult for Wilson who openly criticised the non-progressive hospital committee. Nonetheless, Wilson did manage to make small inroads at the Children's Hospital such as gaining approval for trainee nurses to receive a nominal wage. However, she resigned after two years service and purchased a private hospital, *Somerset House*, in East Melbourne which gave her the autonomy she sought.[65]

Private hospitals were on a par with public hospitals with respect to recruitment and training of probationer nurses. Many private hospitals were ATNA approved and a number of distinguished Australian nurses trained in private hospitals. Wilson held a prominent and influential position within the nursing fraternity and while operating at Somerset House she was awarded the Florence Nightingale Medal for distinguished nursing service in 1929.[66]

However, one of the major hospitals in Melbourne, The Alfred, was actively recruiting a matron in 1933. The position was highly sought after with a salary of £350 per annum, and forty highly qualified nurses from Australia and New Zealand applied. Grace Wilson finally agreed to accept the position with a number of provisos. She wanted £400 per annum and to be in charge of catering and housekeeping. Wilson's commitment to nurse training is apparent, as she stipulated that the three most senior managers in the hospital, the medical superintendent, secretary and herself, serve on the nurse training school sub-committee. She also insisted a tutor sister be appointed and, as all her requests were met, she took up the post on 18 January 1933.[67]

Within a week she implemented The Alfred's first Preliminary Training School (PTS). PTS was system of introductory nurse training, which was still in place in the 1970s, prior to the introduction of tertiary education for nurses. Matron Wilson's nurses were not paid during these eight weeks, and if they were found to be unsuitable they were immediately dismissed. Grace recruited her tutor sister, Miss Newnham, and sister-in-charge of PTS, Gwen Burbidge, from the Melbourne

Hospital, much to the chagrin of Matron Jane Bell. Grace Wilson was a probationer when Jane Bell was matron of Brisbane General Hospital but she was now a serious professional competitor, and a marked rivalry between the two hospitals developed.[68] Similar innovations were occurring in other States. Muriel Knox Doherty was the first tutor sister at RPAH when PTS was introduced in 1933.[69]

The emphasis on the training and professional development of staff by Grace Wilson was inspired. In September 1933 a post-graduate course, akin to what is now known as a 'refresher course', was introduced. It was the first in Victoria and attracted nurses from all over the state owing to the quality of the lectures. The course proved to be extremely popular and added to the kudos of The Alfred. Wilson's initial time at The Alfred was met with resistance by a number of nurses who had grown complacent, so she dismissed them. She had high standards and as the board wanted to restore The Alfred's reputation they supported the matron during every step of her restructuring.

Grace Wilson was also a council member of the RVTNA. When State registration was introduced in August 1934 the RVTNA ceased to exist, but the Royal Victorian College of Nursing (RVCN) came into being and took over the professional development and educational role of the RVTNA. Grace was the first Chairman of the Education Committee of the RVCN and was instrumental in introducing a two-year part-time Diploma in Nursing at the now University of Melbourne in March 1935.[70]

Apart from her civilian roles, Grace Wilson was the Matron-in-Chief of the AANS from 1925–41 – a part-time position for most of this period.[71] In 1937 she led a contingent of the First World War AANS nurses to London for the coronation of King George VI.[72] When the Second World War was declared, Grace Wilson was once again the most senior nurse leader in the AANS. She left The Alfred in May 1940 to devote herself to the AANS full-time; one of her students recorded how *...privileged we were to have Grace Wilson ... as our matron. She was tall, erect, always dignified and a magnificent person in every way. We were particularly proud of her on Anzac Day wearing her Australian Army Nursing Service uniform and going from The Alfred to attend Commemorative services.*[73]

World War Two: Grace Wilson

In 1940 Matron-in-Chief Grace Wilson was dispatched to the Middle East where she served for a year, returning to familiar ports of call including Palestine, Gaza, Alexandria and Cairo.[74] As the 'Rats of Tobruk' dug in against the offensive of the German General Erwin Rommel, Australian nurses like Wilson were ever-present. By this time she was 61 years old and had held senior nursing positions during the interval between the two world wars. In October 1941 she was forced to resign from the AANS as ill-health necessitated her return to Australia. [75] Initially the diagnosis was *...impaired constitution and anaemia...* but this was soon replaced with a less sympathetic diagnosis of *...overage, impaired constitution, anaemia.*[76] Despite this diagnosis the same month she was discharged from the AANS she was appointed Executive Officer, Nursing Control Section, Manpower Directorate in the Department of Labour and National Service, Melbourne, for the remainder of the war.

After the war and during her so-called retirement years Wilson continued to contribute through committee work. Apart from nursing committees and organisations already mentioned she was thrice President of the Returned Nurses' Club, Trustee of the Edith Cavell Trust Fund, Trustee of the Shrine of Remembrance, a life member of the Returned Sailors', Soldiers' and Airmen's Imperial League (1953), (a precursor to the RSL) and an active member of the Australian Red Cross Association and the Girl Guides' Association.

On a more personal note she visited London in 1954, where she married Robert Wallace Bruce Campbell at Holy Trinity Parish Church, Roehampton.[77] Hopefully she fitted a great deal of happiness into her late marriage because she died on her third wedding anniversary, 12 January 1957, at 115 General Hospital, Heidelberg, Victoria.

Arthur Boyd

Ironically, it was in this same hospital fifteen years earlier during the Second World War that Arthur Boyd endured the diagnosis of neurasthenia. His admission included a humiliating test of endurance as he, a good and gentle man like his father

Merric, had *...to produce drawings...* for analysis by psychiatrists. They ridiculed his art and enjoyed placing Freudian interpretations on his work. Fortunately, he continued to paint, to create, and in 1987 he produced one of his finest and most dramatic works, *Australian Scapegoat,* which was exhibited at the 1988 Venice Biennale. A painting which generates the emotions of war without trying to analyse or justify the complexities of it: It is real and it is revolting.

While Arthur Boyd left a legacy of artworks and land to the nation, he had a small and inconspicuous funeral.[78] Grace Wilson, a nurse, was farewelled with a great deal of fanfare. Her husband outlived her when she died aged 77 and she was given a funeral with full military honours at Christ Church, South Yarra.[77] Military histories and newspaper articles often refer to civilian trained Australian nurses who joined the AANS during the 1914-18 conflict to care for the sick and war wounded as 'angels'. However, they were flesh and blood women who endured the same deprivations as soldiers; and while they did not endure the injuries of battle, they endured the horror which comes from being a witness to such suffering. Recently (2007) a Queensland newspaper article was headlined 'An Angel Honoured' when reporting on the establishment of the Grace Wilson Estate at McDowall near the Enoggera Army Base (Turrbal Country) where 4,750 ADF members are stationed. The Grace Wilson Estate consists of fifty homes for Army personnel and it was built at a cost of $A17.5 million. It is a fitting tribute to a practical woman and an outstanding nurse leader.[80]

Jane Bell Legacy

Jane Bell managed to outlive Grace Wilson, who had shadowed her war and civilian nursing career. She retired to an apartment in South Yarra in 1934, aged 61 years. In 1942 she was awarded an OBE for her contribution to nursing. She lived in Melbourne for a further 25 years and died on 6 August 1959. Following a service at Scots Church, the cortege moved through Melbourne and passed the previous and present site of the now Royal Melbourne Hospital. Nurses assembled and paid silent homage to a woman who is synonymous with 'The Royal'. Following a tribute by the Returned Sailors' & Soldiers' Imperial League of Australia the bodily remains of

Jane Bell were cremated.[81] Her fortitude during personal and professional adversity was underscored by her absolute conviction in the professionalism of nurses and nursing.

34 The Final Word

If I should die, think only this of me:
That there's some corner of a foreign field
That is for ever England …
– Rupert Brooke

Rupert Brooke penned these words when death during war was considered to be glorious. [1] Opinions changed during the 1914-18 war. Vera Brittain was a feminist who came to nursing through patriotism in wartime. There is no doubt that she hated nursing – it was not a calling but a duty which had to be endured just as soldiers, who were once poets, endured the ugliness of war. However, she changed her view of Nightingale when she read her essay 'Cassandra' and *…realised the contrast between her rebellious spirit, her administrator's grasp of essentials, and the bigoted narrowness of some of her successors.*[2] When Nightingale's reforms are viewed within an historical and social context they are extraordinary. She provided the impetus for the dissemination of trained nurses who established hospital reforms in diverse parts of the world. The reforms included a prescribed system of ongoing education at a time when, in the main, education of women was considered a waste of time and resources.

In 2008 Brigadier John Caligari (Australian Army) claimed that the present-day military environment necessitated the development of an army of soldiers who thought for themselves. He believes this can be achieved by education as opposed to training *…Training is characterised by what to think. Education is characterised by how to think.*[3] Australian nurses who served in the South African War and the First World War were educated women. They did undertake a period of training in hospitals but essentially they brought to the war an expansive knowledge-base.

Some, like Nellie Gould, had a high-level formal education at Cambridge University as well as vast life experiences through social misfortune and extensive travel. Others, like Rose Creal and Jane Bell, endured difficult family events to develop an emotional maturity which brought self-discipline and empathy to the training hospitals of Australia. After the First World War, when training became the centrepiece of nursing, there was a more rigid ideal of 'the nurse', socially, educationally and intellectually.

The creation of unions, colleges and university courses promoted the professional development of nurse leaders but there began a decline in the community reverence for nurses, who were now workers in an industry. Initially, it had been this idea of belonging to a group of educated women who had a devotion to service which had attracted nurses within the Colonies and later in the States at the turn of the century. Their actions during the war and the influenza pandemic confirmed in the minds of the community that nurses were, indeed, special women. It confirmed in the minds of nurses that they would be treated with respect within the community but often with disdain in their work environment. It was not until the 1970s that the NSW Nurses' Association convinced nurses that it was not a crime to down tools and strike. The pay for a first-year trainee was less than that of a factory worker at the time but within a day of striking their salary more than doubled. This was eight decades after Margaret Graham was nearly dismissed for suggesting to her nurses that a union of nurses brought with it power.

Nightingale was a reformer of public health, of women in the workplace, of education and training for women, of colonial health services but most importantly of military health services. It was war which enabled the military and civilian nurse to be one and the same. It was war which identified the worth of qualified nurses in the CCSs and the civilian hospitals.[4] The shared experience of war gave a number of the First World War nurses a common point of reference when they returned to Australia and they introduced reforms and policy initiatives locally and nationally. They were extremely effective communicators because they were well aware of the power of the media during the First World War. They were also politically astute, as they were from one of the few countries involved in the war where they were able to vote on important issues such as conscription.

The decline of the profession occurred when the economic depression of the 1930s necessitated a change in employment conditions for nurses and most other trades and professions. The ideals and lessons learnt during the adversity of war by the leaders of the previous generation were quickly lost because nurses did not record their history and have failed to value it. The present curriculum for nurses does not have a specific history component. For example, the specialty of public health or infection control has no point of reference for the 1919 influenza pandemic. Nurses around the world know of Nightingale and some may be aware of Edith Cavell but few Australian nurses would think of their history in terms of the initiatives of Bell, Creal, Harvey, Graham, Wilson or Miles Walker. This is despite nurse training being replaced with nurse education - what to think being replaced with how to think. It is not possible to create a future generation of original thinkers without reference to role models who did so a century ago.

Monuments to war nurses commemorate the myth not the reality.[5] Those who survived often came out of the war with residual disabilities - physical, social, psychological - which were dealt with in an ad hoc manner by the authorities. Often it was left to the profession itself to provide for the needs of returning nurses.

The social circumstances of each of the nurses who died during the First World War were as diverse as the families which constituted Australian society at the time. There is no such institution as the typical family nor is there a typical soldier, nurse or casualty. The lesson from the nurses who died is that the war statistics are made up of individuals. Individuals who had personal and family histories and who, if they had not died, would have been at the centre of the next generation's history.

The mere outline of the lives and subsequent deaths of Australian nurses who served overseas during the war provides a glimpse into the lives of one cohort directly involved in the war. It is not the gender of the nurses which makes the details of their lives and deaths worthy of a record, because the loss of a daughter is no more or less grievous than the loss of a son. Nor is it their non-combatant status, because many men did not want to take up arms but an amalgam of social pressures forced them into a situation of having to kill or be killed.

The nurses who died represent a distinct group made up of individuals who shared a number of characteristics - gender (female), education (ATNA qualified), marital status (single or widowed), age (25-40 at the time of their death) and religion (Christian). Despite these characteristics, the most significant was that they died from the effects of nursing overseas during the war; each of their deaths was as unique as their lives. By considering the deaths at an individual level it is possible to view the often-quoted phrase 'twenty million dead' in a different light.

Ironically, Gavrilo Princip, who triggered the chain of events resulting in the First World War by assassinating Archduke Franz Ferdinand, suffered from tuberculosis.[6] He died as the war neared its end, in 1918, while imprisoned in a small section of a Czech fortress town. The location has had a number of different names, but during the Second World War it was a Jewish concentration camp known as *Theresienstadt*.[7]

During 'great' wars it is easy to paint history with a broad brush-stroke but the danger is in missing the details of the picture. The life and subsequent death of Australian nurses was such a detail. Their contribution to those for whom they cared - family, patients, nurses, soldiers and community - was appreciated and noted at the time. Nursing was primarily merit-based and there is no evidence that nurses were themselves anything but egalitarian in their approach, but they did not choose their leaders at this time. Politicians, board directors, leaders of the community and medical practitioners determined which nurses would become leaders at the turn of the twentieth century. Nurses who obtained positions of authority ensured that they did not waste the opportunity and many of the nursing organisations which exist today were founded at this time. The political and social environment into which they were born was as varied as the soldiers and civilians for whom they cared.

The separation of powers between Church and State may be easily articulated but the separation of political influence from matters of personal belief and religion are not - especially during times of war. The concept of divorce was considered a serious moral matter, but nonetheless, divorce rates in Australia steadily rose after the war and into the 1920s.[8] Feuerbach claimed that *...religion is the relation of man to his own nature...*in which case Australian nurses were true to their convictions.[9]

The interval between the First and Second World Wars was a time of progress through attitudinal changes in the fields of medicine, nursing and psychology. Just as the South African War nurses served in the First World War there were a number of civilian nurses who served in both world wars — Grace Wilson being the most notable.

This followed the depression. Life in the 1930s was...*the grey and tragic present.* It was a stark contrast to Rupert Brooke's pre-war life. The emerging dominance of Nazism in Europe and the Japanese Imperial Army in the Pacific meant the tragedy of war was about to be repeated. It is not possible to know if the poet would still ...*have thought that Holiness and Nobleness and Honor describe the causes for which those sacrifices of youth, and work and immortality were offered.*[10]

Socrates, while facing his own mortality, gave due consideration to what happens to a pure soul. He concluded that...*soul, I say, herself invisible, departs to the invisible world – to the divine and immortal and rational: thither arriving, she lives in bliss and is released from the error and the folly of men, their fears and wild passions and all other human ills.*[11]

Endnotes

1 Nursing in Australia 1788-1867

1. Robert Hughes, *The Fatal Shore: A History of the Transportation of Convicts to Australia 1787-1868*, Vintage, London, 2003, p.2.

2. *ibid.*, p.90.

3. Sarah Murgatroyd, *The Dig Tree: The Story of Burke and Wills*, The Text Publishing Company, Melbourne 2002, pp.104, 252-3.

4. Frederick Watson, *The History of the Sydney Hospital from 1811 to 1911*, Government Printer, Sydney, 1911, pp.7-8; 15-15; 29; 36.

5. Bartz Schultz, *A Tapestry of Service: The evolution of Nursing in Australia - Foundation to Federation 1788-1900*, Vol 1, Churchill Livingstone, Melbourne, 1991, p.22.

6. Alice L. Price, *The Art, Science and Spirit of Nursing*, W. B. Saunders Company, Philadelphia, 1965, p.4.

7. Juliet Piggott, *Queen Alexandra's Royal Army Nursing Corps*, Lee Cooper Ltd, London, 1975, p.2.

8. *ibid.*, p.3.

9. *ibid.*

10. B.M.Dossey, *Florence Nightingale Mystic, Visionary, Healer*, Springhouse Corporation, Pennsylvania, 2000, p.110. Studies of the life and work of the English nurse Edith Cavell in Belgium revealed there was a great deal of resistance to secular nursing prior to the First World War - see A.E.Clark-Kennedy, *Edith Cavell*, Faber and Faber, London, 1965.

11. Cecil Woodham-Smith, *Florence Nightingale 1820-1910*, The Reprint Society Ltd, London, 1950, pp.1-2.

12. K. Marx & F. Engels, *The Communist Manifesto*, Oxford University Press, Oxford, 1992, p.vii.

13. Woodham-Smith, *Florence Nightingale*, p.1.

14. Robert G. Richardson (ed.), *Nurse Sarah Anne: with Florence Nightingale at Scutari*, John Murray (Publishers) Ltd, London, 1977, p.114.

15. L.Strachey, *Eminent Victorians*, Chatto and Windus, London, 1919, p.117.

16. Woodham-Smith, *Florence Nightingale*, pp.59-60.

17. Strachey, p.117.

18. Woodham-Smith, *Florence Nightingale*, p.64.

19. Joan Daryl Lindsay, *The Story of the Red Cross: Australian Red Cross Society*, McLaren & Co Pty Ltd, Melbourne, circa 1939 (no page numbers). There is no reference to the publication of his book on nursing in his biographical details but he underwent his medical training in 1828 and the publication of a book on nursing may not have been considered a significant event in his life - McLean, Denis 'Dieffenbach, Johann Karl Ernst 1811-1855' *Dictionary of New Zealand Biography*, updated 22 June 2007 [online 28 March 2009].

20. German Literature Companion, *The Oxford Companion to German Literature*, © 2008, The Oxford University Press [online 29 March 2009].

21. Woodham-Smith, *Florence Nightingale*, p.69.

22. Barry Jones, *Dictionary of World Biography*, Information Australia, Melbourne, 1994, p.275.

23. Woodham-Smith, *Florence Nightingale*, p.69.

24. Florence Nightingale cited in Woodham-Smith, *Florence Nightingale*, p.69.

25. Woodham-Smith, *Florence Nightingale*, p.69.

26. *ibid.*, p.73.

27. Florence Nightingale cited in Woodham-Smith, *Florence Nightingale*, pp.73-4.

28. *ibid.*, p.80.

29. Letter to Mary Clarke from Florence Nightingale (20 August 1853) quoted in Woodham-Smith, *Florence Nightingale*, p.86.

30. Woodham-Smith, *Florence Nightingale*, pp.91-2.

31. Strachey, p.121.

32. Woodham-Smith, *Florence Nightingale*, p.108.

33. K. Fewster, *Gallipoli: The Turkish Story*, Vecihi Başarm, Hatice Hürmüz Başarm, Allen & Unwin, Sydney, 1985, p.36.

34. Richardson (ed.), *Nurse Sarah Anne: with Florence Nightingale at Scutari*, p.66.

35. *ibid.*, p.139.

36. Woodham-Smith, *Florence Nightingale*, pp.107-09.

37. Richardson (ed.), *Nurse Sarah Anne: with Florence Nightingale at Scutari*, p.85.

38. *ibid.*, pp.90-1.

39. Woodham-Smith, *Florence Nightingale*, p.107.

40. *ibid.*, p.108.

41. *ibid.*, p.128.

42. Richardson (ed.), *Nurse Sarah Anne: with Florence Nightingale at Scutari*, pp.84, 86-7, 151-3.

43. Australasian Trained Nurses' Association, Examination for Members, 'Medical Nursing' & 'Obstetric Nursing and Care of Infants' section, June 1914, Mitchell Wing of the State Library of NSW, ML MSS 4144(33) 56 ATNA Examinations (ATNA Records) in (Ruth Rae Collection, ACN Archive, Canberra).

44. Woodham-Smith, *Florence Nightingale*, pp.124-5.

45. *ibid.*, p.131.

46. C. Woodham-Smith, *Queen Victoria: Her Life and Times: Volume One 1819-1861*, Book Club Associates, London, 1972, pp.415 & 419; Richardson (ed.), *Nurse Sarah Anne: with Florence Nightingale at Scutari*, p.61.

47. Elspeth Huxley, *Florence Nightingale*, Weidenfeld and Nicholson Ltd, London, 1975, p.84; Dossey, *Florence Nightingale Mystic, Visionary, Healer*, p.109.

48. R.L.Russell, *From Nightingale to Now: Nurse Education in Australia*, W.B.Saunders/Bailliere, Sydney, 1990, p.9.

49. Woodham-Smith, *Florence Nightingale*, pp.274 & 276.

2 Nightingale Nurses in Australia 1867-1899

1. Cecil Woodham-Smith, *Florence Nightingale 1820-1910*, The Reprint Society Ltd, London, 1950, pp.434-5; E.Burchill, *Australian Nurses since Nightingale 1860-1990*, Spectrum Publications Pty Ltd, Melbourne, 1992, p.18.

2. Frederick Watson, *The History of the Sydney Hospital from 1811 to 1911,* Government Printer, Sydney, 1911, pp.134-5.

3. R. L. Russell, 'We worked hard, but we enjoyed it! General nurse training in NSW - The First 50 Years', *The Lamp*.May 1981, p.58. During this period (1880-1930) Australian nurse leaders had a variety of titles so for ease of narrative the author will use the title 'matron' when referring to the most senior nurse in a civilian hospital. The existing Sydney Hospital also underwent a number of name changes throughout this period but will be referred to as 'Sydney Hospital' for the same reason.

4. John Griffith, 'Osburn, Lucy (1836 - 1891)', *Australian Dictionary of Biography,* National Centre of Biography, Australian National University, Volume 5, 1974, pp.377-8.

5. D.G. Bowd, 'Lucy Osburn c.1836-1891: Founder of the Nightingale System of Nursing at Sydney Hospital', Hawkesbury Press Pty Ltd, Windsor, 1968, p.4.

6. Burchill, *Australian Nurses since Nightingale 1860-1990,* pp.10-2.

7. Manning Clark, *A History of Australia: the earth abideth for ever1851-1888,* Vol 4, Melbourne University Press, Melbourne, 1978, pp.248, 254 - 55.

8. Dorothy Mary Armstrong, *The First Fifty Years: A History of Nursing at the Royal Prince Alfred Hospital, Sydney from 1882 to 1932,* The Royal Prince Alfred Hospital Graduate Nurses' Association, Sydney, 1965, pp.23-4. The Prince Alfred Hospital Board of Directors decided to accept the offer of the 'Royal' prefix on 21 October 1903 as it was prior to the First World War the 'RPAH'is used throughout this book - electronic correspondence, Helen Croll to Ruth Rae, 9 April 2008 (*Ruth Rae Collection,* National Nursing Archives, Canberra). The author gratefully acknowledges Helen Croll's assistance in verifying the date of the royal prefix.

9. Watson, *The History of the Sydney Hospital from 1811 to 1911,* pp.36, 133-5, 202.

10. B. Schultz, *A Tapestry of Service: The evolution of nursing - Foundation to Federation 1788-1900,* Vol 1, Churchill Livingstone, London, 1991, p.219.

11. Watson, *The History of the Sydney Hospital from 1811 to 1911,* p.140.

12. Bowd, 'Lucy Osburn c.1836-1891, pp.12, 18.

13. John Griffith, 'Osburn, Lucy (1836 - 1891)', pp.377-8.

14. Schultz, *A Tapestry of Service,* p.220.

15. Watson, *The History of the Sydney Hospital from 1811 to 1911,* p.139.

16. Bowd, Lucy Osburn c.1836-1891, p.22.

17. Watson, *The History of the Sydney Hospital from 1811 to 1911,* p.168; Schultz, *A Tapestry of Service,* p.87.

18. Schultz, *A Tapestry of Service* p.87.

19. Perdita McCarthy, 'Ellen Julia Gould' in *Australian Dictionary of Biography,* National Centre of Biography, Australian National University, National Centre of Biography, Australian National University, Volume 9, Melbourne, 1983, pp. 59-60.

20. Barry Jones, *Dictionary of World Biography,* Information Australia, Melbourne, 1994, pp.75-6.

21. Armstrong, *The First Fifty Years,* p.24.

22. *ibid.,* p.16; Watson, *The History of the Sydney Hospital from 1811 to 1911,* pp.172, 180. The new Sydney Hospital which rose '*to be a monument of pride to the people of Sydney*' was not completed until 1894 and it was not until 1909 that University of Sydney medical students undertook clinical placements at Sydney Hospital.

23. Perdita McCarthy, 'Ellen Julia Gould' in *Australian Dictionary of Biography,* National Centre of Biography, Australian National University, Volume 9, Melbourne, 1983, p.60.

24. Watson, *The History of the Sydney Hospital from 1811 to 1911,*p.153, 173.

25. L. Potter (Pres), *A Passion to Care: Nursing and Nurses Western Suburbs Hospital 1984-1982,* The Western Suburbs Hospital Graduate Nurses' Association, Sydney, 2008, p.106.

26. Watson, *The History of the Sydney Hospital from 1811 to 1911,*p.178.

27. H. Paterson, *'5.30, Nurse!' The Story of the Alfred Nurses,* History Books, Melbourne, 1996, p.4.

28.Bowd, Lucy Osburn c.1836-1891, pp.20-3.

29. The royal prefix was gazetted in 1939, after the First World War so the present day 'Royal Adelaide Hospital' will be referred to as 'the Adelaide Hospital' throughout this book. J. Durdin, *Eleven Thousand Nurses - A History of Nurse Education at the Royal Adelaide Hospital 1889-1993,* Royal Adelaide Hospital, 1999, p.87.

30. ATNA Rules and Regulations & Schedule of Study, clause (iv) reprinted in V.Hobbs, *But Westward Look - Nursing in Western Australia 1829-1979,* University of Western Australia Press for the Royal Australian Nursing Federation (WA Branch), Perth, 1980, p.236; Durdin, *Eleven Thousand Nurses,* p.24.

31. Durdin, *Eleven Thousand Nurses,* p.25.

32. Nurses' Memorial Foundation of South Australia Incorporated, *Nursing –150 years of Caring in South Australia,* The South Australian Trained Nurses' Centenary Committee, Adelaide,1938 (Reprinted with 1939-1945 supplement in 1989), pp.279-80.

33. Max Griffiths, *Straight from the Heart–Tale of Tragedy and Triumph from the Nurse of the Australian Outback,* Kangaroo Press, Sydney, n/d, p.6; Mary Ann Latto Bett *Military Forces of the Commonwealth Papers,* NAA, Canberra.

34. Griffiths, *Straight from the Heart,* pp. 7, 9, 12.

35. Mary Ann Latto Bett, *Military Forces of the Commonwealth Papers;* Griffiths, *Straight from the Heart,* pp.13 & 81 (photograph).

36. Nurses' Memorial Foundation of South Australia Incorporated (Part 1), pp.288-92.

37. Hobbs, *But Westward Look - Nursing in Western Australia 1829-1979,* pp.12, 62.

38. *ibid.,* p.13; Durdin, *Eleven Thousand Nurses,* p.227.

39.Cited in Judith Cornell AM, Conference Paper, 2nd Annual Australian Nurse Practitioners Conference, Gold Coast, Queensland, 12-14 October 2006. The author gratefully acknowledges the late Judith Cornell AM for providing a transcript of the conference paper.

3 Australasian Trained Nurses' Association (ATNA) 1899

1. B.Kingston, *My Wife, My Daughter and Poor Mary Ann,* Thomas Nelson Australia Pty Ltd, Melbourne, 1975, pp.74-5.

2. ATNA minutes (26 May 1899) cited in Bartz Schultz, *A Tapestry of Service: The evolution of Nursing in Australia - Foundation to Federation 1788-1900,* Vol 1, Churchill Livingstone, Melbourne, 1991, p.350.

3. ATNA Historical Background', in ATNA Records, MLMSS 4144 23(56), Mitchell Wing, State Library of NSW, Sydney.

4. Schultz, *A Tapestry of Service,* pp.351-2.

5. Frederick Watson, *The History of the Sydney Hospital from 1811 to 1911,* Government Printer, Sydney, 1911, p.168; Schultz, *A Tapestry of Service,* p.351.

6. R. Lynette Russell, 'We worked hard, but we enjoyed it! General Nurse Training in NSW - The First 50 Years', *The Lamp.*1981, p.60.

7. Schultz, *A Tapestry of Service,* p.351; Ann M Mitchell 'Kellett, Adelaide Maud (1873 - 1945)', *Australian Dictionary of Biography,* National Centre of Biography, Australian National University,

Volume 9, Melbourne University Press, Melbourne,1983, pp.549-550.

8. Schultz, *A Tapestry of Service*, p.194; 'Australasian Trained Nurses' Association Historical Background', ATNA Records, MLMSS 4144 23 (56), State Library of NSW, Sydney, January 1969. While ATNA included New Zealand trained nurses, New Zealand had addressed the need to differentiate trained nurses from untrained nurses with the introduction of a Nurses' Registration Act as early as 1901 (see Anna Rogers, *While You're Away: New Zealand Nurses at War 1899-1948,* Auckland University Press, Auckland, 2003, p.14).

9. The birth record states her name as 'Lettitia Gladwys Moreton' born at Warracknabeal, Victoria but the spelling and location of her birth have been accepted as that hand written by Miss Moreton at the time of her enlistment; Letitia Gladys Moreton, *Military Forces of the Commonwealth Papers,* NAA, Canberra; Digger-Federation Index.Victoria 1889-1901 [online 18 August 2006].

10. Letitia Gladys Moreton, *Military Forces of the Commonwealth Papers.*

11. Reminiscences of Eleanor Harrald cited in Nurses' Memorial Foundation of South Australia Incorporated, *Nursing –150 years of Caring in South Australia,* The South Australian Trained Nurses' Centenary Committee, Adelaide,1938 (Reprinted with 1939-1945 supplement in 1989), p.47.

12. *ibid;* J Durdin, *Eleven Thousand Nurses – A History of Nurse Education at the Royal Adelaide Hospital 1889-1993,* pp.40-41.

13. Durdin, *Eleven Thousand Nurses,* pp.40-41, 57.

14. ATNA Register of Nurses cited in R.L.Russell, *From Nightingale to Now: Nurse Education in Australia,* W.B. Saunders/Bailliere, Sydney, 1990, p.19.

15. D.G. Bowd, 'Lucy Osburn c.1836-1891: Founder of the Nightingale System of Nursing at Sydney Hospital', Hawkesbury Press Pty Ltd, Windsor, 1968, p.20.

16. Watson, *The History of the Sydney Hospital from 1811 to 1911,* p.143.

17. The name change occurred in 1934 so the present day 'Prince Henry Hospital' will be referred to as the 'Coast Hospital' throughout this book – M.Cordia, *Nurses at Little Bay,* Prince Henry Trained Nurses' Association, Sydney, 1990, pp.13, 129.

18. W. Smith, *Blessed are They – The Story of the Bowral & District Hospital, Bowral, NSW 1889-1989,* Weston and Co. Print, Kiama, 1989, p.28; Potter, p.96.

19. V.Hobbs, *But Westward Look – Nursing in Western Australia 1829-1979,* University of Western Australia Press for the Royal Australian Nursing Federation (WA Branch), Perth, 1980, pp.29-30. The Royal Perth Hospital has undergone a number of name changes and did not adopt the 'Royal' prefix until 1948 so will be referred to as 'Perth Public Hospital' throughout this book – G.C. Bolton & P. Joske, *History of Royal Perth Hospital,* Royal Perth Hospital, Perth, 1982, p.136.

20. Bolton & Joske, *History of Royal Perth Hospital,* p.61.

21. A. Gregory, *The Ever Open Door – A History of the Royal Melbourne Hospital 1848-1998,* Hyland House, Melbourne, 1998, p.96.

22. D.M.Armstrong *The First Fifty Years – A History of Nursing at The Royal Prince Alfred Hospital, Sydney from 1882-1932,* Royal Prince Alfred Graduate Nurses Association, Sydney 1965, p.20.

23. Bolton & Joske, *History of Royal Perth Hospital,* pp.61, 78.

24. Armstrong, *The First Fifty Years,* p.21.

25. Watson, *The History of the Sydney Hospital from 1811 to 1911,* pp.144, 178.

26. Florence Nightingale, *Notes on Nursing – What it is and what it is not,* D.Appleton and Company, New York, 1860, pp.63-79.

27. Narrative, Principal Matron Jessie McHardy White *Records of A.G. Butler: Official Historian of Australian Army Medical Services – Nurses' Narratives.*

28. Cordia, *Nurses at Little Bay,* p.75.

29. Australasian Trained Nurses' Association, Examination for Members, 'Mental Nurses' section, 1911, Mitchell Wing of the State Library of NSW, ML MSS 4144(33) 56 ATNA Examinations (ATNA Records) (copy in possession of the author now in *Ruth Rae Collection*, National Nursing Archives, Canberra).

30. M Dickens, *An Open Book*, Heinemann, London, 1978, pp.70-5.

31. Gregory, *The Ever Open Door,* pp.95-7.

32. Cecil Woodham-Smith, *Florence Nightingale 1820-1910*, The Reprint Society Ltd, London, 1950, pp.414-7.

33. Armstrong, *The First Fifty Years,* p.93; Jan Bassett, *Guns and Brooches: Australian Army Nursing from the Boer War to the Gulf War,* Oxford University Press, Melbourne, 1992, p.9; Woodham-Smith, *Florence Nightingale 1820-1910*, p.413.

34. Rogers, *While You're Away,* pp.14, 43.Details and research relating to this topic have been previously published in R.Rae (2007) 'A comparative analysis of the development of the Australian Army Nursing Service and the New Zealand Army Nursing Service (1899-1918)', *nursing.aust*, Journal of the College of Nursing, 8(2):14-17.

35. P.A. Sargison 2006, 'Maclean, Hester 1859-1932' in *Dictionary of New Zealand Biography,* updated 7 April 2006. URL: http://www.dnzb.govt.nz/; Rogers, *While You're Away,* p.14.

36. Ethel Turner, *Seven Little Australians,* Penguin Group Australia, Melbourne, 1994, pp.1-2.

37. Research relating to Rose Creal has been published in R. Rae, 'Nursing in War and Peace: the life of Matron Rose Creal (1865-1921)', *Journal of the Royal Australian Historical Society,* 95 (1), 2009.

38. Manning Clark, *A History of Australia: The Beginnings of an Australian Civilisation 1824-1851,* Vol 3, Melbourne University Press, Melbourne, 1973, p.454.

39. A. Atkinson, *The Europeans in Australia A History:* Democracy (Vol 2), Oxford University Press, Melbourne, 2004, p.312.

40. Manning Clark, *A History of Australia: The earth abideth for ever 1851-1888,* Vol 4, Melbourne University Press, Melbourne, 1978, p.141.

41. Joanne Ewin, *Meet the Pioneers: Early Families of the Milton-Ulladulla District with Photographs,* (ISBN 0 646 01711 X), 1991, p.177.

42. Sydney Hospital 1915 Annual Report, Printed by WE Smith Ltd., Bridge St, Sydney, 1916, p.106.

43. Ewin, p.177; R.Rae 'The other Matron Porter' *The Milton-Ulladulla Times,* 8 January 2003.

44. Sydney Hospital 1915 Annual Report, p.106.

4 A Short Clinical History of Nursing and Medicine

1. Robert G Richardson (ed.), *Nurse Sarah Anne: with Florence Nightingale at Scutari,* John Murray (Publishers) Ltd, London, 1977, p.158.

2. L. Potter (Pres), *A Passion to Care: Nursing and Nurses Western Suburbs Hospital 1984-1982,* The Western Suburbs Hospital Graduate Nurses' Association, Sydney, 2008, p.48.

3. Barbara F. Cape, *Baillière's Nurses' Dictionary,* Baillière, Tindall and Cox, London, 1956, pp.47, 149, 201.

4. H. Gregory & C. Brazil, *Bearers of the Tradition: Nurses of the Royal Brisbane Hospital 1888-1993,* Boolarong Publications, Brisbane, 1993, p.xi (*n*).

5. P. Garrick and C. Jeffery, *Fremantle Hospital: A Social History to 1987,* Fremantle Hospital, Perth, 1987, p.130.

6. Guy R. Williams, *The Age of Miracles: Medicine and Surgery in the Nineteenth Century,* Constable,

London, 1981, pp.122-3, 125-7.

7. A.G. Butler, *The Official History of the Australian Army Medical Services in the war of 1914-1918 The Western Front*, Vol 2, Australian War Memorial, Canberra, 1940, p.355.

8. Dinning cited in M. Barker, *Nightingales in the Mud,* Allen and Unwin, Sydney, 1989, pp.126-7; Williams, *The Age of Miracles*, pp.122-3.

9. Elsie Tranter diary, 29 January 1918, in G. M. Gillings and J. Richards (eds) ... *in All those Lines: The diary of Sister Elsie Tranter 1916-1919*, s/p.2008, p.91.

10. Garrick & Jeffery, *Fremantle Hospital: A Social History to 1987*, p.130.

11. Potter, *A Passion to Care*, p.63.

12. Jackie Campbell cited in Stephanie Pain, 'The Pharaoh's Pharmacist' in *New Scientist* No. 2634, 15 December 2007, p.42.

13. Williams, *The Age of Miracles*, pp.57-8

14. Florence Nightingale, *Notes on Nursing: What It Is and What It Is Not*, p.94; A. Gregory, *The Ever Open Door – A History of the Royal Melbourne Hospital 1848-1998*, p.52.

15. Gregory, *The Ever Open Door*, p.52.

16. Ann Stafford Bird (aka Mrs Arthur H Garnsey), *Scarlet Pillows: An Australian Nurse's Tales of Long Ago*, Hesperian Press, Perth, 1984, p.132.

17. Gregory, *The Ever Open Door*, pp.55-6, 241. The royal prefix was gazetted in 1935 so the present day 'Royal Melbourne Hospital' will be referred to as 'the Melbourne Hospital' throughout this book.

18. Williams, *The Age of Miracles*, p.59.

19. Death certificate, Rose Ann Creal, *Births, Deaths and Marriages Registration Act 1995* (No 1921/009915), copy in *Ruth Rae Collection*, National Nursing Archives, Canberra.

20. Author photograph, September 2005 and oral history, Doubtful Sound, New Zealand in *Ruth Rae Collection*, National Nursing Archives, Canberra.

21. Winn cited in Butler, *The Western Front*, p.63.

22. Narrative, Principal Matron Gertrude Davis, *Records of A.G. Butler: Official Historian of Australian Army Medical Services – Nurses' Narratives,* AWM 41, File 373.2, Canberra.

23. L. Bickel, *Florey – The Man who Made Penicillin*, (originally published as *Rise up to Life* in 1972) Sun Books Pty Ltd, Melbourne, 1983, pp.11, 35, 244-6.

24. H. Paterson, *'5.30, Nurse!' The Story of the Alfred Nurses*, History Books, Melbourne, 1996, p.38.

25. Jamie Shreeve 'The killer that came in from the cold', 1 July 2006 in *The Good Weekend – Sydney Morning Herald Magazine*, Sydney, pp.36-7; Walter Isaacson, *The Code Breaker: Jennifer Doudna, gene editing, and the future of the human race,* Simon & Schuster (Australia)Pty Ltd, Sydney, 2021.

26. Narrative, K.M. Taylor *Records of A.G. Butler: Official Historian of Australian Army Medical Services – Nurses' Narratives,* p.3.

27. Alice Hope Moulton cited in M.Cordia, *Nurses at Little Bay*, Prince Henry Trained Nurses' Association, Sydney, 1990, pp.84-5.

28. Doherty, Sirl & Ring, *Modern Practical Nursing Procedures,* Dymocks Book Arcade Ltd, Sydney, 1944, pp.ix, 528-9. This was a recommended reading text for a number of years and the foreword was written by Australian nurse leader Rose Kirkcaldie (QAIMNSR). The first Australian nursing text was written by Matron Gwen N. Burbidge, *Lectures for Nurses*, Australasian Medical Publishing Co Ltd, Glebe, circa 1935 (1st ed). The author gratefully acknowledges Judith Godden and the (late) Judith Cornell AM, who brought this information to my attention.

29. Terrot in Richardson, *Nurse Sarah Anne*, p.158.

30. A. G. Butler, *The Official History of the Australian Army Medical Services in the War of 1914-1918 Gallipoli, Palestine and New Guinea*, Vol 1, (2nd ed.), Australian War Memorial, Melbourne, 1938, pp.26, 40; B.F. Miller & C.B. Keane, *Encyclopedia and Dictionary of Medicine and Nursing*, W. B. Saunders Co, London, 1972, pp.55, 470, 1020.

31. Butler, *Gallipoli, Palestine and New Guinea*, p.247.

32. Miller & Keane, *Encyclopedia and Dictionary of Medicine and Nursing*, pp.55 & 470.

33. Butler, *Gallipoli, Palestine and New Guinea*, p.456.

34. Herbert E. Cuff & W.T. Gordon Pugh, *Practical Nursing including Hygiene and Dietetics* (7th ed.), William Blackwood & Sons Ltd, London, 1928, pp.243-4; Cape, *Baillière's Nurses' Dictionary*, p.330.

35. Butler, *Gallipoli, Palestine and New Guinea*, pp.456-7.

36. Williams, *The Age of Miracles*, pp.198-202; B. Jones, *Dictionary of World Biography*, Information Australia, Melbourne, 1994, p.634.

37. Diary entry (13 June 1915) in narrative, E.J. Tucker *Records of A.G. Butler: Official Historian of Australian Army Medical Services - Nurses' Narratives.*

38. Narrative, Alma Bennett, *Records of A.G. Butler: Official Historian of Australian Army Medical Services - Nurses' Narratives.*

39. Narrative, A.N. Smith, *Records of A. G. Butler: Official Historian of Australian Army Medical Services - Nurses' Narratives.*

40. Williams, *The Age of Miracles*, pp.204, 207.

41. John M. Wall, 'Nicholas, George Richard Rich (1884 - 1960)', *Australian Dictionary of Biography*, National Centre of Biography, Australian National University, Volume 11, Melbourne University Press, 1988, pp.18-20.

42. Williams, *The Age of Miracles*, pp.208-11.

43. Brenda Maddox, *Rosalind Franklin: The Dark Lady of DNA*, Harper Collins Publishers, London, 2003, p.134.

44. Williams, *The Age of Miracles*, pp.220-22; Jones, *Dictionary of World Biography*, pp.58, 186.

45. Williams, *The Age of Miracles*, pp. 49-50.

46. Cape, *Baillière's Nurses' Dictionary*, p.111.

47. Williams, *The Age of Miracles*, pp.42-9; Jones, *Dictionary of World Biography*, pp.196, 247, 447.

48. Cape, *Baillière's Nurses' Dictionary*, p.111.

49. Williams, *The Age of Miracles*, p.52.

50. HM Queen Victoria cited in C. Woodham-Smith, *Queen Victoria: Her Life and Times - Volume One 1819-1861*, Book Club Associates, London, 1972, p.388.

51. Gregory, *The Ever Open Door*, p.32.

52. A. Hyslop, *Sovereign Remedies: A History of Ballarat Base Hospital 1850s to 1980s*, Allen and Unwin Australia Pty Ltd, Sydney, 1989, p.38.

5 Colonial Army Nursing in the South African War 1899-1902

1. C. Woodham-Smith, *Florence Nightingale 1820-1910*, Constable and Company Ltd, London, 1950, pp.260-1, 318-21, .343.

2. F. Nightingale, *Notes on Nursing - What it is and what it is not*, D. Appleton and Company, New York, 1860, pp.8-9.

3. R. Goodman, *Our War Nurses: The History of the Royal Australian Army Nursing Corps 1902-1988,* Boolarong Publications, Brisbane, 1988, p.70.

4. Sheila Gray, *The South African War 1899-1902: service records of British and colonial women: a record of the service in South Africa of military and civilian nurses, laywomen and civilians.* ISBN: 0-473-01926-4, Auckland, 1993, self-published, p.13.

5. A.J. Hill, 'Williams, Sir William Daniel Campbell (1856-1919)', *Australian Dictionary of Biography,* National Centre of Biography, Australian National University, Volume 12, Melbourne University Press, 1990, pp.506-508.

6. Correspondence, 'Miss E.J. Gould to Colonel A.G. Butler,' (Gould Letter), 29 June 1933, AWM 41 975, Papers of Historian of Australian Army Medical Services, AWM, Canberra.

7. Gray, *The South African War 1899-1902,* p.13; J.Bassett, *Guns and Brooches,* Oxford University Press, Melbourne, 1992, pp.8-9.

8. Bassett, *Guns and Brooches,* pp.8-9.

9. Gray, *The South African War 1899-1902,* p.13; Ellen Gould, Report titled 'Assistance asked in Connection with the Collection of Historical Material for AANS, AIF' (Gould Report), n/d, Papers of Historian of Australian Army Medical Services (Butler Papers), file 4364/34/6, AWM, Canberra, pp.1-2.

10. B. Tuchman, *The Proud Tower,* Hamish Hamilton, London, 1966, p.32.

11. Manning Clark, *A History of Australia: The People Make Laws 1888-1915,* Vol 5, Melbourne University Press, Melbourne, 1981, p.172; Bassett, *Guns and Brooches,* p.9.

12. Anna Rogers, *While You're Away: New Zealand Nurses at War 1899-1948,* Auckland University Press, Auckland, 2003, p.16.

13. Bassett, *Guns and Brooches,* p.10.

14. Perdita M. McCarthy, 'Pocock, Mary Anne (Bessie) (1863-1946)', *Australian Dictionary of Biography,* National Centre of Biography, Australian National University, Volume 11, Melbourne University Press, 1988, pp.251-2.

15. AWM Nominal Roll: http://www.awm.gov.au/database/[online 7 July 2005]; AWM Honours and Awards: http://www.awm.gov.au/database/[online 8 July 2005]; Bassett, pp.13-6, 21, 22, 24, 27.

16. P. Adam-Smith, *Australian Women at War,* Penguin Books Australia Ltd., Melbourne, 1996, p.10; Bassett, *Guns and Brooches,* p.214.

17. Adam-Smith, *Australian Women at War,* p.10.

18. Photograph of the grave of Fanny Hines at AWM: http://cas.awm.gov.au/photograph/P04544.004 [online 12 January 2008].

19. Julia Anderson cited in Bassett, *Guns and Brooches,* p.24.

20. Australasian Trained Nurses' Association (founded 1899), 'Register of Members 1916', Websdale, Shoosmith Ltd, Sydney, p.87.

21. Woodham-Smith, *Florence Nightingale 1820-1910,* p.193.

22. Alice Terrot cited in Robert G Richardson (ed.), *Nurse Sarah Anne: with Florence Nightingale at Scutari,* John Murray (Publishers) Ltd, London, 1977, p.165.

23. J. Piggott, *Queen Alexandra's Royal Army Nursing Corps,* Leo Cooper Ltd, London, 1975, p.35; Taprell Dorling in assoc. with F Guille *Ribbons and Medals,* George Phillip and Son Ltd., London, 1960, p.39.

24. Dorling, *Ribbons and Medals,* p.19; R.Rae, *First World War Commemorative Nominal Roll,* ACN Trilogy, Canberra, 2015. Note: The aforementioned Nominal Roll includes honours and awards.

25. Stuart Braga, *Anzac Doctor: the Life of Sir Neville Howse, VC,* Hale & Iremonger, Sydney, 2000, p.52.

26. A.G. Butler, *The Official History of the Australian Army Medical Services in the war of 1914-1918: Special Problems and Services*, Vol 3, Australian War Memorial Canberra, 1943, p.455.

27. Tuchman, *The Proud Tower*, pp.57-8.

28. Clark, *The People Make Laws*, p.170.

29. Rogers, *While You're Away*, p.13.

30. V. Hobbs, *But Westward Look–Nursing in Western Australia 1829-1979*, University of Western Australia Press for the Royal Australian Nursing Federation (WA Branch), Perth, 1980, p.17.

31. Bassett, *Guns and Brooches*, pp.9-11.

32. Rogers, *While You're Away*, pp.16, 30.

33. Piggott, *Queen Alexandra's Royal Army Nursing Corps*, p.33.

34. B. Jones, *Dictionary of World Biography*, Information Australia, Melbourne, 1994, p.502.

35. Braga, *Anzac Doctor*, pp.20-1, 88; Treves cited in Piggott, *Queen Alexandra's Royal Army Nursing Corps*, p.33.

36. Jones, *Dictionary of World Biography*, p.13.

37. Piggott, *Queen Alexandra's Royal Army Nursing Corps*, pp.42-3.

38. Piggott, *Queen Alexandra's Royal Army Nursing Corps*, p.41; Nurses' Memorial Foundation of South Australia Incorporated, *Nursing – 150 years of Caring in South Australia*, The South Australian Trained Nurses' Centenary Committee, 1938 (Reprinted with 1939-1945 supplement in 1989), Adelaide, p.214.

39. Piggott, *Queen Alexandra's Royal Army Nursing Corps*, pp.40-5.

40. Y. McEwen *"It's a Long Way to Tipperary": British and Irish nurses in the Great War*, Cualann Press, Dunfermline, 2006, pp.200-08.

41. Narrative, E. Vickers Foote, *Records of A.G. Butler: Official Historian of Australian Army Medical Services - Nurses' Narratives*, AWM 41, File 373.2, Canberra.

42. Rogers, *While You're Away*, pp.32-3.

43. *The New Zealand Army: A History from 1840's to 1990's*, Public Relations of the New Zealand Army, Christchurch, 1990, pp.78-80.

44. C. Manson & C. Manson, *Doctor Agnes Bennett*, Michael Joseph Ltd, London, 1960, p.55.

45. P.A. Sargison, 'Maclean, Hester 1859-1932' in *Dictionary of New Zealand Biography*, updated 7 April 2006. URL: http://www.dnzb.govt.nz/; Rogers, *While You're Away*, p.44.

46. Manson & Manson, p.55.

47. C.E.W. Bean, *Anzac to Amiens* (5th ed.) Australian War Memorial, Canberra, 1968, p.17; *The New Zealand Army: A History from 1840's to 1990's*, p.80.

48. Rogers, *While You're Away*, p.35.

6 Australian Army Nursing Service (AANS) 1902

1. A.G. Butler, *The Official History of the Australian Army Medical Services in the war of 1914-1918: Special Problems and Services*, Vol 3, Australian War Memorial Canberra, 1943, p.549.

2. Perdita M. McCarthy 'McCarthy, Dame Emma Maud (1859-1949)', *Australian Dictionary of Biography*, National Centre of Biography, Australian National University, Volume 10, Melbourne University Press, 1986, pp.218-9.

3. R. Goodman, *Our War Nurses: The History of the Royal Australian Army Nursing Corps 1902-1988,*

Boolarong Publications, Brisbane, 1988, pp.11,19,117.

4. Juliet Piggott, *Queen Alexandra's Royal Army Nursing Corps*, Lee Cooper Ltd, London, 1975, p.7.

5. E.J. Gould, 'New South Wales Assistance asked in connection with the collection of historical material for Australian Army Nursing Service, AIF. Report by Miss EJ Gould' (Gould Report) AWM 4364/34/6, Australian War Memorial, Canberra, 1933, p.3.

6. Piggott, *Queen Alexandra's Royal Army Nursing Corps*, p.45.

7. Gould Report, pp.2-3.

8. Correspondence, O Haynes, 16 July 1916 cited in M Young (ed) *We Are Here Too – Letters and Diaries of Sister Olive Haynes No. 2 AGH November 1914 to February 1918*, Australian Down Syndrome Assoc Inc, Adelaide, 1991, pp.152-3.

9. Alice Terrot cited in Robert G. Richardson (ed.), *Nurse Sarah Anne: with Florence Nightingale at Scutari*, John Murray (Publishers) Ltd, London, 1977, p.95.

10. Piggott, *Queen Alexandra's Royal Army Nursing Corps*, p.41.

11. Terrot in Richardson, *Nurse Sarah Anne*, p.97.

12. J. Anderson 'Some experiences of a Victorian nurse in South Africa', *Una,* Vol 1, No 2, Melbourne, July 1903, p.32.

13. Narrative, Matron Adelaide Maud Kellett *Records of A. G. Butler: Official Historian of Australian Army Medical Services – Nurses' Narratives.*

14. Anna Rogers, *While You're Away: New Zealand Nurses at War 1899-1948,* Auckland University Press, Auckland, 2003, p.186.

15. C. Moorehead, *Dunant's Dream: War, Switzerland and the History of the Red Cross*, Carroll & Graf Publishers, Inc., New York, 1999, pp.212-3, 216-7.

16. V. Brittain, *Testament of Youth*, Virago Press, London, 2006 (first published by Victor Gollancz Limited 1933), p.132.

17. William Keating Brennan, *Military Forces of the Commonwealth Papers*, NAA, Canberra [online 21 February 2007]; Photograph of gravesite at Welford Road Cemetery includes the name of K. Adele Brennan indicating that she was known as Adele (J00731), AWM, Canberra, http://www.awm.gov.au/database/collection.asp [online 16 February, 2007].

18. Correspondence, Jessie Tomlins to Margaretta Tomlins, 9 December 1917 cited in R. Rae, *The Biography of an Australian World War One Nurse: Jessie Tomlins,* amazon.com.

19. K.A. Brennan was not a member of the AANS as indicated in McEwen, p.200 and AWM Commemorative Roll http://www.awm.gov.au/database/croll.asp [online 16 February 2007]; Photograph of Kathleen Adele Brennan in VAD ward uniform (PO5074.002), AWM, Canberra, http://www.awm.gov.au/database/collection.asp [online 16 February, 2007].

20. Kathleen Adele Brennan (VAD), *Military Forces of the Commonwealth Papers,* NAA, Canberra, [online 21 February 2007].

21. Jennifer Horsfield, *Rainbow: The Story of Rania Macphillamy*, Ginninderra Press, Canberra, 2007, pp.47, 49, 56.

22. 'Extract from Standing Orders' cited in Goodman, *Our War Nurses*, p.15.

23. J. Bassett, *Guns and Brooches: Australian Army Nursing from the Boer War to the Gulf War*, Oxford University Press, Melbourne, 1992, pp.27-30.

24. Stuart Braga, *Anzac Doctor: the Life of Sir Neville Howse, VC*, Hale & Iremonger, Sydney, 2000, pp.49-50.

25. Barbara F. Cape *Baillière's Nurses' Dictionary,* Baillière, Tindall and Cox, London, 1956, p.191.

26. M.K. Doherty, M. B. Sirl, O. I. Ring, *Modern Practical Nursing Procedures,* Dymocks Book Arcade

Ltd, Sydney, 1944, p.530; Cape, p.100; A.Maud Kellett interview (no. 128) of Miss A. Young, AWM, Canberra,1919. Miss Young provides the only account of a masseuse included in the interviews of A.Maud Kellett.

27. A.G. Butler, *The Official History of the Australian Army Medical Services in the War of 1914-1918 Gallipoli, Palestine and New Guinea*, Vol 1, (2nd ed.), Australian War Memorial, Melbourne, 1938, p.419.

28. Narrative, E.H. Cuthbert, *Records of A. G. Butler: Official Historian of Australian Army Medical Services - Nurses' Narratives.*

29. A. Hill, *Soldier Boy: The true story of Jim Martin The youngest Anzac,* Penguin Books Australia, Melbourne, 2001.

30. Narrative, Leila Brown, *Records of A. G. Butler: Official Historian of Australian Army Medical Services - Nurses' Narratives.*

31. Frederick Watson, *The History of the Sydney Hospital from 1811 to 1911,* Government Printer, Sydney, 1911, p.178.

7 Preparing for War

1. Juliet Piggott, *Queen Alexandra's Royal Army Nursing Corps*, Lee Cooper Ltd, London, 1975, p.46.

2. E.J. Gould, 'New South Wales Assistance asked in connection with the collection of historical material for Australian Army Nursing Service, AIF. Report by Miss EJ Gould' (Gould Report) AWM 4364/34/6, Australian War Memorial, Canberra, 1933, p.2.

3. A.G. Butler, *The Official History of the Australian Army Medical Services in the war of 1914-1918: Special Problems and Services*, Vol 3, Australian War Memorial Canberra, 1943, p.891 (table 22).

4. Kirsty Harris, *More than Bombs and Bandages: Australian Army Nurses at Work in World War 1*, The Army History Unit, Big Sky Publishing Pty Ltd, Sydney, 2011, p.3.

5. Eliza Harvey, 'World War 1: Thousands of nurses missed out on recognition', www.abc.net.au/news/2014-08-04.

6. Australian War Memorial website - http://www.awm.gov.au/database/roh_eligibility.htm [online 16 February 2006]. The criteria for inclusion in the AWM Roll of Honour are specific and include *'people who have died as a direct result of active service with Australian forces, or while on transfer, and within specified periods in a war or warlike operation in which Australians were involved'* - Australian War Memorial website - http://www.awm.gov.au/database/roh_intro.htm [online 16 February 2006]. The author identified Pearl Goodman as eligible for inclusion (her service record met the criteria) and she is now included in the Roll of Honour. The AIF was disbanded on 31 March 1921 and anyone who died after this date is not eligible for inclusion.

7. Elizabeth Rothery joined the AIF on 22 August 1916 and RTA on 20 July 1917 but this does not include her subsequent tours of transport duty; AWM Nominal Roll: http://www.awm.gov.au/database/133/index.asp [online 17 May 2005].

8. R Kirkcaldie *In Gray and Scarlet* Alexander McCubbin, Melbourne, 1922.

9. Nora Kathleen Fletcher Papers, Mitchell Library, ML MSS 1546 at http://libapp.sl.nsw.gov.au/ [online 8 April 2008].

10. M.Cordia, *Nurses at Little Bay*, Prince Henry Trained Nurses' Association, Sydney, 1990, pp.73 & 377.

11. Photograph and caption 'Portrait of Sister May Dickson, QAIMNS' (PO5159.001) AWM, Canberra, http://www.awm.gov.au/database/collection.asp [online 16 February, 2007].

12. Y. McEwen, *"It's a Long Way to Tipperary": British and Irish nurses in the Great War*, Cualann Press, Dunfermline, 2006, pp.200-08 (no record of service); Name included on AWM Commemorative Roll

http://www.awm.gov.au/database/[online 21 February 2007]; there is no record of her burial with the Commonwealth War Graves Commission: http://www.cwgc.org/debt_of_honour.[online 21 February 2007].

13. Butler, *Special Problems and Services*, p.538 (*n*).

14. Anna Rogers, *While You're Away: New Zealand Nurses at War 1899-1948,* Auckland University Press, Auckland, 2003, p.55.

15. Butler, *Special Problems and Services*, p.538 (*n*).

16. L. Potter (Pres), *A Passion to Care: Nursing and Nurses Western Suburbs Hospital 1984-1982,* The Western Suburbs Hospital Graduate Nurses' Association, Sydney, 2008, pp.97-8, 134, 172.

17. Lieutenant A. T. White, an English clerk to General Birdwood, first used the acronym ANZAC when the Australian and New Zealand troops were still in Cairo, but the term did not gain common usage until after the landing at the Dardanelles - C.E.W. Bean, *Anzac to Amiens* (5th ed.) Australian War Memorial, Canberra, 1968, pp.120-1.

18. Correspondence, O. Haynes, 16 July 1916 cited in M. Young (ed), *We Are Here, Too: The Diaries and Letters of Sister Olive L. C. Haynes November 1914 to February 1918,* Australian Down Syndrome Association Inc, Adelaide, 1991, p.9.

19. Narrative, Leila Smith, *Records of A.G. Butler: Official Historian of Australian Army Medical Services - Nurses' Narratives.*

20. Rose Creal, *Military Forces of the Commonwealth Papers*, NAA, Canberra.

21. P. Adam-Smith, *The ANZACs*, Penguin Books Australia Ltd, Melbourne, 1991, p.44; M Barker, *Nightingales in the Mud: the Digger Sisters of the Great War 1914-1918*, Allen and Unwin, Sydney, 1989, p.12.

22. Australian War Memorial 224, Unit History Manuscripts, MS 384, No.3 AGH cited in . J. Bassett, *Guns and Brooches: Australian Army Nursing from the Boer War to the Gulf War,* Oxford University Press, Melbourne, 1992, p.48.

23. B Rayner, 'Nurse Elizabeth Rothery' in Myrtleford Mail, n/d. The author gratefully acknowledges Eric Barton, Myrtleford and District Historical Society, who provided background information on Elizabeth Rothery. Correspondence, 29 March 2005 in *Ruth Rae Collection*, National Nursing Archives, Canberra.

24. B Rayner, 'Nurse Elizabeth Rothery', Myrtleford Mail, n/d. Henry Norman Rothery DOE: 31 March 1915 KIA: 29 November 1915; AWM websites:
http://www.awm.gov.au/database/roh_intro.htm [online 17 May 2005] and
http://www.awm.gov.au/database/133/index.asp [online 17 May 2005].

25. Elizabeth Rothery joined the AIF on 22 August 1916 and RTA on 20 July 1917 but this does not include her subsequent tours of transport duty; AWM Nominal Roll:
http://www.awm.gov.au/database/133/index.asp [online 17 May 2005].

26. 'Extract from Standing Orders' cited in Goodman, *Our War Nurses*, p.15.

27. A. Hyslop, *Sovereign Remedies: A History of Ballarat Base Hospital 1850s to 1980s*, Allen and Unwin Australia Pty Ltd, Sydney, 1989, p.214.

28. Photograph courtesy of Joan Durdin, Royal Adelaide Hospital and Heritage Committee (*Ruth Rae Collection*, National Nursing Archives, Canberra).

29. Captain F.H. Wickham cited in Goodman, *Our War Nurses*, p.76.

30. Butler, *Special Problems and Services*, p.570.

31. T.A. (Muriel) Robertson (QAIMNSR), NAA record file, NAA, Canberra. Gertrude Muriel Norton Robertson (AANS) was also known as 'Muriel Robertson' but her service record clearly indicates she was RTA on HMAT *Wiltshire* (September 1918) as a casualty and admitted to 11 AGH, Melbourne, where she remained until at least May 1920. Gertrude Muriel Norton Robertson, *Military Forces of the*

Commonwealth Papers, NAA, Canberra [online 10 April 2008].

32. Australian Archives, Victoria, MP 367, Department of Defence correspondence files, 527/1/122, section 7, pp.7-8 cited in Bassett, p.75. The list compiled by Burke has been incorporated in R.Rae, *First World War Commemorative Nominal Roll,* ACN Trilogy, Canberra, 2015; E.K. Burke, *With Horse and Morse in Mesopotamia,* Arthur McQuilty, Sydney, 1927, pp.198-200.

33. Captain F. H. Wickham cited in Goodman, *Our War Nurses*, pp.70, 76.

34. S. Pope & E. A. Wheal, *Dictionary of the First World War,* Macmillan Reference Books, London, 1995, pp.7-8.

35. R. Goodman, *Queensland Nurses: Boer War to Vietnam*, Boolarong Publications, Brisbane, 1985, p.44; J. Gill, 'The Origins of the Australian Army Nursing Service and its involvement in the First World War', *Australian National University Historical Journal 1981-87*, Vol. 15, Canberra, 1981, p.60.

36. Rose Creal, *Military Forces of the Commonwealth Papers.*

37. Goodman, *Our War Nurses*, p.27; Bassett, *Guns and Brooches*, p.101.

39. 'Extract from standing orders - syllabus of qualifications necessary to become members of the Australian Army Nursing Service' cited in Goodman, *Our War Nurses*, pp.15, 27.

39. Rose Creal, *Military Forces of the Commonwealth Papers.*

40. H. Gregory & C. Brazil, *Bearers of the Tradition: Nurses of the Royal Brisbane Hospital 1888-1993*, p.5; J Durdin, *Eleven Thousand Nurses - A History of Nurse Education at the Royal Adelaide Hospital 1889-1993*, p.52.

41. Correspondence from Mrs J. McNeece (C/ - Tatura State School) to Officer-in-Charge Base Records in Irene McPhail, *Military Forces of the Commonwealth Papers,* NAA, Canberra; H. Paterson, *'5.30, Nurse!' The Story of the Alfred Nurses*, History Books, Melbourne, 1996, p.227.

42. B. Tuchman, *The Proud Tower*, Hamish Hamilton, London, 1966, p.119.

43. M. Clark, *A History of Australia: The People Make Laws 1888-1915*, Vol 5, Melbourne University Press, Melbourne, 1981, pp.90-94.

44. Digger-Pioneer Index, Victoria 1836-1888; Digger-Federation Index, Victoria 1889-1901. The author gratefully acknowledges Heather Rendle, Echuca Historical Society, who provided background information on nurses Moorhouse and McPhail. Electronic correspondence, Heather Rendle to Ruth Rae, 11 January 2005 (*Ruth Rae Collection*, National Nursing Archives, Sydney).

45. M. Cannon, *The Human Face of the Great Depression*, Today's Australia Publishing Company, Mornington, 1996, p.266.

46. *The Echuca Advertiser,'*Auctions', 30 March 1896.

47. *The Echuca Advertiser* 'Auctions', 14 May 1896.

48. *The Riverine Herald* 'Echuca Police Court', 17 October 1896. The article details the case of John Chadwick who sued Michael Donohue for labour done at a weekly rate of 15 shillings per week.

49. *The Echuca Advertiser* 'Echuca Police Court - Larceny', 20 October 1896.

50. *The Riverine Herald* 'Accident at Deniliquin', October 1898.

51. *The Riverine Herald*, February 1898, cited in correspondence, Heather Rendle to Ruth Rae, 11 January 2005 (*Ruth Rae Collection*, National Nursing Archives, Canberra).

52. Digger-Federation Index,Victoria 1889-1901.

8 Feminism and AANS Leadership

1. B.F. Miller & C.B. Keane, *Encyclopedia and Dictionary of Medicine and Nursing*, W.B. Saunders Co.,

London, 1972, pp.103 & 987.

2. W. Howard James, *Home Nursing and Ailments of Children: A Handbook for Mothers*, Signs Publishing Company, Melbourne, 1923, p.418.

3. Miller & Keane, *Encyclopedia and Dictionary of Medicine and Nursing*, p.988.

4. M. Cochrane & R. Cochrane *Housekeeping with Dorothy Wordsworth at Dove Cottage* Highgate Publications (Beverley) Limited, Beverley, 2001, p.29.

5. Lyndsay Gardiner 'Bell, Jane (1873 - 1959)', *Australian Dictionary of Biography*, National Centre of Biography, Australian National University, Volume 7, Melbourne University Press, 1979, p.257.

6. A. Atkinson, *The Europeans in Australia: A History: Democracy* (Vol 2), Oxford University Press, Melbourne, 2004, p.292.

7. *The Bulletin*, 26 May 1883 cited in Manning Clark *A History of Australia: the earth abideth for ever 1851-1888,* Vol 4, Melbourne University Press, Melbourne, 1978, p.391.

8. J.A. Williams & R.D. Goodman, *Jane Bell, O.B.E. 1873-1959*, The Royal Melbourne Hospital Graduate Nurses' Association, Melbourne, 1988, pp.4-5.

9. B. Kingston, *My Wife, My Daughter and Poor Mary Ann*, Thomas Nelson Australia Pty Ltd, Melbourne, 1975, p.879. Sydney Hospital Annual Report 1915 'List of Graduates of the Training School Since 1894', printed 1916, p.104.

10. D.G. Bowd, *Lucy Osburn c.1836-1891: Founder of the Nightingale System of Nursing at Sydney Hospital*, Hawkesbury Press Pty Ltd, Windsor, 1968, p.23; F.G. Holden, 'Trained Nursing' paper cited in C.Chambers, *Lessons for Ladies - A Social History of Girls' Education in Australasia 1870-1900*, Hale and Iremonger, Sydney, 1986, p.166.

11. Certificate of Registration, ATNA, Jane Bell, cited in Williams & Goodman, *Jane Bell, O.B.E. 1873-1959*, pp.2,3,6; D.M.Armstrong *The First Fifty Years - A History of Nursing at The Royal Prince Alfred Hospital, Sydney from 1882-1932*, Royal Prince Alfred Graduate Nurses Association, Sydney 1965, pp.92-93.

12. S.B. McGahey, letter (1 January 1900) cited in Williams & Goodman, *Jane Bell, O.B.E. 1873-1959*, p.5.

13. Williams & Goodman, *Jane Bell, O.B.E. 1873-1959*, p.7. The Royal Brisbane Hospital has undergone a number of name changes and adopted the 'Royal' prefix in 1967 so for ease of narrative it will be referred to as 'the Brisbane Hospital' throughout this book - . H. Gregory & C. Brazil, *Bearers of the Tradition: Nurses of the Royal Brisbane Hospital 1888-1993*, Boolarong Publications, Brisbane, 1993, p.150.

14. Janice McCarthy 'Wilson, Grace Margaret (1879-1957)', *Australian Dictionary of Biography*, National Centre of Biography, Australian National University, Volume 12, Melbourne University Press, 1990, pp.522-3; R. Rae 'The conflicts of Grace Wilson (1879-1957) and the emergence of a professional nurse leader in the early twentieth century' presented at Royal College *of* Nursing, *Australia* (Queensland Chapter) History Breakfast, Brisbane, 1 November 2007.

15. Williams & Goodman, *Jane Bell, O.B.E. 1873-1959*, pp.7-9 & 124; http://www.nhs.uk/England/Hospitals/showHospital.aspx?id=RQN03 [online 14 March 2006].

16. A. Gregory, *The Ever Open Door: A history of the Royal Melbourne Hospital 1848-1998*, Hyland House, Melbourne, 1998, pp.120-1.

17. There is a contradiction regarding the correct date of birth of Grace Wilson. The 25 June 1879 date is supported by her birth registration and the *Australian Dictionary of Biography* entry - Janice McCarthy, 'Wilson, Grace Margaret (1879-1957)', *Australian Dictionary of Biography*, National Centre of Biography, Australian National University, Volume 12, Melbourne University Press, 1990, pp.522-3. However, her attestation papers, which were signed by Grace Wilson, states she was born on 25 June 1880 - Grace Wilson *Military Forces of the Commonwealth Papers*, NAA, Canberra.

18. http://www.ccsy.org.au/index.htm Hosted by Carringbush.Net and maintained by Fr Paul.

[online 8 September 2007].

19. Births, Deaths and Marriages [online 14 June 2007].

20. Gregory & Brazil, *Bearers of the Tradition*, pp.18-21 & 222. Grace Wilson was awarded her certificate in 1908 but was awarded the inaugural gold medal for highest marks in a three-year course in 1907.

21. Janice McCarthy, 'Wilson, Grace Margaret (1879-1957)', *Australian Dictionary of Biography*, National Centre of Biography, Australian National University, Volume 12, Melbourne University Press, 1990, pp.522-3; Gregory & Brazil, *Bearers of the Tradition*, p.21; http://www.nhs.uk/England/Hospitals/showHospital.[online 14 March 2006].

22. G.C. Bolton & P. Joske, *History of Royal Perth Hospital*, Royal Perth Hospital, Perth, 1982, p.60. The authors record that a '*somewhat older man, Dr H.F. Harvey, became Perth's first specialist gynaecologist*'.

23. V. Hobbs, *But Westward Look – Nursing in Western Australia 1829-1979*, University of Western Australia Press for the Royal Australian Nursing Federation (WA Branch), Perth, 1980, p.236; J. Durdin, *Eleven Thousand Nurses – A History of Nurse Education at the Royal Adelaide Hospital 1889-1993*, Royal Adelaide Hospital, 1999, p.61.

24. R. Rae (2002), 'Reading between unwritten lines: Australian Army nurses in India, 1916-19', *Journal of the Australian War Memorial*, [online]. Available: awm.gov.au/journal/j36 [25/09/03].

25. Hobbs, *But Westward Look*, pp.61-2.

26. P. Garrick and C. Jeffery, *Fremantle Hospital: A Social History to 1987*, Fremantle Hospital, Perth, 1987, pp.128-9.

27. Williams & Goodman, *Jane Bell, O.B.E. 1873-1959*, pp.123-4.

28. Gregory, *The Ever Open Door*, pp.141-2.

29. Kingston, *My Wife, My Daughter and Poor Mary Ann*, p.88.

30. Williams & Goodman, pp.4-5.

31. Gregory, *The Ever Open Door*, p.241.

32. Williams & Goodman, *Jane Bell, O.B.E. 1873-1959*, p.98.

33. E. Burchill, *Australian Nurses since Nightingale 1860-1990*, Spectrum Publications Pty Ltd, Melbourne, 1992, pp.38-39.

34. D. Aitkin, D. Jinks & J. Warhurst, *Australian Political Institutions*, 4th Edition, Longman Cheshire Pty Ltd, Melbourne, 1980, pp.132-3, 148.

35. L.F. Crisp *The Australian Federal Labour Party 1901-1951*, Hale and Iremonger, Sydney, 1978, pp.73, 215-6.

36. S. Prasser, J. R. Nethercote & J. Warhurst (eds) *The Menzies Era: A Reappraisal of government, politics and policy*, Hale & Iremonger, Sydney, 1995, p.262.

37. J. Horsfield, *Rainbow: The story of Rania Macphillamy*, Ginninderra Press, Canberra, 2007, pp.39, 41, 43, 45.

38. Merrilyn Lincoln, 'Graham, Margaret (1860 – 1942)', *Australian Dictionary of Biography*, National Centre of Biography, Australian National University, Volume 9, Melbourne University Press, 1983, pp.68-69.

39. R. Rae, 'Australian World War One Nurse Leaders – Missing in Action' presented at 'Mars and Minerva: Intellectuals and War in Australia and New Zealand', (Second Trevenna Conference), University of New England, Armidale, 5 February 2006.

40. Durdin, *Eleven Thousand Nurses*, pp.30-1.

41. Merrilyn Lincoln, 'Graham, Margaret (1860 – 1942)', *Australian Dictionary of Biography*, National Centre of Biography, Australian National University, Volume 9, Melbourne University Press, 1983, pp.68-69, 79.

42. S. Rimtoul, 'Dark Tale of Villainous Bone Collector' *The Australian*, 9 May 2003, p.2.

43. Reminiscences of Eleanor Harrald cited in Nurses' Memorial Foundation of South Australia Incorporated, *Nursing –150 years of Caring in South Australia*, The South Australian Trained Nurses' Centenary Committee, Adelaide,1938 (Reprinted with 1939-1945 supplement in 1989), p.44.

44. Rimtoul, 'Dark Tale of Villainous Bone Collector', p.2.

45. Nurses' Memorial Foundation of South Australia Incorporated, p.226.

46. Birth records are in the name of 'Walker' not 'Miles-Walker'; Tasmania Pioneers Index 1788-1888 [3 June 2005]; M Barker, *Nightingales in the Mud: the Digger Sisters of the Great War 1914-1918*, Allen and Unwin, Sydney, 1989, p.112 (photograph).

47. Jean Roberto Walker, born 9 August 1881 in Hobart, Tasmania, was occasionally referred to as Benson-Walker; Jean Roberto Walker, *Military Forces of the Commonwealth Papers*, NAA, Canberra [online 3 June 2005]; Birth Registration of Jean Nellie Walker, Tasmania Births, Deaths & Marriages (http://www.linc.tas.gov.au)[online 27 May 2015]. From 1868–76 the birthplace of Jean Nellie Miles (Walker) was known as Hamilton on Forth.

48. Tasmania Pioneers Index 1788-1888 [3 June 2005].

49. J. Bassett 'Walker, Jean Nellie Miles (1878-1918)', *Australian Dictionary of Biography*, National Centre of Biography, Australian National University, Volume 12, Melbourne University Press, 1990, p.362.

9 The not so Ordinary AANS Nurses

1. Dorothea Mackellar, 'My Country' in *My Country – Australian Poems and Australian Short Stories*, Volume 1, Lansdowne Press, Sydney, 1985, pp.472-3.

2. NSW Federation Index–Pioneer Series 1889-1901 [online 18 August 2006].

3. Mary Florence Stafford, *Military Forces of the Commonwealth Papers,* NAA, Canberra.

4. Correspondence, Mary Mackereth to officer-in-charge, Base Records, 5 March 1920 in Mary Florence Stafford *Military Forces of the Commonwealth Papers;* B. Kingston, *My Wife, My Daughter and Poor Mary Ann*, Thomas Nelson Australia Pty Ltd, Melbourne, 1975, pp.79-81.

5. J. Durdin, *Eleven Thousand Nurses – A History of Nurse Education at the Royal Adelaide Hospital 1889-1993*, Royal Adelaide Hospital, 1999, pp.56-7.

6. There is a discrepancy regarding the dates of Mary Stafford's training. One text claims she completed her training in 1911 - Nurses' Memorial Foundation of South Australia Incorporated, *Nursing – 150 years of Caring in South Australia*, The South Australian Trained Nurses' Centenary Committee, 1938 (Reprinted with 1939-1945 supplement in 1989), Adelaide, p.57. Another claims she completed the course in 1914 - Durdin, *Eleven Thousand Nurses,* p.230. The date has been determined to be 1911-14 following examination of the nurses' register by the author in February 2003 - Nurses' Register, Royal Adelaide Hospital Heritage Office, Adelaide. The author gratefully acknowledges Joan Durdin for her assistance. Attestation paper in Mary Florence Stafford, *Military Forces of the Commonwealth Papers.*

7. Narrative, Victor Mitton Ridgway (brother to Doris) dated 22 November 1970, copy given to the author by Mr Ian Ridgway (nephew of Doris) in June 2005 in *Ruth Rae Collection*, National Nursing Archives, Canberra.

8. John McQuilton, *The Kelly Outbreak 1878-80: the Geographical Dimension of Social Banditry,* Melbourne University Press, Melbourne, 1979,p p.45,46, 50-1.

9. Narrative, Victor Mitton Ridgway, 22 November 1970 in *Ruth Rae Collection.*

10. Durdin, *Eleven Thousand Nurses, p.*230; Nurses' Memorial Foundation of South Australia

Incorporated, p.57.

11. Correspondence, Jessie Tomlins to Margaretta Tomlins, 6 October 1917 (copy in possession of author).

12. B.Tipping, *Narromine Public School Centenary 1883-1983*, Narromine Public School Centenary Committee, Dubbo, 1983, p.44.

13. ATNA rules and regulations, *Council for the Year 1915-16*, clauses XIX–XXII in ATNA Records, MLMSS 4144 23(56), State Library of NSW, Sydney.

14. G. Sherington, *The Royal North Shore Hospital 1888-1988: A Century of Caring*, Howitz Grahame Pty Ltd, Sydney, 1988, p.36. Since its foundation the RNSH has had the royal prefix–Sherington, pp.12-3, 17; M. Rice, *The Close of an Era: A History of Nursing at the RNSH 1887-1987*, The RNSH of Sydney Graduate Nurses Assoc, Sydney, 1988; Sarah Margaret White, 'A World War 1 nurse remembers ...', 31 October 1973, *The Australian Women's Weekly*, 31 October 1973.

15. Ada Mildred Thompson, *Military Forces of the Commonwealth Papers*, NAA, Canberra; NSW Pioneer Index - Pioneer Series 1788-1888 [online 18 August 2006].

16. N. Brennan, *Dr Mannix*, Rigby Limited, Adelaide, 1964, p.23.

17. *The Northern Miner*, 'Charters Towers great pioneering owner/editor died a century ago', 22 May 1990, p.1.

18. Brennan, *Dr Mannix*, pp.26, 47,133-4.

19. June Stoodley, H.J. Gibbney 'O'Kane, Thadeus (1820-1890)', *Australian Dictionary of Biography*, National Centre of Biography, Australian National University, Volume 5, Melbourne University Press, 1974, p.362. The author gratefully acknowledges David Kent, Professor in History, UNE, who provided background information on 'Whiteboyism' - electronic correspondence, David Kent to Ruth Rae, 8 August 2006 in *Ruth Rae Collection*, National Nursing Archives, Canberra.

20. *The Northern Miner*, 'Charters Towers great pioneering owner/editor died a century ago' 22 May 1990, p.1.

21. Rosa O'Kane, *Military Forces of the Commonwealth Papers*, NAA, Canberra.

22. June Stoodley, H.J. Gibbney 'O'Kane, Thadeus (1820-1890)' *Australian Dictionary of Biography*, p.362.

23. Correspondence from Mrs M.J. Hall (aunt), cited in I. Darroch, *The Boonah Tragedy*, Access Press, Bassendean, 2004, p.159; P. Garrick and C. Jeffery, *Fremantle Hospital: A Social History to 1987*, Fremantle Hospital, Perth, 1987, pp.118-9.

24. Digger-Pioneer Index, Victoria 1836-1888 [online 16 June 2005]; Digger-Federation Index, Victoria 1889-1901 [online 18 August 2006].

25. Telephone interview, Ruth Rae with John Sargent (nephew of Hilda Williams and son of Edith Lillian Sargent née Williams), 27 November 2004 (transcript, *Ruth Rae Collection*, National Nursing Archives, Canberra; Correspondence, John Sargent to Ruth Rae, 7 December 2004 in *Ruth Rae Collection*, National Nursing Archives, Canberra.

26. V. Hobbs, *But Westward Look - Nursing in Western Australia 1829-1979*, University of Western Australia Press for the Royal Australian Nursing Federation (WA Branch), Perth, 1980, p.207.

27. R. Pearce, 'The tragic destiny of Sister Rosa O'Kane' in John Pearn & Peggy Carter (eds), *Bridgeheads of Northern Health*, Department of Child Health, Brisbane, 1996, p.50.

28. Telephone interview, Ruth Rae with John Sargent, 27 November 2004 (transcript, *Ruth Rae Collection*, National Nursing Archives, Canberra).

29. Hobbs, *But Westward Look*, p.207; Digger-Federation Index, Victoria 1889-1901[online 18 August 2006].

30. Telephone interview, Ruth Rae with John Sargent, 27 November 2004 & Correspondence, John

Sargent to Ruth Rae, 7 December 2004 in *Ruth Rae Collection*, National Nursing Archives,Canberra.

31. Telephone interview, Ruth Rae with John Sargent, 27 November 2004 transcript in *Ruth Rae Collection*, ACN, Canberra; Australian War Memorial Roll of Honour: http://www.awm.gov.au/database/roh_eligibility.htm [online 15 June 2005].

10 War

1. B.H. Liddell Hart, *History of the First World War*, Cassell and Co. Ltd., London, 1970, p.17; B. Jones, *Dictionary of World Biography*, Information Australia, Melbourne, 1994, p.268; H. Strachan, *The First World War: A new Illustrated History*, Simon & Schuster, London, 2003, p.3.

2. D. Denholm (ed), *Behind the Lines: One Woman's War 1914-18 Ethel Cooper*, Collins, Sydney, 1982, p.22.

3. C.E.W. Bean, *Anzac to Amiens* (5th ed.), Australian War Memorial, Canberra, 1968, p.22.

4. R. Rae, 'Reading between unwritten lines: Australian Army nurses in India, 1916-19', *Journal of the Australian War Memorial*, Canberra, 2002 [online]. Available: awm.gov.au/journal/j36 [25/09/03]

5. Liddell Hart, *History of the First World War*, p.2.

6. C. Moorehead, *Dunant's Dream: War, Switzerland and the History of the Red Cross*, Carroll & Graf Publishers, Inc., New York, 1999, pp.60-1, 67.

7. B. Tuchman, *The Guns of August*, Macmillan Publishing Co, New York, 1962, pp.18-9, 98, 122-23, p.128.

8. Liddell Hart, *History of the First World War*, pp.52,56, 132.

9. Bean, *Anzac to Amiens*,p.197.

10. Cooper cited in Denholm (ed), *Behind the Lines*, pp.106 & 200.

11. K. Fewster, *Gallipoli: The Turkish Story*, Vecihi Başarm, Hatice Hürmüz Başarm, Allen & Unwin, Sydney, 1985, pp.xi, 11-12, 32-4, 36-38, 40.

12. *ibid.*, p.43; Strachan, *The First World War*, pp.105-6

13. A.Maud Kellett interview Gladys Walter, AWM, Canberra, 1919.

14. Manning Clark, *A History of Australia: The People Make Laws 1888-1915*, Vol 5, Melbourne University Press, Melbourne, 1981, p.311.

15. *ibid.*, p.300; L.F. Crisp, *The Australian Federal Labour Party 1901-1951*, Hale and Iremonger, Sydney, 1978, p.23(*n*).

16. Fred Tomlins, *Military Forces of the Commonwealth Papers*, NAA, Canberra.

17. J. Beaumont (ed), *Australia's War 1914-1918*, Allen and Unwin,Sydney,1995, p.5; Correspondence, Fred Tomlins to George Tomlins, 30 April 1915 in R. Rae, *The Biography of an Australian Light Horseman: Fred Tomlins*, 2023, Amazon.com.

18. C. Fallows, *Love and War: Stories of War Brides from the Great War to Vietnam*, Bantam Books, Sydney, 2002, p.31.

19. Diary, Fred Tomlins, 5 November 1914 in R. Rae *The Biography of an Australian Light Horseman: Fred Tomlins*.

11 Australian Nurses in German New Guinea

1. A.G. Butler, *The Official History of the Australian Army Medical Services in the War of 1914-1918: Gallipoli, Palestine and New Guinea*, Vol 1, (2nd ed.), Australian War Memorial, Melbourne, 1938, p.782.

2. Stuart Braga, *Anzac Doctor: the Life of Sir Neville Howse, VC*, Hale & Iremonger, Sydney, 2000, p.99.

3. S.S. Mackenzie, *Official History of Australia in the War of 1914-18: the Australians at Rabaul*, Vol X, Angus and Robertson Ltd, Sydney, 1942, pp.58-9.

4. R. Kirkcaldie, *In Gray and Scarlet*, Alexander McCubbin, Melbourne, 1922, p.24.

5. D. M. Armstrong, *The First Fifty Years: A History of Nursing at the Royal Prince Alfred Hospital, Sydney from 1822 to 1932*, Royal Prince Alfred Hospital Graduate Nurses' Association, Sydney, 1965, p.129.

6. R. Rae, 'Soldiers of the ANZAC Mounted Division and nurses of the 14th Australian General Hospital - desert correspondents in World War One', *Australian Defence Force Journal*, 149:53, Canberra, 2001.

7. A.W. Jose, *Official History of Australia in the War of 1914-18 – The Royal Australian Navy*, Vol. 9 (11th ed), Angus and Robertson Ltd., Sydney, 1943, pp.1-46. For ease of narrative the term 'Australian soldier' includes naval personnel and the term 'Australian nurse' includes all Australian nurses irrespective of whether they were bona fide members of the AANS.

8. Braga, *Anzac Doctor*, p.100.

9. Kirkcaldie, *In Gray and Scarlet*, pp.10-15.

10. J. Bassett, *Guns and Brooches: Australian Army Nursing from the Boer War to the Gulf War*, Oxford University Press, Melbourne, 1992, p.32; Kirkcaldie, *In Gray and Scarlet*, p.19 & photograph caption opposite page 18.

11. Narrative, Sarah de Mestre, *Records of A. G. Butler: Official Historian of Australian Army Medical Services – Nurses' Narratives*, AWM 41, File 373.2, Canberra, p.1.

12. Kirkcaldie, *In Gray and Scarlet*, pp.17, 23& 27, 29-30, 36-7.

13. H. Gregory & C. Brazil, *Bearers of the Tradition: Nurses of the Royal Brisbane Hospital 1888-1993*, p.18; R. Goodman, *Queensland Nurses: Boer War to Vietnam*, Boolarong Publications, Brisbane, 1985,p.38. AWM Nominal Roll: http://www.awm.gov.au/database/[online 9 April 2008]; AWM Honours and Awards: http://www.awm.gov.au/database/[online 9 April 2008].

14. G. Robinson, *The Forgotten Women*, self-published, 1989, Mt Gravatt, Queensland, pp.12-3; Goodman *Our War Nurses*, pp.22-3. The identity of the nurses is stated in a photograph (JO 1866) held within the collection database of the AWM– http://cas.awm.gov.au/ [online 9 April 2008].

15. Anna Rogers, *While You're Away: New Zealand Nurses at War 1899-1948*, Auckland University Press, Auckland, 2003, p.38.

16. Braga, *Anzac Doctor*, p.102.

17. B.F. Miller & C.B. Keane, *Encyclopedia and Dictionary of Medicine and Nursing*, W.B. Saunders Co., London, 1972, p.556.

18. Braga, *Anzac Doctor*, pp.102-3.

19. Letherbridge cited in Robinson, *The Forgotten Women*, pp.12-3.

20. Kirkcaldie, *In Gray and Scarlet*, pp.10 & 39.

21. Butler, *Gallipoli, Palestine and New Guinea*, p.795 (*n*). Goodman claims that five nurses from RPAH were sent via the *Grantala* and were stationed at Rabaul during the war in a civilian capacity. It would appear he has confused Kirkcaldie and the *Grantala* nurses with May Gibbon and her colleagues who left Australia in December 1914. Butler clearly states they were AANS and there is scant reference to them or their service with the AWM – R. Goodman, *Our War Nurses: The History of the Royal Australian Army Nursing Corps 1902-1988*, Boolarong Publications, Brisbane, 1988, p.22.

22. Bassett, *Guns and Brooches*, pp.139-140; For an excellent account by a nurse who was interned, see Betty Jeffrey *White Coolies*, Angus and Robertson, Sydney, 1954.

23. P. Adam-Smith, *Prisoners of War: From Gallipoli to Korea*, Penguin Books Australia Ltd, Melbourne, 1992, p.22.

24. *ibid.*, pp.5 & 84. Winston Churchill was captured during the South African War and recorded that *'... you are in the power of the enemy. You owe your life to his humanity, your daily bread to his compassion. You must obey his orders, await his pleasure, possess your soul in patience.'*

12 The First AANS Contingent to Egypt 1914-15

1. R. Goodman, *Our War Nurses: The History of the Royal Australian Army Nursing Corps 1902-1988*, Boolarong Publications, Brisbane, 1988, p.22.

2. Correspondence, Dr Sheldon, undated in Jean Nellie Miles Walker, *Military Forces of the Commonwealth Papers*, NAA, Canberra.

3. The service record of Miss Jean Nellie Miles Walker includes official documents which list her mother as next-of-kin while others list her brother as next-of-kin; Correspondence in Jean Nellie Miles Walker *Military Forces of the Commonwealth Papers.*

4. Gould, E. J., 'New South Wales assistance asked in connection with the collection of historical material for Australian Army Nursing Service, AIF. Report by Miss EJ Gould' (Gould Report) AWM 4364/34/6, Australian War Memorial, Canberra, 1933, p.2.

5. The AWM Roll of Honour lists Jean Nellie Miles Walker's place of enlistment as Hobart. Jean Roberto Benson-Walker was born and enlisted in Hobart. However, Jean Nellie Miles Walker signed her oath to the AIF in Egypt as did a number of AANS nurses who sailed with the first contingent; AWM, Roll of Honour, http://www.awm.gov.au/database/roh.asp [online 3 June 2005]; Jean Nellie Miles Walker, *Military Forces of the Commonwealth Papers.*

6. J. Bassett, *Guns and Brooches: Australian Army Nursing from the Boer War to the Gulf War*, Oxford University Press Australia, Melbourne, 1992, pp.12-3.

7. Narrative, Matron A. Maud Kellett, *Records of A.G. Butler, Official Historian of Australian Army Medical Services – Nurses' Narratives,* AWM, Canberra.

8. AWM database of gazetted honours and awards; R.Rae, *First World War Commemorative Nominal Roll,* ACN Trilogy, Canberra, 2015. Note: Caution is advised in accepting the gazetted awards as complete. For example, Clementina Hay Marshall was MID for her service on transport duty during the Gallipoli Campaign but the only gazetted decoration listed with the AWM is the ARRC – *Sydney Morning Herald, 'Nurse Honoured'*, 14 January 1916, p.3.

9. R. Rae 'Ellen Julia Gould: a civilian nurse and founder of the military nursing tradition in Australia (1860-1941)', *Journal of the Royal Australian Historical Society*, 92 (2), 2006, p.175.

10. A.G. Butler, *The Official History of the Australian Army Medical Services in the war of 1914-1918: Special Problems and Services*, Vol 3, Australian War Memorial, Canberra, 1943, p.549.

11.'The Lady Superintendents Reports No.1 (Miss Jane Bell)', Royal Melbourne Hospital archives, The Royal Melbourne Hospital, Melbourne (reviewed by author February 2003).

12. A.G. Butler, *Special Problems and Services*, p.495.

13. J. Durdin, *Eleven Thousand Nurses – A History of Nurse Education at the Royal Adelaide Hospital 1889-1993*, Royal Adelaide Hospital, 1999, p.227.

14. J.A. Williams & R.D. Goodman, *Jane Bell, O.B.E. 1873-1959*, The Royal Melbourne Hospital Graduate Nurses' Association, Melbourne, 1988, pp.12-13; Nurses' Memorial Foundation of South Australia Incorporated, *Nursing –150 years of Caring in South Australia*, The South Australian Trained Nurses' Centenary Committee, Adelaide,1938 (Reprinted with 1939-1945 supplement in 1989), p.197.

15. Hilda Mary Knox, *Military Forces of the Commonwealth Papers,* NAA, Canberra.

16. Correspondence, Greg Kirk to Ruth Rae, 2005 in *Ruth Rae Collection*, National Nursing Archives, Canberra. The author gratefully acknowledges Greg Kirk.

17. John McQuilton, *The Kelly Outbreak 1878-80: the geographical dimension of social banditry,* Melbourne University Press, Melbourne, 1979, pp.5, 171-4. Australian born (Edward) Ned Kelly (1855-1880) was of Irish decent. He became an infamous bushranger and debate about the justice or injustice of his hanging continues today. The activities of his gang in North Eastern Victoria resulted in the area being known as 'Kelly country'.

18. Narrative, V. Woniarski, *Records of A.G. Butler, Official Historian of Australian Army Medical Services - Nurses' Narratives*, p.1.

19. Williams and Goodman, *Jane Bell, O.B.E. 1873-1959*, pp.15-6.

20. Barrett & Deane, *Australian Army Medical Corps in Egypt,* H.K. Lewis and Co, London, 1918, pp.22-3.

21. M. Barker, *Nightingales in the Mud: the Digger Sisters of the Great War 1914-1918,* Allen and Unwin, Sydney, 1989, p.34.

22. Diary, O Haynes, 13 March 1915 cited in M Young (ed) *We Are Here Too - Letters and Diaries of Sister Olive Haynes No. 2 AGH November 1914 to February, 1918*, Australian Down Syndrome Assoc Inc, Adelaide, 1991, p.33.

23. Narrative, Emma Cuthbert, *Records of A.G. Butler, Official Historian of Australian Army Medical Services - Nurses' Narratives.*

24. Narrative, Leila Smith, *Records of A.G. Butler, Official Historian of Australian Army Medical Services - Nurses' Narratives.*

25. Stuart Braga, *Anzac Doctor: the Life of Sir Neville Howse, VC,* Hale & Iremonger, Sydney, 2000, pp.210-1.

26. Williams & Goodman, *Jane Bell, O.B.E. 1873-1959*, p.25.

27. Surgeon-General Ford, DMS Egypt, cited in Williams and Goodman, *Jane Bell, O.B.E. 1873-1959*, p.23.

28. Barrett &Deane, *Australian Army Medical Corps in Egypt,* p.22.

29. A.G. Butler, *The Official History of the Australian Army Medical Services in the War of 1914-1918: Gallipoli, Palestine and New Guinea*, Vol 1, (2nd ed.), Australian War Memorial, Melbourne, 1938, pp.276-7.

30. Narrative, Grace Burns, *Records of A.G. Butler, Official Historian of Australian Army Medical Services - Nurses' Narratives.*

31. AWM Embarkation roll: http://www.awm.gov.au/cms_images/awm8/

32. Newspaper article 'Called Home!' *The Elmore Standard*, 3 July 1915. The author acknowledges Mr David Cotton, Research Officer, Australian Institute of Genealogical Studies Inc, Bendigo Area, who provided background information on nurses Bicknell, Hennessy and Tyson. Correspondence dated 19 January 2005 in *Ruth Rae Collection,* National Nursing Archives, Canberra.

33. Norma Mowbray, *Military Forces of the Commonwealth Papers,* NAA, Canberra.

34. Olive Haynes, diary entry, 30 September 1915 in M. Young (ed), *We Are Here, Too: The Diaries and Letters of Sister Olive L. C. Haynes November 1914 to February 1918*, p.39.

35. The Gould Report, p.6; Bassett, *Guns and Brooches*, p.41; R. Rae, 'Ellen Julia Gould: a civilian nurse and founder of the military nursing tradition in Australia (1860-1941)', *Journal of the Royal Australian Historical Society*, 92 (2), 2006, p.176.

36. Barrett & Deane, *Australian Army Medical Corps in Egypt,* p.22.

37. Bassett, *Guns and Brooches,* p.44.

38. C.E.W. Bean, *Official History of Australia in the War of 1914-1918 – The Story of ANZAC: The First Phase,* Vol 2, Angus and Robertson Ltd., Sydney, 1935, p.571; Butler, *Special Problems and Services,* pp.587-8.

39. Haynes in Young, *We Are Here, Too,* p.55.

40. Bassett, *Guns and Brooches,* p.44.

41. Haynes in Young, *We Are Here, Too,* pp.33, 47.

42. Bassett, *Guns and Brooches,* pp.44-45; R. Goodman, *Queensland Nurses: Boer War to Vietnam,* Boolarong Publications, Brisbane, 1985, p.50.

43. Goodman, *Our War Nurses,* p.41.

13 A Sexual Revolution and the Impact on Military Nursing

1. J.Horsfield, *Rainbow: The story of Rania Macphillamy,* Ginninderra Press, Canberra, 2007, pp.56-7, 67.

2. Letter, 11 November 1918, cited by Monica Sinclair in Department of Veterans' Affairs, *Simply Hell let Loose: Stories of Australians at war,* ABC Books, Sydney, 2002, pp.48-9.

3. M. Barker, *Nightingales in the Mud: the Digger Sisters of the Great War 1914-1918,* Allen and Unwin, Sydney, 1989, p.3.

4. A.G. Butler, *The Official History of the Australian Army Medical Services in the war of 1914-1918: Special Problems and Services,* Vol 3, Australian War Memorial, Canberra, 1943, pp.530-1.

5. V. Brittain, *Testament of Youth,* Virago Press, London, 2006 (first published by Victor Gollancz Limited 1933), p.143.

6. J. Piggott *Queen Alexandra's Royal Army Nursing Corps,* Leo Cooper Ltd, London, 1975, p.35.

7. M.Cordia, *Nurses at Little Bay,* Prince Henry Trained Nurses' Association, Sydney, 1990, p.102.

8. Butler, *Special Problems and Services,* pp.172-3,152.

9. B.F. Miller & C.B. Keane, *Encyclopedia and Dictionary of Medicine and Nursing,* W.B. Saunders Co., London, 1972, pp.931-2.

10. L. Potter (Pres), *A Passion to Care: Nursing and Nurses Western Suburbs Hospital 1984-1982,* The Western Suburbs Hospital Graduate Nurses' Association, Sydney, 2008, p.75.

11. Cordia, *Nurses at Little Bay,* pp.101-3.

12. Australasian Trained Nurses' Association (founded 1899) 'Register of Members 1916', Websdale, Shoosmith Ltd, Sydney; Butler, *Special Problems and Services,* p.537 *(n).*

13. Correspondence, Neville Howse (DMS–AIF) to General Birdwood, 4 June 1917, Howse Papers, 2 DRL, 1351, Australian War Memorial, Canberra; Australian Army Journal 'Royal Australian Army Nursing Corps', Editorial, Vol 57, February 1954, p.39.

14. J. Bassett, *Guns and Brooches: Australian Army Nursing from the Boer War to the Gulf War,* Oxford University Press, Melbourne, 1992, p.41.

15. R. Kearney, *Silent Voices: The story of the 10th Battalion, AIF,* New Holland, Sydney, 2005, p.62. The author gratefully acknowledges the Late Janet Uhr who brought this publication to my attention.

16. AWM Roll of Honour: http://www.awm.gov.au/database/roh.asp[online 18 August 2006]; Phillip de Quetteville Robin also had three cousins who were killed in France - Kearney, *Silent Voices,* p.62.

17. Cordia, *Nurses at Little Bay,* pp.105-6.

18. Butler, *Special Problems and Services,* p.159-62.

19. A.G. Butler, *The Official History of the Australian Army Medical Services in the War of 1914-1918: Gallipoli, Palestine and New Guinea,* Vol 1, (2nd ed.), Australian War Memorial, Melbourne, 1938, p.264; C. Fallows, *Love and War: Stories of War Brides from the Great War to Vietnam,* Bantam Books, Sydney, 2002, p.15.

20. Stuart Braga, *Anzac Doctor: the Life of Sir Neville Howse, VC,* Hale & Iremonger, Sydney, 2000, p.233.

21. Fallows, *Love and War,* p.20.

22. M. Tilton, *The Grey Battalion,* Angus and Robertson Ltd, Sydney, 1933, p.79.

23. H. Strachan, *The First World War: A New Illustrated History,* Simon & Schuster, London, 2003, p.230.

24. H. Campbell, *Aids to Pathology* (4 ed), Baillière, Tindall and Cox, London, 1920, p.13.

25. Stephanie Pain, 'The Pharaoh's Pharmacist' in *New Scientist* No. 2634, 15 December 2007, p.43.

26. B. Kingston, *My Wife, My Daughter and Poor Mary Ann,* Thomas Nelson Australia Pty Ltd, Melbourne, 1975, pp.8-10, 70.

27. Cordia, *Nurses at Little Bay,* p.105.

28. Fallows, *Love and War,* p.16.

29. Butler, *Special Problems and Services,* p.157-9.

30. Campbell, *Aids to Pathology,* p.13.

31. Bassett, *Guns and Brooches,* p.80.

32. Brittain, *Testament of Youth,* p.419.

33. 'Extract from Standing Orders' cited in R. Goodman, *Our War Nurses: The History of the Royal Australian Army Nursing Corps 1902-1988,* Boolarong Publications, Brisbane, 1988, p.15.

34. Correspondence, Principal Matron Jane Bell to Surgeon-General Ford (British DMS – Egypt), 8 August 1915 cited in Bassett, *Guns and Brooches,* pp.37 & 40.

35. Goodman, *Our War Nurses,* p.85.

36. Bassett, *Guns and Brooches,* p.40.

37. A. Rogers, *While You're Away: New Zealand Nurses at War 1899-1948,* Auckland University Press, 2003, pp.59, 185-7.

14 Gallipoli and the Reality of War

1. J. Lee, *A Soldier's Life: General Sir Ian Hamilton 1853-1947,* Macmillan Publishers Limited, London, 2000, p.231.

2. H. Strachan, *The First World War: A New Illustrated History,* Simon & Schuster, London, 2003, p.275.

3. B.H. Liddell Hart, *History of the First World War,* Cassell and Co. Ltd., London, 1970, p.137.

4. C.E.W. Bean, *Anzac to Amiens* (5th ed.), Australian War Memorial, Canberra, 1968, pp.120-1.

5. V. Brittain, *Testament of Youth,* Virago Press, London, 2006 (first published by Victor Gollancz Limited 1933), p.124.

6. K. Fewster, *Gallipoli: The Turkish Story,* Vecihi Başarm, Hatice Hürmüz Başarm, Allen & Unwin, Sydney, 1985, pp.49-53, 55-6.

7. R. McMullin, *Pompey Elliott,* Scribe Publications Pty Ltd, Melbourne, 2002, pp.58, 62-3, 64-7, 118.

8. Hamilton cited in Lee, *A Soldier's Life,* p.162; Fewster, *Gallipoli: The Turkish Story,* p.76

9. Abdul Rahman cited in Fewster, *Gallipoli: The Turkish Story*, p.75.

10. A.G. Butler, *The Official History of the Australian Army Medical Services in the war of 1914-1918: Gallipoli, Palestine and New Guinea*, Vol 1, (2nd ed.), Australian War Memorial, Melbourne, 1938, pp.101, 122, 144, 150.

11. (Late) E. Wrobel (curator), 'Those who served 1914-1918' file, Lucy Osburn - Nightingale Foundation, Sydney Hospital & Sydney Eye Hospital, Sydney. The author gratefully acknowledges the assistance of (Late) Elinor Wrobel during the research of nurses who trained at Sydney Hospital. Sister Katherine Minnie Porter is occasionally referred to in the records of the AWM as Sister Donaldson after her marriage. She is not to be confused with Katherine Lawrence Porter who also trained at Sydney Hospital - R. Rae, 'The other Matron Porter' *The Milton-Ulludulla Times*, 8 January 2003.

12. Diary, 25 April 1915 in Narrative, E. Tucker, *Records of A.G. Butler: Official Historian of Australian Army Medical Services - Nurses' Narratives*, AWM 41, Australian War Memorial, Canberra.

13. Brittain, *Testament of Youth*, p.171.

14. M. Barker, *Nightingales in the Mud: the Digger Sisters of the Great War 1914-1918*, Allen and Unwin, Sydney, 1989, pp.35-6.

15. Narrative, Evelyn Vickers Foote, *Records of A.G. Butler: Official Historian of Australian Army Medical Services - Nurses' Narratives*, p.2.

16. Kathleen Power, *Military Forces of the Commonwealth Papers*, NAA, Canberra.

17. The voyage on the *Mongolia* came to an abrupt end when the ship hit a mine forty miles off Bombay. This incident is referred to in greater detail in Ruth Rae, *Scarlet Poppies*.

18. Kathleen Power, *Military Forces of the Commonwealth Papers*, Attestation Paper, 9 March 1916.

19. R. Goodman, *Our War Nurses: The History of the Royal Australian Army Nursing Corps 1902-1988*, Boolarong Publications, Brisbane, 1988, p. 57.

20. G.P. Walsh 'Kirkpatrick, John Simpson (1892 - 1915)', *Australian Dictionary of Biography*, National Centre of Biography, Australian National University, Volume 9, Melbourne University Press, Melbourne, 1983, pp. 612-3.
21. Kathleen Power, *Military Forces of the Commonwealth Papers*.

22. Narrative, Pauline E. Pierre Humbert, *Records of A.G. Butler: Official Historian of Australian Army Medical Services - Nurses' Narratives*, p.1,8.

23. After the First World War the Red Crescent Societies were formalised - C. Moorehead, *Dunant's Dream: War, Switzerland and the History of the Red Cross*, Carroll & Graf Publishers, Inc., New York, 1999, pp.126, 295.

24. Letitia Gladys Moreton, *Military Forces of the Commonwealth Papers*, NAA, Canberra; B.F. Miller & C.B. Keane, *Encyclopedia and Dictionary of Medicine and Nursing*, WB Saunders Co, London, 1972, p.470.

25.Agnes Beryl, Corfield *Military Forces of the Commonwealth Papers*, NAA, Canberra.

26. R. Goodman, *Queensland Nurses: Boer War to Vietnam*, Boolarong Publications, Brisbane, 1985, p.vi.

27. The electoral roll (1903) lists Peter Berrie as an Engineer in Cairns and his wife Agnes as a domestic worker at the Shamrock Hotel. The electoral roll (1913) states her father was 'a miner' (telephone conversation Helen Kindt, Mareeba History Society, with Ruth Rae, 23 February 2007). The author acknowledges Helen Kindt for her assistance.

28. H. Gregory & C. Brazil, *Bearers of the Tradition: Nurses of the Royal Brisbane Hospital 1888-1993*, Boolarong Publications, Brisbane, 1993, p.19.

29. *ibid; Military Forces of the Commonwealth Papers* [online 21 February 2007]. (Photograph AWM P11098.001)

30. Mary Florence Stafford, *Military Forces of the Commonwealth Papers*, NAA, Canberra; AWM Roll of

Honour: http://www.awm.gov.au/database/roh.asp.AWM Nominal Roll: http://www.awm.gov.au/database.

31. Graeme Lang Wilson, *Military Forces of the Commonwealth Papers,* NAA, Canberra; Grace Wilson, *Military Forces of the Commonwealth Papers,* NAA, Canberra.

32. Bassett, *Guns and Brooches,* p.46.

33. Norman John Wilson, *Military Forces of the Commonwealth Papers,* NAA, Canberra; Roy Wilson, *Military Forces of the Commonwealth Papers,* NAA, Canberra.

34. Graeme Lang Wilson, *Military Forces of the Commonwealth Papers.*

35. Bean, *Anzac to Amiens,* pp.140-1, 148-9.

36. Wilson cited in Goodman, *Our War Nurses,* pp.41-2; C.E.W. Bean, *Official History of Australia in the War of 1914-1918 - The Story of ANZAC: The First Phase,* Vol 2, Angus and Robertson Ltd., Sydney, 1935, p.390(*n*).

37. Selwyn-Smith cited in Goodman, *Queensland Nurses,* p.54.

38. A.Maud Kellett interview (no. 41) F.M. Howitt, AWM, Canberra, 1919.

39. H. Weatherhead cited in M.E. Clampett, *My Dear Mother,* Muriel Clampett, Melbourne, 1992, p.150; Rae, *Scarlet Poppies,* pp.102-3

40. Wilson cited in Bassett, p.67.

41. A.Maud Kellett interview (no. 18) C. Donnelly, AWM, Canberra, 1919.

42. A.Maud Kellett interview (no. 41) F.M. Howitt, AWM, Canberra, 1919.

43. Diary, Olive Haynes, 30 September 1915 in M Young (ed), *We are here, too: The diaries and letters of Sister Olive LC Haynes November 1914 to February 1918,* Australian Down Syndrome Association Incorp. Adelaide, 1991, p.81.

44. Bean, , *Anzac to Amiens,* p.165.

45. Lee, *A Soldier's Life,* p.220.

46. Butler, *Gallipoli, Palestine and New Guinea,* p.350 (*n*).

47. AWM Embarkation Roll: http://www.awm.goc.au/cms_images/awm8/26-66-3/pdf/151-175.pdf [online 28 February 2006]; Goodman suggests L.G. Moreton was a Queensland casualty but there is no evidence for this claim whereas Beatrice Lilian Moreton was born at Gayndah, Queensland- Goodman, *Queensland Nurses,* p.vi; Beatrice Lilian Moreton, *Military Forces of the Commonwealth Papers,*NAA, Canberra.

48. Narrative, Blodwyn E. Williams, *Records of A.G. Butler: Official Historian of Australian Army Medical Services - Nurses' Narratives.*

49. Correspondence, L.G. Moreton, 27 August 1915, 2 AGH, Cairo, Egypt in Typed Extracts of Correspondence at *AWM File No. 12/11/1398 - 2 DRL 97,* Australian War Memorial, Canberra, p.2.

50. Electronic correspondence, Pearl Collins to Ruth Rae, 6 January 2005 (*Ruth Rae Collection,* National Nursing Archives, Canberra). The author gratefully acknowledges Pearl Collins, Research Manager, Echuca/Moama Family History Group Inc, who provided background information on nurses Moorhouse and McPhail.

51. Electronic correspondence, Heather Rendle to Ruth Rae, 11 January 2005 (*Ruth Rae Collection,* National Nursing Archives, Canberra).

52. *The Riverine Herald,* 'Died on service', Echuca, 10 December 1918.

53. Leslie James Moorhouse, *Military Forces of the Commonwealth Papers,* NAA, Canberra.

54. Edith Ann Moorhouse, *Military Forces of the Commonwealth Papers,* NAA, Canberra.

55.Correspondence, L.G. Moreton, 6 August, 1915, 2 AGH, Cairo, Egypt, *AWM File No. 12/11/1398 - 2*

DRL 97, p.1. J. Bassett, 'Walker, Jean Nellie Miles (1878-1918)' *Australian Dictionary of Biography*, National Centre of Biography, Australian National University, Volume 12, Melbourne University Press, 1990, p.362.

56. Edith Ann Moorhouse, *Military Forces of the Commonwealth Papers*; Goodman, *Our War Nurses*, p.40; Barker, *Nightingales in the Mud*, p.22.

57. Butler, *Gallipoli, Palestine and New Guinea*, p.401.

58. Bean, *Anzac to Amiens*, pp.165, 171-2, 179-81.

59. A. Donnell, *Letters of an Australian Army Nursing Sister*, Angus and Robertson Ltd, Sydney, 1920, pp.98-9.

60. The number of MID attributed to Grace Wilson varies from different sources including Goodman, *Our War Nurses*, p.68 and Janice McCarthy, 'Wilson, Grace Margaret (1879-1957)', *Australian Dictionary of Biography*, National Centre of Biography, Australian National University,Volume 12, Melbourne University Press, 1990, pp.522-3. However, the Australian War Memorial website indicates the following awards to Grace Wilson were gazetted in London on the following dates - RRC (1st class) 21 September 1916; MID 5 May 1916, 21 June 1916, 13 July 1916, 31 December 1918. Wilson also received two recommendations for an Order of the British Empire but was awarded the higher award of Commander of the British Empire which was gazetted on 1 January 1919 - AWM Honours and Awards: http://www.awm.gov.au/honours/honours/ [online 11 November 2007].

15 War Wounds and Disease

1. Campbell cited in A.G. Butler, *The Official History of the Australian Army Medical Services in the war of 1914-1918: Special Problems and Services*, Vol 3, Australian War Memorial, Canberra, 1943, pp.62, 78-9.

2. Perditta McCarthy, 'Ellen Julia Gould' in *Australian Dictionary of Biography*, National Centre of Biography, Australian National University, Volume 9, Melbourne University Press, Melbourne, 1983, p.60; A. Rogers, *While You're Away: New Zealand Nurses at War 1899-1948*, Auckland University Press, 2003, p.43; Butler, *Special Problems and Services*, p.64.

3. Butler, *Special Problems and Services*, p.72.

4. Register of Australasian Trained Nurses' Association (ATNA) Members 1916, Websdale, Shoosmith Ltd., Sydney.

5. Perdita McCarthy, 'Ellen Julia Gould', *Australian Dictionary of Biography*, p.60; Rogers, *While You're Away*, p.43.

6. Jung cited in Anthony Storr, *Jung*, Fontana/Collins, London, 1973, pp.20-21.

7. Oppenheimer cited in P. Singer, *Pushing Time Away*, Harper Perennial, Sydney, 2003, pp.285-6.

8. Butler, *Special Problems and Services*, p.61.

9. Campbell cited in Butler, *Special Problems and Services*, p.84.

10. Butler, *Special Problems and Services*, p.76 & (*n*).

11. Research relating to this topic has been previously published in R. Rae, 'An historical account of shell-shock during the First World War and reforms in mental health in Australia 1914-1939', *International Journal of Mental Health Nursing*, 2007, 16: 266-273; Butler, *Special Problems and Services*, p.74.

12. C.E.W. Bean, *Anzac to Amiens* (5th ed.), Australian War Memorial, Canberra, 1968, pp.77, 287-8, 294.

13. Butler, *Special Problems and Services*, pp.59, 86-7, 99.

14. M. B. Wright, 'Psychological Emergencies in War Time' in *War Wounds and Air Raid Casualties*,

Articles from the British Medical Journals, H.K. Lewis and Co. Ltd., London, 1939, pp.174-5.

15. Perdita McCarthy, 'Ellen Julia Gould', *Australian Dictionary of Biography*, p.60.

16. Butler, *Gallipoli, Palestine and New Guinea*, p.417.

17. Campbell cited in Butler, *Special Problems and Services,* p.83.

18. Woollard cited in Butler, *Special Problems and Services,* p.106.

19. A.Maud Kellett interview (no. 11) L. Comber, AWM, Canberra, 1919; Rae, *Scarlet Poppies* pp.80-2

20. Narrative, E.W. King, *Records of A. G. Butler, Official Historian of Australian Army Medical Services – Nurses' Narratives.*

21. Violet Young, *Outlines of Nursing,* The Scientific Press Ltd, London, 1914, pp.15, 21, 23.

22. Narrative, V. Woniarski, *Records of A.G. Butler, Official Historian of Australian Army Medical Services – Nurses' Narratives;* A.Maud Kellett interview (no.14) Matron-in-Chief Evelyn Conyers, AWM, Canberra, 1919, p.4.

23. Newspaper article 'Called Home!' *The Elmore Standard*, 3 July 1915.

24. Y. McEwen, *"It's a Long Way to Tipperary": British and Irish nurses in the Great War*, Cualann Press, Dunfermline, 2006, p.200.

25. Correspondence, David Cotton to Ruth Rae, 19 January 2005, *Ruth Rae Collection,* National Nursing Archives, Canberra.

26. Florence MacKenzie, *Military Forces of the Commonwealth Papers*, NAA, Canberra.

27. Correspondence, Mrs I. McNabb, Denmark, WA to Paymaster, 5 MD, AIF in Florence MacKenzie, *Military Forces of the Commonwealth Papers*; http://www.outbackfamilyhistory.com.au [15.5.2025].

28. B.F. Miller & C.B. Keane, *Encyclopedia and Dictionary of Medicine and Nursing*, W.B. Saunders Co, London, 1972, pp.279-280.

29. A.Maud Kellett interview (no. 103) E.A.M. Riordon, AWM, Canberra, 1919.

30. Butler, *Gallipoli, Palestine and New Guinea*, p.247.

31. Correspondence, Fred Tomlins to Jessie Tomlins, 6 December 1916 (copy in possession of author).

32. Butler, *Special Problems and Services*, pp.925-7. It is not possible to ascertain the number of Australian soldiers who suffered from cholera because Neville Howse ordered that all medical records be destroyed to ostensibly protect the privacy of the soldiers; Butler, *Special Problems and Services*, pp.925 & (*n*).

33. Butler, *Gallipoli, Palestine and New Guinea*, pp.349-350.

34. A.G. Butler, *The Official History of the Australian Army Medical Services in the war of 1914-1918: The Western Front*, vol 2, Australian War Memorial, Canberra, 1940, p.581.

35. Miller & Keane, *Encyclopedia and Dictionary of Medicine and Nursing*, pp.293-4.

36. Miller & Keane, *Encyclopedia and Dictionary of Medicine and Nursing*, p.196; World Health Organization website: http://www.who.int/topics/cholera/[online 26 October 2025]; S. Singer & H. R. Hilgard, *The Biology of People*, W.H. Freeman and Company, San Francisco, 1978, pp.318-9.

37. Miller and Keane, *Encyclopedia and Dictionary of Medicine and Nursing*, p.196.

38. Narrative, Evelyn Vickers Foote, *Records of A.G. Butler, Official Historian of Australian Army Medical Services – Nurses' Narratives*, p.3.

39. W. Gordon Sears, *Materia Medica for Nurses: a text-book of drugs and therapeutics* (4th ed.), Edward Arnold (Publishers) Ltd., London, 1959, pp.46-7.

40. World Health Organization website: Cholera prevention and control http://www.who.int/topics/cholera/control/en/index.html [online 29 October 2025].

41. Butler, *Gallipoli, Palestine and New Guinea*, pp.349-350.

42. Miller & Keane, *Encyclopedia and Dictionary of Medicine and Nursing*, p.707.

43. Butler, *Gallipoli, Palestine and New Guinea*, p. 456.

44. Miller & Keane, *Encyclopedia and Dictionary of Medicine and Nursing*, p.992.

45. Narrative, Matron Adelaide Maud Kellett, *Records of A.G. Butler, Official Historian of Australian Army Medical Services - Nurses' Narratives,* p.9.

46. P. Adam-Smith, *Australian Women at War*, Penguin Books Australia Ltd., Melbourne, 1996, p.65.

47. Matron Rose Creal 'No 14 Australian General Hospital, Report of Nursing Services from 23 September 1916 to 30 September 1917', Medical History File of the Official Medical Historian A.G. Butler, AWM, Canberra, p.4.

48. J. Bassett, *Guns and Brooches: Australian Army Nursing from the Boer War to the Gulf War*, Oxford University Press, Melbourne, 1992, pp.88-9.

49. Narrative, A.M. Kellett, *Records of A. G. Butler, Official Historian of Australian Army Medical Services - Nurses' Narratives,* p.9; Correspondence, LG Moreton, 30 July 1916, c/o DMS, Indian Medical Services, Bombay in Typed Extracts of Correspondence at *AWM File No. 12/11/1398 - 2 DRL 97,* Australian War Memorial, Canberra, p.8.

50. A. Hill, *Soldier Boy: The true story of Jim Martin The youngest Anzac,* Penguin Books Australia, Melbourne, 2001, pp.121-2.

51. Miller & Keane, *Encyclopedia and Dictionary of Medicine and Nursing*, p.379.

52. K. Fewster, *Gallipoli: The Turkish Story*, Vecihi Başarm, Hatice Hürmüz Başarm, Allen & Unwin, Sydney,1985, pp.84-5.

53. Narrative, Victor Mitton Ridgway (brother to Doris) dated 22 November 1970, copy given to author by Mr Ian Ridgway (nephew of Doris) in June 2005 (*Ruth Rae Collection*, National Nursing Archives, Canberra).

16 Nursing in Egypt 1915-16

1. Ruth Rae, *The Biography of an Australian Light Horseman: Fred Tomlins*, amazon, 2023, pp.190-201.

2. Correspondence, L.G. Moreton, 9 January 1916, Nurses Red Cross Rest Home, Zizinia, Bacos Remlah via Alexandria, *AWM File No. 12/11/1398 - 2 DRL 97*, p.2.

3. J. Bassett, *Guns and Brooches: Australian Army Nursing from the Boer War to the Gulf War*, Oxford University Press, Melbourne, 1992, p.44; A.G. Butler, *The Official History of the Australian Army Medical Services in the war of 1914-1918 Gallipoli, Palestine and New Guinea*, Vol 1, (2nd ed.), Australian War Memorial, Melbourne, 1938, pp.74-5.

4. Diary, Sister Agnes Isambert cited in R. Goodman, *Our War Nurses: The History of the Royal Australian Army Nursing Corps 1902-1988,* Boolarong Publications, Brisbane, 1988, p.47. The AANS nurses who were official mourners were Agnes Isambert, Maud Isobel Baker, Mary Florence Whipham, Annie Scott, Beatrice Louise Gibbon, Gladys Ivy Echlin; AWM Nominal Roll [online 22 November 2006].

5. Norma Mowbray, *Military Forces of the Commonwealth Papers*, NAA, Canberra.

6.Diary, Sister Isambert, 3 February 1916 cited in R. Goodman, *Queensland Nurses: Boer War to Vietnam*, Boolarong Publications, Brisbane, 1985, p.58.

7. Wallets of letters from Lizzie Ryland to Agnes Berrie, https://www.awm.gov.au/collection/C2601511.

8. 'The Chronicle' at www.lighthorse.org.au [online February 2007] © Australian Light Horse Ltd; S &

T McIvor, *Salute the Brave: a pictorial history of Queensland war memorials*, Queensland University Press, Brisbane, 1994, p.187.

9. Y. McEwen, *"It's a Long Way to Tipperary": British and Irish nurses in the Great War*, Cualann Press, Dunfermline, 2006, p.203. Goodman, *Queensland Nurses*, p.59.

10. Goodman, *Queensland Nurses*, pp.129 & 125; Commemorative War Graves Commission [online 21.2.07] http://www.cwgc.org/search/casualty; AWM Commemorative Roll (no record) [online 20 April 2007].

11. Correspondence, Fred Tomlins to Margaretta Tomlins, 6 July 1915, copy in possession of author.
12. Elsie Tranter diary, 27 October 1917, in G. M. Gillings and J. Richards (eds), *...in all those lines: The diary of Sister Elsie Tranter 1916-1919*, s/p.2008, p.81.

13. Australian War Memorial: http://www.unsw.adfa.edu.au/~rmallett/Transports.html [online 6 March 2006] and [last update 09 October 2003].

14. A. Donnell, *Letters of an Australian Army Nursing Sister*, Angus and Robertson Ltd, Sydney, 1920, p.106.

15. Elsie Rose Grant, *Military Forces of the Commonwealth Papers*, NAA, Canberra.

16. AWM Embarkation Roll: http://www.awm.gov.au/cms_images/[online 23 May 2005].

17. 'Casualty Form - Active Service' in Elsie Rose Grant, *Military Forces of the Commonwealth Papers*.

18. May Tilton, *The Grey Battalion*, Angus and Robertson Limited, Sydney, 1933.

19. 'Casualty Form - Active Service' in Elsie Rose Grant, *Military Forces of the Commonwealth Papers*.

20. Correspondence, Ellen Grant to Officer-in-Charge (AIF, Melbourne) 22 January 1916 in Elsie Grant *Military Forces of the Commonwealth Papers*.

21. A. Rogers, *While You're Away: New Zealand Nurses at War 1899-1948*, Auckland University Press, 2003, p.104; Details and research relating to this topic have been previously published in R. Rae (2007) 'A comparative analysis of the development of the Australian Army Nursing Service and the New Zealand Army Nursing Service (1899-1918)', *nursing.aust*, Journal of the College of Nursing, 8(2):14-17.

22.Rogers, *While You're Away*, pp.94-7, 104.

23. W.H. Menadue *Ballarat Base Hospital Nurse Training Registers 1888-1988*, Ballarat Base Hospital Trained Nurses' League, Ballarat, 1993, p.2.The author gratefully acknowledges W. Menadue for her assistance with research relating to nurses who trained at Ballarat Base Hospital.

24. Rogers, *While You're Away*, p.106.

25 Marie Cameron, *Military Forces of the Commonwealth Papers*, NAA, Canberra.

26. Narrative E. Tucker, *Records of A.G. Butler, Official Historian of Australian Army Medical Services - Nurses' Narratives*; Diary, Alice Kitchen cited in P. Adam-Smith, *Australian Women at War*, Penguin Books Australia Ltd., Melbourne, 1996, p.22; J. Lee *A Soldier's Life: General Sir Ian Hamilton 1853-1947*, Macmillan Publishers Limited, London, 2000, pp.230-2.

27. Bassett, *Guns and Brooches*, p.58.

28. J. Bassett, 'Walker, Jean Nellie Miles (1878-1918)' *Australian Dictionary of Biography*, Volume 12, Melbourne University Press, 1990, p.362.

29. Letitia Gladys Moreton, *Military Forces of the Commonwealth Papers*, NAA, Canberra; AWM Embarkation Roll: http://www.awm.goc.au/cms_images/ [online 28 February 2006]. For example, Sister Smeaton-White boarded the *Kyarra* on 13 April 1915 and stated the time taken for her to reach Suez was seven weeks and three days although additional time was needed to pick up troops in Queensland and to call into Townsville to unload a soldier who required surgery; A.Maud Kellett interview (no. 106) E.J. Smeaton-White, AWM, Canberra, 1919.

30. Ross Mallett Transport home page for Australian Defence Force Academy, UNSW

http://www.unsw.adfa.edu.au/~rmallett/Transports.html [last update 09.10.2003] [online 26 January 2006].

31. Digger–Pioneer Index.Victoria 1836-1888 [18 August 2006].

32. Beatrice Middleton Watson, *Military Forces of the Commonwealth Papers,* NAA, Canberra; Digger–Pioneer Index.Victoria 1836-1888[online 18 August 2006].

33. Beatrice Middleton Watson, *Military Forces of the Commonwealth Papers.*

34. AWM Embarkation Roll: http://www.awm.gov.au/cms_images/ [online 16 August 2006].

35. J. Bassett, 'Walker, Jean Nellie Miles (1878-1918)' *Australian Dictionary of Biography,* National Centre of Biography, Australian National University, Volume 12, Melbourne University Press, 1990, p.362.

36. Mary Florence Stafford, *Military Forces of the Commonwealth Papers (Medical Board Report),* NAA, Canberra.

37. Beatrice Middleton Watson, *Military Forces of the Commonwealth Papers.*

38. Herbert E. Cuff & W.T. Gordon Pugh, *Practical Nursing including Hygiene and Dietetics* (7th ed.), William Blackwood & Sons Ltd, London, 1928, p.438.

39. B.F. Miller & C.B. Keane, *Encyclopedia and Dictionary of Medicine and Nursing,* W.B. Saunders Co., London, 1972, pp.570-1.

40. Narrative, Sister G. A. Grewar, *Records of A.G. Butler, Official Historian of Australian Army Medical Services – Nurses' Narratives,* p.3.

41. A.G. Butler, *The Official History of the Australian Army Medical Services in the war of 1914-1918: The Western Front,* Vol 2, Australian War Memorial, Canberra, 1940, p.932.

42. Cuff & Pugh, *Practical Nursing including Hygiene and Dietetics,* p.438.

43. Beatrice Middleton Watson, *Military Forces of the Commonwealth Papers.*

44. R. Reid, *Just Wanted to be there – Australian Service Nurses 1899-1999,* Department of Veteran's Affairs, Commonwealth of Australia, 1999, p.43 (photograph); AWM Embarkation Roll: http://www.awm.gov.au/cms_images/ [online 16 August 2006].

45. C. Fallows, *Love and War: Stories of War Brides from the Great War to Vietnam,* Bantam Books, Sydney, 2002, p.94.

46. J. Horsfield, *Rainbow: The story of Rania Macphillamy,* Ginninderra Press, Canberra, 2007, p.66.

47. John Rickard,'White, Vera Deakin (1891-1978)', Australian Dictionary of Biography, National Centre of Biography, Australian National University, published in hardcopy 2002, accessed online 26 October 2025; Ruth Rae, *The Biography of an Australian Light Horseman: Fred Tomlins,* amazon, 2025, p.326.

48.AWM online 26 October 2025, Accession Number ARTVO5498.

49. A. J. Smithers, *Sir John Monash: A Biography of Australia's Most Distinguished Soldier of the First World War,* Angus and Robertson, Sydney, 1973, pp.139-140; C.E.W. Bean, *Anzac to Amiens* (5th ed.), Australian War Memorial, Canberra, 196, pp.192-3.

50. Bean, *Anzac to Amiens,* pp.188, 271, 391.

51. H.S. Gullett, *Official History of Australia in the War of 1914-18 Sinai and Palestine* (12th ed), Vol 7, Angus and Robertson Ltd, Sydney, 1944, p.645.

52. J Beaumont (ed), *Australia's War 1914-1918,* Allen and Unwin, Sydney,1995, p.151.

53. Correspondence, L.G. Moreton, 29 April 1916, No. 4 Aux, Abbassia, Egypt *AWM File No. 12/11/1398 – 2 DRL 97,* p.4.

54. May Tilton, *The Grey Battalion*, Angus and Robertson Limited, Sydney, 1933, pp.88-9. The long suffering 'baby donkey' was also taken for a meal in a fashionable restaurant in Cairo by two Anzacs to the chagrin of a number of Englishmen.

55. Correspondence, L.G. Moreton, 29 April 1916, No. 4 Aux, Abbassia, Egypt *AWM File No. 12/11/1398 – 2 DRL 97*, pp.4-5.

56. Correspondence, L.G. Moreton, 15 May 1916, No. 4 Aux, Abbassia, Egypt, *AWM File No. 12/11/1398 – 2 DRL 97*, p.5.

57. Correspondence, Jessie Tomlins to Margaretta Tomlins, 27 April 1919 in Ruth Rae, *The Biography of an Australian First World War nurse: Jessie Tomlins*, amazon.com. 2025.

17 Australian Nurses in Europe 1914-16

1. The official war diary of the Matron-in-Chief, British Expeditionary Force, The National Archives, WO95/3988,3989,3990 & 3991 [on-line 4 June 2025].

2. Electronic correspondence, Selena Williams to Ruth Rae, 18 December 2006 in *Ruth Rae Collection*, National Nursing Archives, Canberra; Electronic correspondence, Mike Moore to Ruth Rae, 1 January 2007 in *Ruth Rae Collection*, National Nursing Archives, Canberra. The author gratefully acknowledges Mike Moore, Fitzroy History Society who provided background information on the early life of Myrtle Wilson. Trove, nla.gov.au/newspaper/article/20061961 [on-line 4 June 2025].

3. Bundaberg Genealogical Association Inc, 'Bundaberg and District Pioneers: A Biographical Index to 1901', p.328.

4. *Bundaberg Mail*, 'Advertisement Mrs Boyles High School for Girls', March 1893.

5. *Bundaberg Mail*, 'High School for Girls', 15 December 1893.

6. Bundaberg Genealogical Association Inc, 'Obituaries in the Bundaberg Newspapers', vol. 8, n/d, p.71.

7. H. Gregory & C. Brazil, *Bearers of the Tradition: Nurses of the Royal Brisbane Hospital 1888-1993*, Boolarong Publications, Brisbane, 1993, p.18. The author gratefully acknowledges (Late) Judith Cornell, archivist, The College of Nursing, Sydney and Cecilia Brazil, curator, Brisbane Hospital Museum for their assistance. Queensland Electoral Roll 1913 in Queensland data search version 7.1 Queensland Family History Society for 1913; The author acknowledges Jan Hegert, Bundaberg Genealogical Association Inc who provided background information on the life of Myrtle Wilson in Bundaberg – Electronic correspondence, Jan Hegert to Ruth Rae, January 2007 in *Ruth Rae Collection*, National Nursing Archives, Canberra.

8. 1. The official war diary of the Matron-in-Chief, British Expeditionary Force, The National Archives, WO95/3988,3989,3990 & 3991 [on-line 4 June 2025].

9. Commonwealth War Graves website: http://www.cwgc.org/ [online 24 January 2007].

10. Y. McEwen, *"It's a Long Way to Tipperary": British and Irish nurses in the Great War*, Cualann Press, Dunfermline, 2006, p.204; *Bundaberg Mail*, obituary 'Nurse Myrtle Wilson', 28 December 1915. Service Record of Myrtle Wilson, The National Archives, Kew. The official war diary of the Matron-in-Chief, British Expeditionary Force, The National Archives, WO95/3988,3989,3990 & 3991 [on-line 4 June 2025], The National Archives Website, UK].British Jouranl of Nursing , 15 January 1916 {on-line 6 June 2025]. AWM Photograph on-line with Myrtle back row 3rd from right. No record with AWM on 6 June 2025.

11. When war was declared Andrew Fisher was the Australian Prime Minister but he resigned in October 1915, two months prior to the successful Gallipoli evacuation. He was Prime Minister three times (1908-9, 1910-13 and 1914-15) but found the burden of responsibility for leading a country during a war too high. He continued to serve Australia as the High Commissioner to London from 1916 to 1921 – L.F. Crisp *The Australian Federal Labour Party 1901-1951*, Hale and Iremonger, Sydney,

1978, p.31(*n*). Sir Joseph Cook, the father-in-law of Australian nurse Elsie Cook, was appointed to the position from 1921-7 – Crisp, *The Australian Federal Labour Party 1901-1951,* p.124(*n*).

12. Sarah Margaret White, 'A World War 1 nurse remembers …' 31 October 1973, The Australian Women's Weekly, 31 October 1973. The author gratefully acknowledges Tony Cornell who brought this article to my attention.

13. C. Moorehead *Dunant's Dream: War, Switzerland and the History of the Red Cross*, Carroll & Graf Publishers, Inc., New York, 1999, p.209.

14. Chris Cuneen 'Dudley, Lady Rachel (1867-1920)', *Australian Dictionary of Biography*, National Centre of Biography, Australian National University, Volume 8, Melbourne University Press, 1981, pp.347-8.

15. The Royal Australian and New Zealand College of Radiologists, 'The Australian Voluntary Hospital and Herschel Harris' in *Inside News*, Vol 3 (no. 2) March 2007, pp.6-7.

16. Kevin Brady (ed) *Streets of Condobolin & the Historical Significance of their Names* Condobolin Historical Society, s/p, 2002, n/p. Una and Margaret married and remained in the district.

17. John Norton, Family history file of Elizabeth McGregor, copy sent to author in November 2007 in *Ruth Rae Collection*, National Nursing Archives, Canberra. The author gratefully acknowledges John Norton (grand-nephew of Elizabeth McGregor) for providing copies of relevant material relating to the life of Elizabeth McGregor and her sisters.

18. Memorial Service for Elizabeth McGregor, Condobolin Presbyterian Church (15 December 1918) and reported in full in 'The Lachlander', 25 December 1918 in *Ruth Rae Collection*, National Nursing Archives, Canberra.

19. Brady, *Streets of Condobolin & the Historical Significance of their Name,* n/p.

20. John Norton, Family history file of Elizabeth McGregor in *Ruth Rae Collection*, National Nursing Archives, Canberra; ATNA Register, The College of Nursing archives, Sydney. It was commonplace for hospitals to insist the second trainee from the same family use their mother's maiden surname to differentiate two nurses from the same family, but Helen was known as 'Nurse Cameron'.

21. John Norton, Family history file of Elizabeth McGregor in *Ruth Rae Collection*, National Nursing Archives, Canberra.

22. ATNA Register, The National Nursing Archives, Canberra.

23. Australian War Memorial Record 371/93 'Nominal Roll of Nursing Staff, Australian Voluntary Hospital, Wimereux, January 1915' in *Ruth Rae Collection*, National Nursing Archives, Canberra; H. Strachan, *The First World War: A New Illustrated History*, Simon & Schuster, London, 2003, p.152.

24. Strachan, *The First World War*, 2003, pp.152-5.

25. John Norton, Family history file of Elizabeth McGregor in *Ruth Rae Collection*, National Nursing Archives, Canberra.

26. Memorial Service for Elizabeth McGregor, Condobolin Presbyterian Church (15 December 1918) and reported in full in '*The Lachlander*', 25 December 1918 in *Ruth Rae Collection*, National Nursing Archives, Canberra. The only reference to her award is the 'Serbian Cross' but the closest decoration of this description, at the time, is the Serbian Cross of Mercy '*This decoration was in the form of a Maltese cross with an inscription in the centre of the face 'For Nursing the Wounded and Sick', and on the other side the Serbian Royal Arms. The ribbon was ordinarily sky blue, but all crosses awarded during the First World War had the red moiré ribbon*' in Taprell Dorling in assoc. with F. Guille, *Ribbons and Medals*, George Phillip and Son Ltd., London, 1960, p.256.

27. Personal collection of John Norton, with copy in Family history file of Elizabeth McGregor in *Ruth Rae Collection*, National Nursing Archives, Canberra.

28. Christine E. Hallett, 'The personal writings of First World War nurses: a study of the interplay of authorial intention and scholarly interpretation', *Nursing Inquiry* 2007, 14(4):320-329, p.325.

29. Florence Farmborough, *Nurse at the Russian Front: A Diary 1914-1918,* Constable, London, 1974, pp.19, 21-2, 27-8.

30. B.H. Liddell Hart, *History of the First World War*, Cassell and Co. Ltd., London, 1970, p.146.

31. Diary, Florence Farmborough, 17 April 1915 in Florence Farmborough, *Nurse at the Russian Front: A diary 1914-1918,* Constable, London, 1974, p.33.

32. Diary, Florence Farmborough, 22 April 1915, p.36.

33. Liddell Hart, *History of the First World War*, p.147.

34. Diary, Florence Farmborough, 22 April 1915, p.36.

35. Strachan, *The First World War,* pp.249-50.

36. Correspondence, Alice Cooper, 21 November 1915 in D Denholm (ed), *Behind the Lines: One Woman's War 1914-18 Ethel Cooper*, Collins, Sydney, 1982, p.112.

37. A.E. Clarke-Kennedy, *Edith Cavell*, Faber & Faber, London, 1966, pp.161, 181-2, 207.

38. Clarke-Kennedy, p.225.

18 Global Changes 1916-1918

1. B.H. Liddell Hart, *History of the First World War*, Cassell and Co. Ltd, London, 1970, p.305; Manning Clark *A History of Australia: The Old Dead Tree and the Young Tree Green 1916-35*, Vol 6, Melbourne, 1987, p.84.

2. H. Strachan, *The First World War: A New Illustrated History*, Simon & Schuster, London, 2003, p.256.

3. N. Brennan, *Daniel Mannix*, Rigby Ltd., Adelaide, 1964, p.115.

4.Patrick Pearse, Speech 'Proclamation of the Irish Republic', 24 April 1916 quoted in Brian MacArthur (ed) *The Penguin Book of Twentieth Century Speeches*, London, 1992, pp.46-8.

5. B.E. Escott *Twentieth Century Women of Courage*, Sutton Publishing Limited, London, 1999, p.7.

6. MacArthur, p.47; Brennan, *Daniel Mannix*, p.127.

7. Brennan, *Daniel Mannix*, pp.126-8.

8. L.F. Crisp, *The Australian Federal Labour Party 1901-1951*, Sydney, 1978, pp.135-6. Crisp correctly asserts that Hughes had not contravened anything written in the Federal Platform but concedes that five of the six States and the spirit of the Federal Labor Party were known to be anti-conscription. Ironically, Hughes could have introduced conscription without a referendum by claiming a 'moral mandate' via normal parliamentary processes - see Crisp, *The Australian Federal Labour Party 1901-1951*, p.211 *(n).*

9. J.T. Lang *The Turbulent Years – The autobiography of J.T.Lang*, Sydney, 1970, pp.40-2.

10. Graham Fricke *Profiles of Power: The Prime Ministers of Australia*, Houghton Mifflin Australia Pty Ltd, Melbourne, 1990, p.73.

11. Crisp, *The Australian Federal Labour Party 1901-1951*, pp 135-6, 211(*n*)

12. Brennan, *Daniel Mannix*, pp.129-30.

13. ANZAC portal, Department of Veterans' Affairs; NAA on line 26/7/2025.
14. Australian Electoral Commission, online 19 July 2025.
15. Crisp, *The Australian Federal Labour Party 1901-1951*, pp.73, 215-6.
16. A. Donnell, *Letters of An Australian Army Sister*, Angus and Robertson Ltd, Sydney, 1920, pp.147-8.

17. D. Aitkin, B. Jinks & J. Warhurst ,*Australian Political Institutions*, 4th ed, Longman Cheshire Pty Ltd, Melbourne, 1980, p.148.

18. Tilton, p.282.

19. C. Clifford, *The Asquiths*, John Murray (Publishers), London, 2002, p.145(*n*).

20. Strachan, *The First World War*, pp.206-8; Liddell Hart, pp.291-4.

21.Scarletfinders online 28 October 2025 'Queen Alexandra's Royal Naval Nursing Service, Staff Members 1884-1928'; Blog *Fascinating Facts of the Great War* 'Reflections on the Battle of Jutland by a nurse on the Hospital Ship "Plassy" (by kind permission of Andrew of the Facebook Page Hospital Ships of the Grand Fleet 1914-18 (Monday May 1916) on line 28 October 2025.

22. Peter Hopkirk, *On Secret Service East of Constantinople; the plot to bring down the British Empire*, John Murray (Publishers) Ltd, London, 1994, p.241.

23. Strachan, *The First World War*, pp.256-7.

24. Diary, Florence Farmborough, early May 1917 in Farmborough, p.266.

25. Liddell Hart, *History of the First World War*, pp.75, 295.

26.Diary, Florence Farmborough, 11 May 1917 in Florence Farmborough *Nurse at the Russian Front: A Diary 1914-1918,* Constable, London, 1974, p.267.

27. V. Brittain, *Testament of Youth*, Virago Press, London, 2006 (first published by Victor Gollancz Limited 1933), p.171.

28. Diary, Florence Farmborough, 4 March 1917 in Farmborough, pp.254-6.

29. Liddell Hart, *History of the First World War*, p.304.

30. D. Miller, *Anarchism,* J. M. Dent and Sons Ltd., London, 1984, p.91; Strachan, p.255.

31. Strachan, *The First World War*, p.255; Diary, Florence Farmborough, 11 May 1917, in Farmborough, p.268.

32. Diary, Florence Farmborough, 13 May 1917 & 28 June 1917 in Farmborough, pp.269-270, 282.

33. C.E.W. Bean, *Anzac to Amiens* (5th ed.), Australian War Memorial, Canberra, 1968, p.358.

34. Liddell Hart, *History of the First World War*, p.305. Manning Clark cites the conversations at Brest-Litovsk which resulted in the negotiation of a peace treaty between Germany and Russia which finally concluded on 5 March 1918 as being the correct date - Manning Clark, *A History of Australia: The Old Dead Tree and the Young Tree Green 1916-35,* p.84.

35. Diary, Florence Farmborough, January 1918 in Farmborough, pp.373, 382-5, 396, p.402.

36. Robert K. Massie, The Romanovs: The Final Chapter, The Random House Publishing Group, New York, 1995, pp.19, 184,186,200,278.

19 Establishing Australian Hospitals and Casualty Clearing Stations in Europe and England 1916-1918

1. B.H. Liddell Hart, *History of the First World War*, Cassell and Co. Ltd, London, 1970, pp.232 & 236.

2. A.G. Butler, *The Official History of the Australian Army Medical Services in the war of 1914-1918: Special Problems and Services*, Vol 3, Australian War Memorial Canberra, 1943, p.397.

3. A.G. Butler, *The Official History of the Australian Army Medical Services in the war of 1914-1918: The Western Front*, Vol 2, Australian War Memorial, Canberra, 1940, pp.438-9; Butler, *Special Problems and Services*, pp.134, 553.

4. Butler, *The Western Front*, pp.829 *(table)*, 364-5, 378, 772.

5. *ibid.*, pp.829 *(table)*, p.371.

6. Narrative Ada Smith, *Records of A.G. Butler: Official Historian of Australian Army Medical Services –*

Nurses' Narratives; A.Maud Kellett interview (no 69) Amy Holloway Mathews, AWM, Canberra, 1919.

7. L. Potter (Pres), *A Passion to Care: Nursing and Nurses Western Suburbs Hospital 1984-1982,* The Western Suburbs Hospital Graduate Nurses' Association, Sydney, 2008, p.70.

8. Joan Daryl Lindsay *The Story of the Red Cross: Australian Red Cross Society*, McLaren & Co Pty Ltd, Melbourne, circa 1939 (no page numbers).

9. Butler, *The Western Front*, pp.368-9.

10. *ibid.*, pp.187-8; 364; 382-7 (*table*).

11. The author acknowledges Peter Rees who kindly shared information about the 'Bluebirds'; Bathurst Historical Society provided information about Sister Fraser Thompson during a visit by the author in 2002; Diary, Elsie Cook (nee Sheppard) 22 February 1915 cited in J. Bassett, *Guns and Brooches: Australian Army Nursing from the Boer War to the Gulf War*, Oxford University Press, Melbourne, 1992, pp.39-40.

12. Elsie Tranter diary, 10 November 1917, in G.M. Gillings and J. Richards (eds) ...*in All those Lines: The Diary of Sister Elsie Tranter 1916-1919*, s/p.2008, p.83.

13. Butler, *The Western Front*, p.775(*n*).

14. Elsie Tranter diary, 24, 26 January 1918 & 1 March 1918, in Gillings and Richards (eds), *in All those Lines,* pp.91 & 95; Elsie May Tranter, *Military Forces of the Commonwealth Papers*, Service Record, NAA, Canberra.

15. Mary Violet Aitken, *Military Forces of the Commonwealth Papers*, Service Record, NAA, Canberra; Beulah Rotherdale McMinn *Military Forces of the Commonwealth Papers*, Service Record, NAA, Canberra.

16. Elsie May Tranter, *Military Forces of the Commonwealth Papers*.

17. Mary Violet Aitken, *Military Forces of the Commonwealth Papers*; Beulah Rotherdale McMinn, *Military Forces of the Commonwealth Papers*.

18. Elsie Tranter diary entries, 16, 18, 20 January, 8 February, 6,16 &17 March 1918 in Gillings and Richards (eds), ...*in All those Lines,* pp.90, 92-4.

19. Gillings and Richards (eds), *in All those Lines,* pp.99-127.

20. Elsie Tranter diary entries, 8, 27 February, 29 March 1918 in Gillings and Richards (eds), *in All those Lines,* pp.92, 94, 100.

21. Potter, *A Passion to Care,* p.42.

20 Australian Army Nursing Service in Europe and England 1916-1918

1. H. Strachan, *The First World War: A new illustrated history*, Simon & Schuster, London, 2003, p.159.

2. *ibid.*, p.160.

3. B.F. Miller & C.B. Keane, *Encyclopedia and Dictionary of Medicine and Nursing*, W.B. Saunders Co., London, 1972, p.379; Strachan, *The First World War*, p.159.

4. J.D. Buxton, 'Injuries of the Lower Limb' in *War Wounds and Air Raid Casualties*, Articles from the *British Medical Journals*, H.K. Lewis and Co. Ltd., London, 1939, pp.81-3; Miller & Keane, *Encyclopedia and Dictionary of Medicine and Nursing*, p.251.

5. Elsie Tranter diary, 2 March 1917, in G.M. Gillings and J. Richards (eds) ...*in All those Lines: The Diary of Sister Elsie Tranter 1916-1919*, s/p.2008, p.44.

6. A.Maud Kellett interview (no.29) S.E. Faulkner, AWM, Canberra, 1919.

7. Sarah Margaret White, 'A World War 1 nurse remembers ...' 31 October 1973, *The Australian Women's Weekly*, 31 October 1973.

8. 'Hospital Committee' *The Cairns Post*, 13 October 1915, p.8.

9. Pearl Stella Goodman, *Military Forces of the Commonwealth Papers,* NAA, Canberra.

10. Enlisted with AIF (AANS) in Brisbane, Queensland on 7 December 1916 and embarked on 29 December 1916 - Record, *Central Army Records Office*, Victoria Barracks, Melbourne (reviewed by author 25 February 2003); Attestation papers (5 March 1917) in Pearl Stella Goodman, *Military Forces of the Commonwealth Papers* ; AWM Embarkation Roll: http://www.awm.gov.au/cms_images/ [online 8 August 2006]; AWM Nominal Roll dates DOE: 12 November 1916 and RTA 16 December 1917 AWM Nominal Roll: http://www.awm.gov.au/database/ [online 8 August 2006]; Active Service Casualty Form (5 March 1917) in Pearl Stella Goodman, *Military Forces of the Commonwealth Papers*.

11. Confidential proceedings of a Medical Board (11 December 1917) in Pearl Stella Goodman *Military Forces of the Commonwealth Papers.*

12. Detailed Medical History of an Invalid (5 March 1918) in Pearl Stella Goodman, *Military Forces of the Commonwealth Papers.*

13. Jessie Tomlins, *Military Forces of the Commonwealth Papers*, NAA, Canberra.

14. Guy R. Williams, *The Age of Miracles: Medicine and Surgery in the Nineteenth Century,* Constable, London, 1981, pp.27-8.

15. Miller & Keane, *Encyclopedia and Dictionary of Medicine and Nursing*, pp.987-8.

16. Doherty, Sirl & Ring, *Modern Practical Nursing Procedures,* Dymocks Book Arcade Ltd, Sydney, 1944, pp.288-290.

17. Confidential proceedings of a Medical Board (11 December 1917) in Pearl Stella Goodman, *Military Forces of the Commonwealth Papers.*

18. Miller & Keane, *Encyclopedia and Dictionary of Medicine and Nursing*, p.988.

19. 'Nurse Deceased' *The Cairns Post*, 8 March 1919.

20. Attestation paper (7 December 1916) in Pearl Stella Goodman, *Military Forces of the Commonwealth Papers.*

21. Last Will and Testament (12 October 1915) and annexed to Probate (8 October 1919) in Pearl Stella Goodman, *Military Forces of the Commonwealth Papers.*

22. AWM Embarkation Roll: http://www.awm.gov.au/cms_images [online 8 August 2006].

23. Correspondence, Mrs. F.H. Tait to Officer-in-Charge Base Records, 30 May 1921 & 1 May 1922 in Pearl Stella Goodman, *Military Forces of the Commonwealth Papers.*

24. Correspondence, Officer-in-Charge Base Records to Mrs. F.H. Tait, 22 June 1921 & 22 May 1922 in Pearl Stella Goodman, *Military Forces of the Commonwealth Papers.*

25. Correspondence, Officer-in-Charge Base Records to Mr A.E. Goodman, 26 July 1921 in Pearl Stella Goodman, *Military Forces of the Commonwealth Papers.*

26. R. Rae, photograph of Cairns RSL Obelisk, Cairns, August 2002 (*Ruth Rae Collection*, National Nursing Archives, Canberra); A notation incorrectly reads that she died on 15 August 1918 in Record, Pearl Goodman, Central Army Records Office, Victoria Barracks, Melbourne (reviewed by author 25 February 2003). AWM Roll of Honour, NAA Service Record, Pearl Goodman, 2025.

21 First Australian General Hospital (1AGH) in Europe and England 1916-1918

1. A.G. Butler, *The Official History of the Australian Army Medical Services in the war of 1914-1918: Special Problems and Services*, Vol 3, Australian War Memorial Canberra, 1943, pp.564, 719.

2. Narrative, Leila Smith, *Records of A.G. Butler: Official Historian of Australian Army Medical Services – Nurses' Narratives*, Australian War Memorial, Canberra, pp.1-2.

3. Mary Florence Stafford, *Military Forces of the Commonwealth Papers,* NAA, Canberra.

4. Mark Day, 'Gallant girls under fire' *The Weekend Australian* (Inquirer) 30-31 August 2008, p.29; Maffra History in consultation with Pauline Hitchens, including image from Family Records, Maffra Library, Gippsland, Victoria.

5. Hilda Mary Knox, *Military Forces of the Commonwealth Papers*, NAA, Canberra.

6. Leslie James Moorhouse, AWM Roll of Honour website: http://www.awm.gov.au/database/roh.asp [online 6 June 2005].

7. AIF Proceedings of a Court of Inquiry, Abbassia, 30 January 1917 into the disappearance of No 15220 Private R.C.D. Knox *Military Forces of the Commonwealth Papers,* NAA, Canberra.

8. Correspondence, Officer-in-Charge Base Records to Mr J.B. Knox, 14 June 1917 in private. R.C.D. Knox, *Military Forces of the Commonwealth Papers.*

9. Correspondence, Officer-in-Charge Base Records to Mr J. B. Knox, 24 May 1921 in private. R.C.D. Knox, *Military Forces of the Commonwealth Papers;* Commonwealth War Graves website: http://www.cwgc.org/.

10. Commonwealth War Graves website: http://www.cwgc.org/.

11. Greg Kirk, correspondence in 'Knox, Hilda Mary. Sister. Australian Army Nursing Service'. Greg Kirk to Ruth Rae, 2005 in *Ruth Rae Collection*, National Nursing Archives, Canberra.

12. May Tilton, *The Grey Battalion*, Angus and Robertson Limited, Sydney, 1933, pp.144-5.

13. Sarah Margaret White, 'A World War 1 nurse remembers …' 31 October 1973, *The Australian Women's Weekly*, 31 October 1973; Tilton, p.197; Elsie Rose Grant *Military Forces of the Commonwealth Papers.*

14. Correspondence, Agnes Cullen Jones cited in J. McQuilton, *Rural Australia and the Great War: From Tarrawingee to Tangambalanga,* Melbourne University Press, Melbourne, 2001, p.190.

15. Tilton, *The Grey Battalion*, p.221, 247.

16. Digger-Pioneer Index. Queensland 1829-1889.

17. AWM Roll of Honour: http://www.awm.gov.au/database/roh.asp [online 18 August 2006].

22 Second Australian General Hospital (2AGH) in Europe and England 1916-1918

1. Correspondence, Agnes Cullen Jones cited in J. McQuilton, *Rural Australia and the Great War: From Tarrawingee to Tangambalanga,* Melbourne University Press, Melbourne, 2001, pp.131-2.

2. Edith Ann Moorhouse, *Military Forces of the Commonwealth Papers*, NAA, Canberra.

3. Narrative, Leila Smith, *Records of A.G. Butler, Official Historian of Australian Army Medical Services – Nurses' Narratives*, AWM, Canberra, pp.2-3.

4. The author has positively identified more than 75 families who had at least two and occasionally three daughters who were members of the AANS, QAIMNSR or the NZANS; R.Rae, *First World War Commemorative Nominal Roll,* ACN Trilogy, Canberra, 2015.

5. Diary, Alice Ross-King, February 1919, AWM, Canberra. Alice Ross-King (AANS) recorded in her

diary '*Topsy Tyson has died of Spanish Flu'*. The diary entry is two months prior to the date of death of Fanny Isobel Catherine Tyson but it was written by Ross-King en route back to Australia on the *City Of York*, so while the dates and cause of death are both incorrect the inaccuracy may be due to the writer re-writing the diary at a later stage and/or inserting an incorrect date. Either way it is symptomatic of the limitations of primary sources as history. R. Rae 'The Limitations of Primary Sources as Historical Data', conference paper, Stories from the Field 2, University of Sydney, 27 September 2001; R. Rae 'Reading between the unwritten lines: Australian Army nurses in India, 1916 - 19', *Journal of the Australian War Memorial*, Canberra, May 2002.

6. NSW Federation Index-Pioneer Series 1889-1901 [online 8 August 2006].

7. R. Goodman, *Our War Nurses: The History of the Royal Australian Army Nursing Corps 1902-1988,* Boolarong Publications, Brisbane, 1988, p.46; Fanny Isobel Catherine Tyson *Military Forces of the Commonwealth Papers.*

8. Casualty Form in Fanny Isobel Catherine Tyson *Military Forces of the Commonwealth Papers*, NAA, Canberra.

9. Casualty Form in Theresa Adelaide Tyson, *Military Forces of the Commonwealth Papers*, NAA, Canberra.

10. M. Barker, *Nightingales in the Mud: the Digger Sisters of the Great War 1914-1918*, Allen and Unwin, Sydney, 1989, p.123.

11. Minnie Kate Porter, *Military Forces of the Commonwealth Papers*, NAA, Canberra.

12. Service and Casualty Form Part 2 (entry dated 10 December 1918) in Fanny Isobel Catherine Tyson *Military Forces of the Commonwealth Papers.*

13. Elsie Tranter diary, 1 January 1918, in G.M. Gillings and J. Richards (eds), *...in all those lines: The diary of Sister Elsie Tranter 1916-1919*, s/p.2008, p.87.

14. Attestation paper in Fanny Isobel Catherine Tyson, *Military Forces of the Commonwealth Papers.*

15. The official history recorded Fanny's death as 'cerebral' but her death certificate specifies 'cerebral haemorrhage'; death certificate and telegram (21 April 1919) from London headquarters to AIF, Australia in Fanny Isobel Catherine Tyson, *Military Forces of the Commonwealth Papers*; A.G. Butler, The *Official History of the Australian Army Medical Services in the war of 1914-1918: Special Problems and Services*, Vol 3, Australian War Memorial Canberra, 1943, p.588.

16. Fanny Isobel Catherine Tyson, *Military Forces of the Commonwealth Papers.*

23 Third Australian General Hospital (3AGH) in Europe and England 1916-1918

1. J. Bassett, *Guns and Brooches: Australian Army Nursing from the Boer War to the Gulf War*, Oxford University Press, Melbourne, 1992, p.58

2. Wilson diary cited in Bassett, *Guns and Brooches*, p.58.

3. Record, Central Army Records Office, Victoria Barracks, Melbourne (reviewed by author 25 February 2003).

4. Correspondence, Julia Dickinson to Officer-in-Charge (Base Records), 18 August 1920 in Ruby Dickinson, *Military Forces of the Commonwealth Papers*, NAA, Canberra. The attestation paper clearly states Julia Dickinson lived in Mosman, NSW, while the AIF burial order form states the address is Mosman, Queensland - Ruby Dickinson *Military Forces of the Commonwealth Papers.*

5. The ATNA entry for Ruby Dickinson claims she worked at Narrabri Hospital from September 1913 until 1916 but the evidence that she embarked for overseas duty in 1915 is beyond doubt - Ruby Dickinson, *Military Forces of the Commonwealth Papers*. The address given for the Ruby Dickinson who registered with ATNA was 39 Spit Road, Mosman, North Sydney, clearly differentiating her from

Ruby Droma Dickinson - ATNA Register, Australian Nursing Archives, Canberra, p.70.

6. J. McKenzie, *Bright Shadows: A History of Medical Services in Narrabri*, United Hospitals Auxiliary NSW Inc, Narrabri, 2001, pp.12, 14.

7. M. Barker, *Nightingales in the Mud: the Digger Sisters of the Great War 1914-1918*, Allen and Unwin, Sydney, 1989, p.164.

8. Correspondence, Jessie Tomlins to Margaretta Tomlins, 14 June 1919, copy in possession of author.

9. Ruby Dickinson, *Military Forces of the Commonwealth Papers.*

10. J. Bassett, 'Walker, Jean Nellie Miles (1878-1918)' *Australian Dictionary of Biography*, National Centre of Biography, Australian National University, Volume 12, Melbourne University Press, 1990, p.362.

11. A.G. Butler, The *Official History of the Australian Army Medical Services in the war of 1914-1918: Special Problems and Service*s, Vol 3, Australian War Memorial Canberra, 1943, p.576; Narrative, Leila Brown, *Records of A.G. Butler, Official Historian of Australian Army Medical Services - Nurses' Narratives*, AWM, Canberra.

12. Narrative, Sister E. H. Cuthbert, *Records of A. G. Butler: Official Historian of Australian Army Medical Services - Nurses' Narratives,* AWM 41, File 373.2, Canberra.

13. Anne Donnell, *Letters from an Australian Army Sister*, Angus and Robertson Ltd, Sydney, 1920, pp.14-18.

14. May Tilton, *The Grey Battalion*, Angus and Robertson Limited, Sydney, 1933, pp.207-8.

15. Narrative, Emma Cuthbert, *Records of A.G. Butler, Official Historian of Australian Army Medical Services - Nurses' Narratives.*

16. Donnell, *Letters from an Australian Army Sister*, pp.216, 225-6.

17. E. Russell, *War and Nature: Fighting Humans and Insects with Chemicals from World War 1 to Silent Spring,* Cambridge University Press, Cambridge, 2001, p.28.

18. Connant cited in Russell, *War and Nature*, p.43.

19. Daily Chronicle cited in P. Vansittart, *Voices from the Great War*, Pimlico, London, 1998, p.63.

20. Lord Moran cited in Vansittart, *Voices from the Great War*, pp.215-6.

21. Barbara F. Cape, *Baillière's Nurses' Dictionary,* Baillière, Tindall and Cox, London, 1956.

22. Narrative, Emma Cuthbert *Records of A.G. Butler, Official Historian of Australian Army Medical Services - Nurses' Narratives.*

23. McWhae cited in A.G. Butler, *The Official History of the Australian Army Medical Services in the war of 1914-1918: The Western Front*, Vol 2, Australian War Memorial, Canberra, 1940, pp.463-4.

24. War Office Committee, Inquiry into Shell-Shock cited in Butler, *Special Problems and Services*, p.125.

25. Donnell, *Letters from an Australian Army Sister*, p.249.

26. Manifold in Butler, *Special Problems and Services*, p.112.

27. L. Gameson cited in L. Macdonald, *The Roses of No Man's Land,* Penguin Books Ltd, London, 1980, pp.216-7.

28. J. Cohen cited in Bill Gammage, *The Broken Years: Australian Soldiers in the Great War,* Penguin Books Australia Ltd, Sydney, 1974, pp.164-5.

29. H. Deardon cited in Macdonald, *The Roses of No Man's Land,* p.222.

30. H. Strachan, *The First World War: A new illustrated history*, Simon & Schuster, London, 2003, p.243 (photograph and caption).

31. Butler, *Special Problems and Services*, pp.74, 576.

32. Narrative, A.M. Kellett, *Records of A. G. Butler: Official Historian of Australian Army Medical Services – Nurses' Narratives.*

33. Butler, *The Western Front*, p.404.

34. Barker, *Nightingales in the Mud*, pp.162-3, 782.

35. Kate Porter, *Military Forces of the Commonwealth Papers,* NAA, Canberra; Minnie Kate Porter, *Military Forces of the Commonwealth Papers,* NAA, Canberra; A. McAndrew, *Milton-Ulladulla in the Wars*, s/p (ISB 0 9596744 6 2), Sydney, 1994, p.109.

36. C.E.W. Bean, *Anzac to Amiens* (5th ed), Australian War Memorial, Canberra, 1968, pp.398-400, 408-9.

37. Miles Walker cited in Barker, *Nightingales in the Mud*, p.140.

38. Evelyn Davies cited in Barker, *Nightingales in the Mud*, p.115.

39. Bassett, *Guns and Brooches*, p.58.

40. 'Report on Nursing Staff, April 1918' by Principal Matron Grace Wilson, Third Australian General Hospital, *Records of A.G. Butler, Official Historian of Australian Army Medical Services,* Australian War Memorial, Canberra.

41. James McPherson, *Battle Cry of Freedom*, Oxford University Press, New York, 1988, p.619.

42. Correspondence, Florence Nightingale to Mary Clarke, 20 August 1853 cited in Cecil Woodham-Smith *Florence Nightingale 1820-1910*, London, 1950, p.86; R. Rae 'Reading between unwritten lines: Australian Army Nurses in India 1916-19' Journal of the Australian War Memorial, Canberra.

43. Narrative, L.E. Young, *Records of A.G. Butler, Official Historian of Australian Army Medical Services – Nurses' Narratives.*

44. Correspondence, Sister Selwyn-Smith cited in R. Goodman, *Queensland Nurses: Boer War to Vietnam*, Boolarong Publications, Brisbane, 1985, p.44.

45. Bassett, *Guns and Brooches*, p.69.

46.Narrative, A. Maud Kellett, *Records of A.G. Butler, Officil Historian of Australian Army Medical Services – Nurses' Narratives.*

47. Butler, *Special Problems and Services*, p.577.

48. Donnell, *Letters from an Australian Army Sister*, p.249.

49. Casualty Form in Ruby Dickinson, *Military Forces of the Commonwealth Papers*, Service Record, NAA, Canberra.

50. Clinical chart in Ruby Dickinson *Military Forces of the Commonwealth Papers.*

51. Burial report in Ruby Dickinson *Military Forces of the Commonwealth Papers.*

52. Correspondence, Julia Dickinson to Major McLean (AIF), 3 December 1918 in Ruby Dickinson, *Military Forces of the Commonwealth Papers.*

53. Correspondence, Officer-in-Charge Base Records to Mr Sydney Rushbrook Dickinson (brother to Ruby Droma Dickinson) in Ruby Dickinson, *Military Forces of the Commonwealth Papers.*

54. There are a number of discrepancies in the spelling of the surname for both nurses but both signed their surname 'Dickinson' not 'Dickenson'; Ruby Droma Dickinson, *Military Forces of the Commonwealth Papers*; Ruby Dickinson, *Military Forces of the Commonwealth Papers.*

24 2 ACCS and a Night of Valour on 22 July 1917

1. Elizabeth Whiteside in Department of Veterans' Affairs, *Simply Hell let Loose: Stories of Australians at war*, ABC Books, Sydney, 2002, p.61.

2. A.G. Butler, *The Official History of the Australian Army Medical Services in the war of 1914-1918 The Western Front*, vol 2, Australian War Memorial, Canberra, p.72.

3. A.Maud Kellett interview (no.58) Kate Laity, AWM, Canberra, 1919; M. Barker, *Nightingales in the Mud: the Digger Sisters of the Great War 1914-1918*, Allen and Unwin, Sydney, 1989, p.165.

4. A.G. Butler, *The Official History of the Australian Army Medical Services in the war of 1914-1918: Special Problems and Services*, Vol 3, Australian War Memorial Canberra, 1943, pp.133-4 (*n*).

5. Barbara F. Cape, *Baillière's Nurses' Dictionary*, Baillière, Tindall and Cox, London, 1956, p.209.

6. Narrative, Mary Dwyer, *Records of A.G. Butler, Official Historian of Australian Army Medical Services - Nurses' Narratives,* AWM, Canberra.

7. Anne Donnell, *Letters from an Australian Army Sister,* Angus and Robertson Ltd, Sydney, 1920, p.253.

8. May Tilton, *The Grey Battalion,* Angus and Robertson Limited, Sydney, 1933.

9. Narrative, Mary Dwyer, *Records of A.G. Butler, Official Historian of Australian Army Medical Services - Nurses' Narratives.*

10. Narrative, Edith E. Simpson, *Records of A.G. Butler, Official Historian of Australian Army Medical Services - Nurses' Narratives.*

11. Barker, *Nightingales in the Mud,* p.113.

12.Butler, *The Western Front,* p.355.

13. Dinning cited in Barker, *Nightingales in the Mud,* p.126.

14. Butler, *Special Problems and Services*, p.558 (*n*).

15.Jacqualine Abbott, 'Davidson, Ethel Sarah (1872-1939)', *Australian Dictionary of Biography,* National Centre of Biography, Australian National University, http://adb.anu.edu.au/biography/davidson-ethel-sarah-5898/text10043,published first in hardcopy1981,accessed online 31 October 2025.

16. Narrative, E.S. Davidson, *Records of A.G. Butler, Official Historian of Australian Army Medical Services - Nurses' Narratives.*

17. Matron E.S. Davidson, *Commonwealth Military Papers,* NAA, Canberra; Barker, *Nightingales in the Mud,* 165.

18. Narrative, E.S. Davidson, *Records of A.G. Butler, Official Historian of Australian Army Medical Services - Nurses' Narratives*; Jacqualine Abbott, 'Davidson, Ethel Sarah (1872-1939)', Australian Dictionary of Biography Note: the ADB entry and the AWM Access Number 41957 have a number of inconsistencies. The author has used the narratives or writings of Ethel Davidson wherever possible.

19. Butler, *The Western Front,* pp.187-8,364,382-7.

20. Barrett J. Carr 'Deacon, Clare (1891- 1952)', *Australian Dictionary of Biography,* National Centre of Biography, Australian National University, Volume 8, Melbourne University Press, Melbourne, 1981, pp.39-41; Jacqueline Abbott 'Cawood, Dorothy Gwendolen (1884 - 1962)', *Australian Dictionary of Biography,* National Centre of Biography, Australian National University, Volume 7, Melbourne University Press, Melbourne, 1979, p.594. Note: Discrepancies between ADB and AWM as she was not sick for all of 1918 and the AWM nominal roll claims she was awarded the MM and ARRC but she received the MM and was MID; Lorna M. Finnie 'Ross-King, Alice (1891 - 1968)', *Australian Dictionary of Biography,* National Centre of Biography, Australian National University, Volume 11, Melbourne University Press, 1988, pp.459-460. Alice Ross King, personal diary, AWM, Canberra; Lt Col. J. Ramsay Webb in Appendix to 2 ACCS Unit Diary, AWM, Canberra; *Commonwealth Military Papers,* NAA, Canberra for Mary Jane Derrer, Dorothy Cawood, Alice Ross-King, Clare Deacon.

21. Lorna M. Finnie 'Ross-King, Alice (1891–1968)', *Australian Dictionary of Biography*, pp.459-460. Alice Ross King, personal diary, AWM, Canberra.

22. Jacqueline Abbott 'Cawood, Dorothy Gwendolen (1884 - 1962)', *Australian Dictionary of Biography*, p.594.

23.Barrett J. Carr 'Deacon, Clare (1891 - 1952)', *Australian Dictionary of Biography*, pp.39-41.

24. Mary Jane Derrer, *Commonwealth Military Records.*

25. M. Collins, & L. George, 'An Alphabetical Listing of Nurses who went overseas with the AIF in World War 1 1914-1918' (unpublished), Australian War Memorial, Canberra,1995. Mervyn Collins and Leanne George were volunteers with the Australian War Memorial. They cross-referenced to the Embarkation Nominal Roll by using a four figure number identifying the embarkation microfiche. There are two embarkation numbers next to the entry for M.J. Derrer, with the assumption being made that the first relates to the first enlistment; R.Rae, *First World War Commemorative Nominal Roll,* ACN Trilogy, Canberra, 2015.

26. Captain F.H. Wickham cited in R. Goodman, *Our War Nurses – The History of the Royal Australian Army Nursing Corps,* Boolarong Publications, Brisbane, 1988, p.70; J. Bassett, *Guns and Brooches: Australian Army Nursing from the Boer War to the Gulf War*, Oxford University Press, Melbourne, 1992, pp.81-2.

27. L.A. Deacon, *Beyond the Call,* Regal Press, Hobart, n/d, pp.42-4.

25 The Valour Continues at CCS

1. Taprell Dorling in assoc. with F. Guille, *Ribbons and Medals*, George Phillip and Son Ltd., London, 1960, pp.40-1, 49.

2. M. Lincoln, 'Pratt, Rachel (1874–1954)', *Australian Dictionary of Biography*, National Centre of Biography, Australian National University, Volume 11, Melbourne University Press, Melbourne, 1988, pp.276-7.

3. R. Pratt, 'Nursing at Lemnos, August - December 1915', *Reveille,* issue 12, vol 6, 1933.

4. Lincoln, 'Pratt, Rachel (1874 - 1954)', *Australian Dictionary of Biography*, pp.276-7.

5. M. Tilton, *The Grey Battalion,* Angus and Robertson Ltd, Sydney, 1933, p.240; J. Bassett, *Guns and Brooches: Australian Army Nursing from the Boer War to the Gulf War,* Oxford University Press, Melbourne, 1992, p.65 - Bassett incorrectly refers to Alicia Mary Kelly as Rachel Kelly but there is little doubt her biographical details relate to Alicia Mary Kelly.

6. L.A. Deacon, *Beyond the Call,* Regal Press, Hobart, n/d, pp.46-7.

7. Correspondence, Pearl Corkhill, 29 July 1918 cited in Deacon, *Beyond the Call,* p.46.

8. Australian War Memorial Collections [REL/17126], AWM, Canberra.

9. Richard E. Reid, 'Corkhill, Elizabeth Pearl (1887-1985)', *Australian Dictionary of Biography,* National Centre of Biography, Australian National University, http://adb.anu.edu.au/biography/corkhill-elizabeth-pearl-12358/text22203published first in hardcopy 2007,accessed online 31 October2025; Photograph AWM AO4728.

10. AWM Honours and Awards: http://www.awm.gov.au/database/; R. Goodman, *Our War Nurses – The History of the Royal Australian Army Nursing Corps,* Boolarong Publications, Brisbane, 1988, p.67.

11. R. Goodman, *Queensland Nurses: Boer War to Vietnam,* Boolarong Publications, Brisbane, 1985, p.117.

12. Goodman, *Our War Nurses,* p.67.

13. Nurses' Memorial Foundation of South Australia Incorporated, *Nursing –150 years of Caring in*

South Australia, The South Australian Trained Nurses' Centenary Committee, Adelaide, 1938 (Reprinted with 1939-1945 supplement in 1989), p.116.

14. Peter James. 'A thoroughly Cordial relationship. A Narrative Account of the French Flag Nursing Corp 1914-1919' in The Bulletin of the UK Association of the History of Nursing, vol.6, Nov. 2017, pp.17-24; Personal details of Louise Dorrington in *Nursing –150 years of Caring in South Australia*, The South Australian Trained Nurses' Centenary Committee, p.116.

15. Maud Morrison, *Military Forces of the Commonwealth Papers*, NAA, Canberra.

16. Christina Morrison, *Military Forces of the Commonwealth Papers*, NAA, Canberra.

17. Newspaper article, *The West Australian*, 11 December 1918, p.7 (copy at Mitchell Library, State Library of NSW, Sydney); email correspondence, Selena Williams to Ruth Rae, 20 January 2008 in *Ruth Rae Collection*, National Nursing Archives, Canberra. The author gratefully acknowledges Selena Williams for bringing this research to my attention.

18. J. Durdin, *Eleven Thousand Nurses – A History of Nurse Education at the Royal Adelaide Hospital 1889-1993*, Royal Adelaide Hospital, 1999.

26 Nursing the Australian Light Horsemen in Egypt 1916-1919

1. C. Clifford, *The Asquiths*, John Murray (Publishers), London, 2002, p.145(*n*).

2. J.A. Williams & R.D. Goodman, *Jane Bell, O.B.E. (1873-1959): Lady Superintendent, The Royal Melbourne Hospital (1910-1934),* Royal Melbourne Graduate Nurses' Association, Melbourne, 1988, pp.26-31.

3. R. Goodman, *Queensland Nurses: Boer War to Vietnam*, Boolarong Publications, Brisbane, 1985, p.55; Bassett, p.53.

4. J. Bassett, *Guns and Brooches: Australian Army Nursing from the Boer War to the Gulf War*, Oxford University Press, Melbourne, 1992, p.53.

5. A.G. Butler, *The Official History of the Australian Army Medical Services in the war of 1914-1918 Gallipoli, Palestine and New Guinea*, Vol 1, (2nd ed.), Australian War Memorial, Melbourne, 1938,p. 550; Bassett, *Guns and Brooches*, pp.26, 54.

6. A. Rogers, *While You're Away: New Zealand nurses at war 1899-1948,* Auckland University Press, 2003, pp.180-1.

7. Diary, O. Haynes, 23 January 1916 cited in M. Young (ed), *We Are Here Too – Letters and Diaries of Sister Olive Haynes No. 2 AGH November 1914 to February,* 1918, Australian Down Syndrome Assoc Inc, Adelaide, 1991, p.115.

8. Conyers cited in P. Adam-Smith, *Australian Women at War*, Penguin Books Australia Ltd., Melbourne, 1996, p.25.

9. Diary, Alice Kitchen cited in M. Barker, *Nightingales in the Mud: the Digger Sisters of the Great War 1914-1918,* Allen and Unwin, Sydney, 1989, p.32; C.E.W. Bean, *Anzac to Amiens* (5th ed), Australian War Memorial, Canberra, 1968, pp.145-9.

10. Diary, 28 December 1915, Alice Kitchen cited in P. Adam-Smith, *The ANZACs*, Penguin Books Australia Ltd, Melbourne, 1991, p.202.

11. Bassett, *Guns and Brooches,* pp.34, 53-4..

12. M. Barker, *Nightingales in the Mud: the Digger Sisters of the Great War 1914-1918,* Allen and Unwin, Sydney, 1989, pp. 21-2, 35-7. Specifically, Sister Pocock was pleased Gould was 'passed over'. Sister Pocock had served with Gould in the Boer War and was Acting Matron of 2 AGH for a short period. Pocock seemed to have staff problems throughout the war with some AANS refusing to work with her.

13. C.E.W. Bean, *Official History of Australia in the War of 1914-1918 – The Story of ANZAC: The First*

Phase, Vol 2, Angus and Robertson Ltd., Sydney, 1935, p.774.

14.P.A. Pedersen *Monash: As Military Commander*, Melbourne University Press, Melbourne, 1985, p.302.

15. B.H. Liddell Hart, *History of the First World War*, Cassell and Co Ltd, London, 1970, pp.432, 435.

16. H.S. Gullett, *Official History of Australia in the War of 1914-18: Sinai and Palestine* (12th ed), vol 7, Angus and Robertson Ltd, Sydney, 1944, p.61.

17. A.J. Hill, 'Chauvel, Sir Henry George (Harry) (1865 – 1945)', *Australian Dictionary of Biography*, National Centre of Biography, Australian National University, Volume 7, Melbourne University Press, Melbourne, 1979.

18. R. Goodman, *Our War Nurses – The History of the Royal Australian Army Nursing Corps*, Boolarong Publications, Brisbane, 1988, p.97.

19. 'The Lady Superintendent Reports No.1 (Miss Jane Bell)', Royal Melbourne Hospital archives, The Royal Melbourne Hospital, Melbourne (reviewed by author February 2003).

20. Gullett, *Sinai and Palestine*, p.62.

21. Frederick Watson, *The History of the Sydney Hospital from 1811 to 1911*, Government Printer, Sydney, 1911, p.202.

22. Australasian Trained Nurses' Association (founded 1899) 'Register of Members 1916', Websdale, Shoosmith Ltd, Sydney, National Nursing Archives, Canberra.

23. Ruth Rae, *Rose Creal: The biography of an Australian nurse leader (1865-1921)*, amazon.com, 2023.

24. Liddell Hart, *History of the First World War*, p.64.

25. Goodman, *Our War Nurses*, p.86.

26. Postcard, Lowrey (AANS) to Campbell (AANS) in Rae, *Rose Creal: The biography of an Australian nurse leader (1865-1921)*, p.76.

27. Rose Creal, *Military Forces of the Commonwealth Papers*, National Archives of Australia, Canberra.

28. Matron Rose Creal 'No. 14 AGH Unit Diary, Report of Nursing Services from 23 September 1916 to 30 September 1917, Egypt', Australian War Memorial, Canberra.

29. S. Pope, *Dictionary of Napoleonic Wars*, Cassell, London, 1999, p.20.

30. Creal 'No. 14 AGH Unit Diary'; Watson, p.178. (See AWM *Photograph 12* for a view of the operating theatre).

31. Creal 'No 14 AGH Unit Diary'.

32. Goodman, *Our War Nurse*, p.86; Correspondence, Jessie Tomlins to Margaretta Tomlins, 18.1.16 [sic]. The date of the letter is incorrect and should read 18.12.16. The letter was sent from Kandy, Ceylon and postcards dated 28.12.16 were also sent from Colombo and letters dated January 1917 were sent from Egypt, copies in possession of author.

33. A.Maud Kellett interview, (no. 119) Jessie Tomlins, AWM, Canberra, 1919; Correspondence, Jessie Tomlins to 'My Dear People', 14 January 1917, copy in possession of author.

34. Ruth Rae, *The biography of an Australian First World War army nurse: Jessie Tomlins*, amazon.com, 2025.

35. Bassett, *Guns and Brooches*, p.83.

36. Gullett, *Sinai and Palestine*, pp. 135, 190.

37. J. Horsfield, *Rainbow: The story of Rania Macphillamy*, Ginninderra Press, Canberra, 2007, pp.69-70.

38. Gullett, *Sinai and Palestine*, p.173.

39. Bean, *Anzac to Amiens*, p.282.

40. Gullett, *Sinai and Palestine,* p.333.

41. Rae, *Jessie Tomlins Biography*, pp120-1.

42. Y. McEwen, *"It's a Long Way to Tipperary": British and Irish nurses in the Great War*, Cualann Press, Dunfermline, 2006, p.72. Photograph of Kathleen Adele Brennan in VAD ward uniform (PO5074.002), AWM, Canberra.

43. Correspondence, Medical Advisor (London) to Base Officer (Melbourne), 3 January 1922 in William Keating Brennan, *Military Forces of the Commonwealth Papers*, NAA, Canberra.

44. Kathleen Adele Brennan (VAD), *Military Forces of the Commonwealth Papers* [online 21 February 2007].

45. William Keating Brennan, *Military Forces of the Commonwealth Papers.*

46. Gullett, *Sinai and Palestine,* pp.246, 342.

47.H. Strachan, *The First World War: A new illustrated history*, Simon & Schuster, London, 2003, p.275.

48. Liddell Hart, *History of the First World War*, p.432.

49. Rae, *Fred Tomlins Biography*; Rae, *Jessie Tomlins Biography.*

50. Photograph AWM PO 8401.015.

51. The average available pubic hospital beds for NSW (30 June 2005) was 21,808 - NSW Health Annual Report 2004/5, NSW Health Department, 2005.

52. Barker, *Nightingales in the Mud,* p.63.

53. Bassett, *Guns and Brooches*, p.83.

54. Gullett, *Sinai and Palestine*, pp.697-8.

55. AWM Commemorative Roll http://www.awm.gov.au/database/croll.asp [online 19 February 2007].

56. H.V. Morton, *In the Step.of the Master*, Methuen & Co. Ltd, London, 1937, p.323. This cemetery is now referred to as the 'Jerusalem War Cemetery, Israel's Commonwealth War Graves Commission http://www.cwgc.org/search/ [online 21 February 2007].

57. Cited in Goodman, *Queensland Nurses,* p.115.

58. Gullett, *Sinai and Palestine,* p.379.

59. Correspondence from Base Records Office, AIF (including extract from Second Supplement No. 31093, to the *London Gazette* dated 1st January 1919 AIF) to Miss E.F. Creal, C/o Miss Turpey, Anson Street, Orange in Rose Creal Service Record, *Military Forces of the Commonwealth Papers.*

27 Australian Nurses on the British Salonika Front 1917-1919

1.Alan Wakefield and Simon Moody, *Under the devil's eye: Britain's forgotten army at Salonika 1915-1918*, 2004 in The Salonika front, 1915-1918, URL: https://nzhistory.govt.nz/media/photo/salonika-front-19151918, (Manatū Taonga — Ministry for Culture and Heritage), update 30-Jul-2014.

2. R. Goodman, *Our War Nurses: The History of the Royal Australian Army Nursing Corps 1902-1988,* Boolarong Publications, Brisbane, 1988, pp.88-90.

3. Perditta M. McCarthy, 'White, Jessie McHardy (1870-1957), Australian Dictionary of Biography, National Centre of Biography, Australian National University, first published in hardcopy 1990, vol 12, Melbourne University Press. Note: The correct spelling of the nurse leader who was Jessie McHardy White has created much confusion, even in the official records. The author has adopted the spelling of McHardy in line with the ADB entry and research. This is despite her service record, written in own hand and signed by her, on occasions, is written McHardie. The ADB entry was informed by the written name on her birth certificate and the maiden name of her mother being

recorded as McHardy as per ADB research. Emails: Stephen Wilks, Acting Managing Editor, ADB, Canberra, 3-8 September 2025; Jessie McHardy-White, *Military Forces of the Commonwealth Papers*, NAA, Canberra.
4. Ethelda Uren photograph AWM P10964.001 and Map H 1576, AWM, Canberra.
5. A.G. Butler, The *Official History of the Australian Army Medical Services in the war of 1914-1918: Special Problems and Service*s, Vol 3, Australian War Memorial Canberra, 1943, p.569; Goodman, *Our War Nurses*, p.90.

6. Narrative L.M. Appleton, *Records of A.G Butler, Official Historian of Australian Army Medical Services - Nurses' Narratives.*

7.A.Maud Kellett interview (no.52), Sister E.D. Jackson, AWM, Canberra, 1919; A. Maud Kellett interview, S. Arnold, AWM, Canberra, 1919; The Medal Hound Website, maintained by Keith Emroll, 5 Sept 2025.

8. Gladys Leila Walter, *Military Forces of the Commonwealth Papers*, NAA, Canberra.

9. The use of nicknames within the AANS was not unusual during the war.

10. A. Hyslop, *Sovereign Remedies: A History of Ballarat Base Hospital 1850s to 1980s*, Allen and Unwin Australia Pty Ltd, Sydney, 1989, p.214.

11. Narrative, Alma Bennett, *Records of A.G Butler, Official Historian of Australian Army Medical Services - Nurses' Narratives.*

12. Gertrude Edith Munro, *Military Forces of the Commonwealth Papers*, NAA, Canberra.

13. Nurses' Registrar, Weekly Times. 26 October 1918 cited in Hyslop, *Sovereign Remedies,* p.214.

14. R. Reid, *Just Wanted to be there – Australian Service Nurses 1899-1999*, Department of Veteran Affairs, Commonwealth of Australia, 1999, p.43.

15. Gertrude Edith Munro, *Military Forces of the Commonwealth Papers.*

16. The AWM Roll of Honour lists her date of death as 10 September 1918 but there is little doubt it was 10 October 1918 in view of the detailed account in her service record which also agrees with the AWM Nominal Roll date: Gertrude Edith Munro *Military Forces of the Commonwealth Papers*; AWM Roll of Honour: http://www.awm.gov.au/database/roh.asp [online 18 August 2006]; AWM Nominal Roll: http://www.awm.gov.au/database/ [online 18 August 2006]; J. Bassett *Guns and Brooches: Australian Army Nursing from the Boer War to the Gulf War*, Oxford University Press, Melbourne, 1992, p.88; Butler, *Special Problems and Service*s, p.588.

16. A.Maud Kellett interview, G. Walter, AWM, Canberra. Note: This interview includes an accompanying letter.

17. Gladys Walter, *Military Forces of the Commonwealth Papers.*

18. A.Maud Kellett interview, G. Walter.

19. Evelyn Grace Ione Nowland, Casualty Form in *Military Forces of the Commonwealth Papers*, NAA, Canberra.

20. Goodman, *Our War Nurses,*p.95; A.M. Kellett interview (no.52), E.D. Jackson, AWM, Canberra; Butler, *Special Problems and Services,* p.588. Note: The number of nurses who were invalided home varies from source to source owing to the absence of reliable statistics. Sister Jackson claims '*75 being boarded for Australia*' but Goodman cites DGMS Howse who claimed 62 were returned to Australia.

21. Elizabeth Rothery, *Military Forces of the Commonwealth Papers*, NAA, Canberra. Note: Elizabeth Rothery joined the AIF on 22 August 1916 and RTA on 20 July 1917 but this does not include her subsequent tours of transport duty; AWM Nominal Roll: http://www.awm.gov.au/database/133/index.asp [online 17 May 2005].

22. B. Rayner, 'Nurse Elizabeth Rothery' in Myrtleford Mail, n/d. The author gratefully acknowledges Eric Barton, Myrtleford and District Historical Society, who provided background information on Elizabeth Rothery. Correspondence, 29 March 2005 in *Ruth Rae Collection,* National Nursing Archives,

Canberra; J McQuilton *Rural Australia and the Great War: From Tarrawingee to Tangambalanga*, Melbourne University Press, Melbourne, 2001, pp.132-3.

23. May Hennessy, *Military Forces of the Commonwealth Papers*, NAA, Canberra.

24. *Mooltan* was built in 1905, P&O, and was torpedoed in the Mediterranean Sea with loss of one life. The vessel was replaced with a ship of the same name; *Encyclopedia of Australian Shipwrecks* at http://oceans1.customer.netspace.net.au/war-wrecks.html [online 8 August 2006].

25. May Hennessy, Casualty form (31 March 1919), *Military Forces of the Commonwealth Papers*.

26. Urgent telegram from S.M.O. Scott, *Novgorod*, to Melbourne based Matron-in-Chief, AANS, 30 March 1919 in May Hennessy *Military Forces of the Commonwealth Papers*.

27. Urgent telegram from S.M.O. Scott, *Novgorod*, to Melbourne based Matron-in-Chief, AANS, 30 March 1919 in May Hennessy *Military Forces of the Commonwealth Papers*; 'Deaths - Hennessy' *Bendigoman*, 11 April 1919; 'Death of Sister Hennessy', *Bendigo Advertiser*, 11 April 1919. Note: Her brother was also in Geelong when she died and she had recently been visited by her cousin, Captain Rentoul, who was a chaplain.

28. 'Late Sister Hennessy' *Bendigo Advertiser*, 12 April 1919; 'Notice' *Bendigo Advertiser*, 11 April 1919.

29. 'Late Sister Hennessy' *Bendigoman*, Thursday 17 April 1919. Correspondence, David Cotton (Research Officer, Australian Institute of Genealogical Studies Inc, Bendigo Area) to Ruth Rae, 19 January 2005 in *Ruth Rae Collection*, National Nursing Archives, Canberra.

30. *Bendigo Advertiser* (untitled) 14 April 1919.

31. 'Late Sister Hennessy' *The Bendigo Advertiser*, 12 April 1919, p.2; 'Late Sister Hennessy' *Bendigoman*, 17 April 1919, p.5.

32. 'Late Sister Hennessy' *Bendigoman*, 17 April 1919, p.5.

33. Leonard Carter, 'letter to the editor', *The Bendigo Advertiser*, 17 April 1919.

28 India and Mesopotamia

1. B. Jones, *Dictionary of World Biography*, Information Australia, Melbourne, 1994, p.752; S. Pope & E. A. Wheal, *Dictionary of the First World War*, Macmillan Reference Books, London, 1995, p.236.

2. E. Denison Ross, 'Gertrude Bell' in *The Post Victorians* (n/ed), Ivor Nicholson & Watson, Ltd., London, 1933, pp.62-66.

3. C. Woodham-Smith, *Florence Nightingale 1820-1910*, Constable and Company Ltd , London, 1950, pp.260-1, 321; B.H. Liddell Hart, *History of the First World War*, Cassell and Co Ltd, London, 1970, p.154.

4. Woodham-Smith, *Florence Nightingale 1820-1910*, pp.260-1.

5. R. Goodman, *Our War Nurses: The History of the Royal Australian Army Nursing Corps 1902-1988*, p.70.

6. Pope and Wheal, *Dictionary of the First World War*, pp.315 & 559.

7.Liddell Hart, *History of the First World War*, pp.154-5.

8. Pope and Wheal, *Dictionary of the First World War*, p.317.

9. Correspondence, L.G. Moreton, 8 August 1916, AANS, Indian Medical Service, Quetta, India in Typed Extracts of Correspondence at *AWM File No. 12/11/1398 – 2 DRL 97*, Australian War Memorial, Canberra, p.8.

10. R.Rae, *First World War Commemorative Nominal Roll*, ACN Trilogy, Canberra, 2015.

11. AWM 224, unit history manuscripts, MS 610, 52/5, F.H. Wickham, 'Report on AANS and AAMC

in India' cited in Bassett, p.76.

12. Australian Archives, Victoria, MP 367, Department of Defence correspondence files, 527/1/122, section 7, pp.7-8 cited in J. Bassett, *Guns and Brooches: Australian Army Nursing from the Boer War to the Gulf War*, Oxford University Press, Melbourne, 1992, p.75; E.K. Burke, *With Horse and Morse in Mesopotamia,* Arthur McQuilty, Sydney, 1927, pp.198-200. Note: The personnel list in Burke contains the names of more than 500 AANS nurses who nursed in India as part or all of their overseas service.

13. Correspondence, L.G. Moreton, 8 August 1916, AANS, Indian Medical Service, Quetta, India in Typed Extracts of Correspondence at *AWM File No. 12/11/1398 – 2 DRL 97*, Australian War Memorial, Canberra, p.8.

14. Burke, *With Horse and Morse in Mesopotamia,* pp.124-5; A.G. Butler, The *Official History of the Australian Army Medical Services in the war of 1914-1918: Special Problems and Service*s, Vol 3, Australian War Memorial Canberra, 1943, p.570.

15. Liddell Hart, *History of the First World War*, p.155.

16. Goodman, *Our War Nurses*, pp.70-1; Burke, *With Horse and Morse in Mesopotamia,* p.124; Butler, *Special Problems and Services*, p.567; Narrative, Principal Matron G.E. Davis, *Records of A.G. Butler, Official Historian of Australian Army Medical Services – Nurses' Narratives*, p.1; *Bio: Emily Hoadley,* Served in the Boer War (NSWANSR) and had offered her services in the Russo-Japanese war (1905) even though Australia was not involved. She may have been Matron at Burrangong District Hospital near Young 1894-1900 and 1902-1904. The break in tenure is in line with the date of her Boer War service. *'Matron Hoadley was at Parkes Hospital in 1910'* – electronic correspondence, Evonne Hutton (Parkes Family History Society) to Ruth Rae, 7 March 2002 in *Ruth Rae Collection,* National Nursing Archives, Canberra. The author gratefully acknowledges Evonne Hutton. During the First World War she was attached to 2 MD, DOE: 5 May 1915 & RTA:not recorded. Senior Sister 3 AGH; highest rank was matron of Trimulgherry Hospital (500 patients) in Secunderabad, Hyderabad, India – Bassett *Guns and Brooches*, 1992, pp. 27, 29-30, 74; Sheila M. Gray, *The South African War 1899-1902: Service Record of British and Colonial Women – A record of the Service in South Africa of Military and Civilian Nurses, Laywomen and Civilians,* s/p.Auckland, 1993, p.70; M. Barker, *Nightingales in the Mud: the Digger Sisters of the Great War 1914-1918*, Allen and Unwin, Sydney, 1989, p.79.

17. 'AIF attestation paper of persons enlisted for service abroad' in Kathleen Power, *Military Forces of the Commonwealth Papers,* NAA, Canberra.

18. Amy Veda O'Grady, *Military Forces of the Commonwealth Papers*, Service Record, NAA, Canberra.

19. Marist Melbourne Province - http://www.maristmelb.org.au/ [online 16 September 2006].

20. Amy Veda O'Grady *Military Forces of the Commonwealth Papers;* Electronic correspondence, Gabriele Haveaux (archivist Royal Melbourne Hospital) to Ruth Rae, 7 March 2006 in *Ruth Rae Collection*, National Nursing Archives, Canberra. The author gratefully acknowledges Gabriele Haveaux.

21. Amy Veda O'Grady *Military Forces of the Commonwealth Papers.*

22. Amy Veda O'Grady, *Military Forces of the Commonwealth Papers*. Question 11 of the AANS enrolment form reads in full *'What is your experience in the execution of medical orders?'* and while it was essential that an AANS nurse be registered with either ATNA or RVTNA, a number of nurses had many years of hospital nursing experience before being in a financial or social position to commence their formal training period. Miss Rose Creal, Matron of Sydney Hospital and 14 AGH in Egypt is a case in point.

23. Woodham-Smith, *Florence Nightingale 1820-1910*, p.320.

24. Barker, *Nightingales in the Mud*, p.76; Narrative, Eileen A. Burke, *Records of A.G. Butler, Official Historian of Australian Army Medical Services – Nurses' Narratives*, p.1.

25. Barker, *Nightingales in the Mud*, p.76; Narrative, Eileen A. Burke, *Records of A.G. Butler, Official Historian of Australian Army Medical Services – Nurses' Narratives*, p.1: *Bio: Eileen A. Burke*, Sister AANS, DOE: 26 Dec 1916 (Melbourne) & RTA: 28 August 1919. Served in a number of locations in India

where she contracted malaria; transport duty between Bombay and Basra; transport duty to Egypt; 31 BGH, Abbassia, Egypt; 1 AGH, Sutton Veny, England.

26. Kathleen Power, *Military Forces of the Commonwealth Papers*; Narrative, Principal Matron G.E. Davis, *Records of A.G. Butler, Official Historian of Australian Army Medical Services - Nurses' Narratives*,p.1; Butler, *Special Problems and Services*, p.588.

27. Narrative, Eileen A. Burke, *Records of A.G. Butler, Official Historian of Australian Army Medical Services - Nurses' Narratives.*

28. A. Donnell, *Letters of An Australian Army Sister*, Angus and Robertson Ltd, Sydney, 1920, p.106.

29. May Tilton, *The Grey Battalion*, Angus and Robertson Limited, Sydney, 1933, p.111.

30. P. Adam-Smith, *Australian Women at War*, Penguin Books Australia Ltd., Melbourne, 1996, p.65.

31. Correspondence to Rev. Father O'Grady in Amy Veda O'Grady, *Military Forces of the Commonwealth Papers.*

32. Kathleen Power, *Military Forces of the Commonwealth Papers.*

33. Burke, *With Horse and Morse in Mesopotamia,* p.127.

34. Pamela Woods, *Dirt: Filth and Decay in a New World Arcadia*, Auckland University Press, Auckland, 2005, pp.216-7.

35. Casualty Form in Kathleen Power, *Military Forces of the Commonwealth Papers.*

36. Correspondence, Michael Power, 12 December 1922 in Kathleen Power, *Military Forces of the Commonwealth Papers.*

37. Amy Veda O'Grady in *Military Forces of the Commonwealth Papers.*

38. Narrative, Principal Matron G.E. Davis, *Records of A.G. Butler, Official Historian of Australian Army Medical Services - Nurses' Narratives.*

39. AWM Embarkation Roll: http://www.awm.gov.au/cms_images/[online 14 March 2006].

40. Burke, *With Horse and Morse in Mesopotamia,* p.125.

41. Narrative, Principal Matron G.E. Davis, *Records of A.G. Butler, Official Historian of Australian Army Medical Services - Nurses' Narratives,* p.2.

42. Bassett, *Guns and Brooches,* pp.77-8.

43.Letitia Gladys Moreton, *Military Forces of the Commonwealth Papers.*

44. Correspondence, L.G. Moreton, 2 August 1916, AANS, Indian Medical Service, Bombay, India in Typed Extracts of Correspondence at *AWM File No. 12/11/1398 - 2 DRL 97*, pp.8-9.

45. A. Atkinson, *The Europeans in Australia A History: Democracy*, Vol 2, Oxford University Press, Melbourne, 2004, p.316.

46. Unit War Diary, 14 AGH, AWM 509/2/25 cited in Goodman, *Our War Nurses*, p.85.

47. Correspondence, L.G .Moreton, 2 August 1916, AANS, Indian Medical Service, Bombay, India in Typed Extracts of Correspondence at *AWM File No. 12/11/1398 - 2 DRL 97*, p.8.

48. Woodham-Smith, *Florence Nightingale 1820-1910*, pp.320-1.

49. Correspondence, L.G. Moreton, 8 August 1916, AANS, Indian Medical Service, Quetta, India in Typed Extracts of Correspondence at *AWM File No. 12/11/1398 - 2 DRL 97*, p.9; Goodman, *Our War Nurses*, p.70.

50. Christine Eliza Morrison, *Military Forces of the Commonwealth Papers.*

51. Letitia Gladys Moreton, *Military Forces of the Commonwealth Papers.*

52. B.F. Miller & C.B. Keane, *Encyclopedia and Dictionary of Medicine and Nursing*, W.B. Saunders Co., London, 1972, p.992.

53. Telegram, 1 November 1916 in Letitia Gladys Moreton, *Military Forces of the Commonwealth Papers.*

54. E. Herbert Cuff & W.T. Gordon Pugh, *Practical Nursing including Hygiene and Dietetics* (7th ed.), William Blackwood & Sons Ltd, London, 1928, pp.421-2; Barbara F. Cape, *Baillière's Nurses' Dictionary,* Baillière, Tindall and Cox, London, 1956, pp.330-1.

55. Telegram, 14 November 1916 in Letitia Gladys Moreton, *Military Forces of the Commonwealth Papers.*

56. Miller & Keane, *Encyclopedia and Dictionary of Medicine and Nursing,* p.992.

57. Letitia Gladys Moreton, *Military Forces of the Commonwealth Papers.*

58. AWM Roll of Honour, http://www.awm.gov.au/database/roh.asp [online 28 February 2006]

59.Correspondence, Joan MacLeod to her mother, 6 April 1968 in Pam Barlow (ed.) *The Longest Mile: A Nurse in the Vietnam War 1968-9,* s/p.Townsville, 2006, p.2.

60. Probate No. 38219, Melbourne, 6 February 1917 in Letitia Gladys Moreton, *Military Forces of the Commonwealth Papers.*

61. Jessie Gibson, *Military Forces of the Commonwealth Papers,* NAA, Canberra.

62. Correspondence, Mr R. Blackburn to 2 September 1970 in *Military Forces of the Commonwealth Papers;* Electronic correspondence, Pearl Collins to Ruth Rae, 6 January 2005 in *Ruth Rae Collection,* National Nursing Archives, Canberra.

63. Kings Park Memorial, Perth, WA (viewed by author February 2003).

64. Bassett, *Guns and Brooches,* p.76; Burke, *With Horse and Morse in Mesopotamia,* pp.125-6.

65. *Table 4* was developed from data in Burke, *With Horse and Morse in Mesopotamia,* pp.125-6; Bassett, *Guns and Brooches,* p.76; Goodman, *Our War Nurses,* p.75; Narrative, Sister Annie Low, *Records of A.G. Butler, Official Historian of Australian Army Medical Services - Nurses' Narratives. Bio:* Low, Annie Lyon, b. circa 1886, C/E, lived at Paddington, NSW prior to enlistment, NOK-Father, Mr A.C. Low of Market Street, Mudgee, NSW, embarked on the *Kashgar* from Sydney on 2 September 1916; AWM Embarkation Roll: http://www.awm.gov.au/cms_images/ [online 18 March 2006].

66. Burke, *With Horse and Morse in Mesopotamia,* p.126; Gwen Robinson, *The Forgotten Women,* s/p.Mt Gravatt, 1989, pp.67-8; Goodman, *Our War Nurses,* p.75. *Bio: Lillian Ella Fletcher,* DOE: 20 July 1915 & RTA: 3 July 1919, Sister AANS, served in India and on transport duty; AWM Nominal Roll, http://www.awm.gov.au/database/[online 14 March 2006]; No honours or awards http://www.awm.gov.au/database/roh_award.asp [online 14 March 2006].

67. Gertrude Muriel Norton Robertson *Military Forces of the Commonwealth Papers.*

68. Taprell Dorling in assoc. with F. Guille, *Ribbons and Medals,* George Phillip and Son Ltd., London, 1960, p.91.

69. Correspondence, Gertrude Davis, 24 February 1923 in Gertrude Muriel Norton Robertson *Military Forces of the Commonwealth Papers.*

70. Correspondence, N. Hobbes, March 1915 in AWM 2 DRL/162, Australian War Memorial, Canberra.

71. NSW Pioneer Index-Pioneer Series 1788-1888 [online 18 August 2006]; M. Oppenheimer, *Oceans of Love: Narrelle - An Australian Nurse in World War 1,* ABC Books, Sydney, 2006, pp.25-6.

72 I. Brodsky, *Sydney's Nurse Crusaders: A Century of Trained Nursing in Australia,* Old Sydney Free Press, Sydney, 1968, p.124 (photograph).

73. D.M. Armstrong, *The First Fifty Years: A History of Nursing at the Royal Prince Alfred Hospital, Sydney from 1822 to 1932,* Royal Prince Alfred Hospital Graduate Nurses' Association, Sydney, 1965, p.87; Bassett, *Guns and Brooches,* p.10.

74. 'ATNA Register 01, General Nursing, Obstetrics, Mental Nurses 1916', National Nursing Archives, Canberra.

75. Correspondence, N. Hobbes to 'My Dearest Smithkins' 26 July 1915 in AWM 2 DRL/162.

76. Correspondence, N. Hobbes, 5 May 1915, AWM 2 DRL/162; Bassett, *Guns and Brooches,* pp.34-6; NSW Pioneer Index-Pioneer Series 1788-1888 [online 18 August 2006]. John Hobbes died of stomach cancer at Port Macquarie while working as a Police Magistrate in 1893 - Oppenheimer, *Oceans of Love,* p.27.

77. Rose Kirkcaldie trained at RPAH and returned from the First World War to become Acting Assistant Matron and later became the highly esteemed Matron of the Royal Alexandra Hospital for Children, Sydney - Armstrong, *The First Fifty Years,* pp.132, 141 & 143; Correspondence, N. Hobbes, May 1915 in AWM 2 DRL/162.

78. Correspondence, N. Hobbes, July 1916 cited in Barker, *Nightingales in the Mud,* p.73.

79. Narrative, E. Vickers Foote, *Records of A.G. Butler, Official Historian of Australian Army Medical Services - Nurses' Narratives;* E. Vickers Foote, *Military Forces of the Commonwealth Papers.*

80. Correspondence, N. Hobbes, 25 September 1916, AWM 2 DRL/162.

81. Correspondence, N. Hobbes, August 1917 cited in Barker, *Nightingales in the Mud,* pp.78-9; Oppenheimer, *Oceans of Love,* pp.211, 215 & 218.

82. Barker, *Nightingales in the Mud* p.69; Oppenheimer, *Oceans of Love,* p.27.

83. Miller & Keane, *Encyclopedia and Dictionary of Medicine and Nursing,* pp.116, 542.

84.The Transplantation Society of Australia and New Zealand: Australian National Organ Allocation Protocols - http://www.racp.edu.au/tsanz/oap3.htm [online 12 September 2006]; http://www.weizmann.ac.il/Biology/ [online 12 September 2006].

85. Oppenheimer, *Oceans of Love,* pp.250, 256-7.

29 Controversy at 34 Welsh General Hospital, Deolali, India 1917 – 1918

1 Ashleigh Wadman, Nursing the British Raj, 28 October 2014, AWM online. Note: The following details of Alma Bennett's experience at 34 WGH are included in a number of the author's publications. The incident is considered to be essential for this publication to understand the undercurrent of secrecy during the war and the impact it had on the welfare of the nurses.

2. Alma Bennet, Commonwealth Military Papers, NAA, Canberra.

3. Narrative, Alma Bennett, *Records of A.G. Butler, Official Historian of Australian Army Medical Services - Nurses' Narratives,* AWM, Canberra.

4. B.F. Miller & C.B. Keane, *Encyclopedia and Dictionary of Medicine and Nursing,* W.B. Saunders Co., London, 1972, pp.774, 885.

5. Narrative, Alma Bennett, *Records of A.G. Butler, Official Historian of Australian Army Medical Services - Nurses' Narratives.*

6. R. Rae 'The Limitations of Primary Sources as Historical Data', conference paper, Stories from the Field 2, University of Sydney, 27 September 2001; R. Rae 'Reading between the unwritten lines: Australian Army nurses in India, 1916 – 19', *Journal of the Australian War Memorial,* Canberra, May 2002 at http://www.awm.gov.au/journal/j36/nurses.htm [online 11 August 2006].

7. Narrative, Alma Bennett, *Records of A.G. Butler, Official Historian of Australian Army Medical Services - Nurses' Narratives.*

8. Letter from Principal Matron G.E. Davis to E.Tracy Richardson, Matron-in-Chief AANS, Victoria Barracks, National Archives of Australia *'False accusations against Australian nurses serving in India'* series MP 367/1, item no. 527 27 516, 26 May 1918. Notation from Colonel Seddon, National Archives of Australia *'False accusations against Australian nurses serving in India'* series MP 367/1, item no. 527 27 515, 7 May 1918; J. Bassett, *Guns and Brooches: Australian Army Nursing from the Boer War to the Gulf War,* Oxford University Press Australia, Melbourne, 1992, pp.78-80.

9. Memorandum for Surgeon Fetherston, DGAAMS, National Archives of Australia *'False accusations against Australian nurses serving in India'* series MP 367/1, item no. 527 27 531, 28 August 1918.
10.Confidential Minute from Surgeon General Fetherston, DGAAMS, National Archives of Australia *'False accusations against Australian nurses serving in India'* series MP 367/1, item no. A.527 27 531, 13 December 1918.
11. Ruth Rae, Rose Creal: The biography of an Australian Nurse Leader (1865-1921), amazon.com.
12. R. Goodman, *Our War Nurses: The History of the Royal Australian Army Nursing Corps 1902-1988,* p.86.
13.Letter from Principal Matron G.E.Davis to Miss E.Tracy Richardson, Matron-in-Chief AANS, Victoria Barracks, National Archives of Australia *'False accusations against Australian nurses serving in India'* series MP 367/1, item no. 527 27 516, 26 May 1918.
14. *ibid;* Correspondence from Ken McColl to Ruth Rae, 27 June 2002, in *Ruth Rae Collection,* National Nursing Archives, Canberra.
15. Memorandum for Surgeon General Fetherston, DGAAMS, National Archives of Australia *'False accusations against Australian nurses serving in India'* series MP 367/1, item no. 527 27 531, 28 August 1918.
16. Narrative, Principal Matron G.E. Davis, Records of A.G.Butler, Historian of Australian Army Medical Services - Nurses' Narratives.
17. Memorandum for Surgeon General Fetherston, DGAAMS, National Archives of Australia *'False accusations against Australian nurses serving in India'* series MP 367/1, item no. 527 27 531, 28 August 1918, attachment A and B.
18. Bassett, *Guns and Brooches,* p.81.
19. Decode of Cablegram received from the Viceroy of India from Simla, 25 May 1918, 8.15pm., National Archives of Australia *'False accusations against Australian nurses serving in India'* series MP 367/1, item no. 527 27 411, 25 May 1918.
20. A.G.Butler (ed.), *Official History of The Australian Army Medical Services 1914-18,* 3 vols, (1st ed.), Australian War Memorial, Canberra, 1938-43.
21. A.Maud Kellett interview (no.84) Miss McLean, AWM, Canberra, 1919.
22. A.Maud Kellett interview (no.13) Miss C. Cadwallader, AWM, Canberra.
23. Letter, Daphne Cadwallader to *Dear Mother & Matey,* 25 May 1918, original letter retained by Ken McColl, Canberra and copy in *Ruth Rae Collection,* National Nursing Archives, Canberra.
24. Butler, Official History of the Australian Army Medical Services 1914-18,vol.3,pp.567-9.
25. Memorandum for Surgeon General Fetherston, DGAAMS from T.Trumble, National Archives of Australia *'False accusations against Australian nurses serving in India'* series MP 367/1, item no. 527 27 516, 7 August 1918.
26.Letter, Fetherston to White, Fetherston papers, bundle 4, item 7 (ii of xiii) 3 DRL 251, 14 March 1916, Australian War Memorial, Canberra.
27. Bassett, *Guns and Brooches,* pp.55-79.
28.Letter, Fetherston to Howse, Australian War Memorial records 370.2, 13 March 1917, AWM, Canberra.
29.Extract from letter dated 6 June 1918, unsigned, National Archives of Australia *'False accusations against Australian nurses serving in India'* series MP 367/1, item no. 527 27 501.
30. Letter signed Arthur Johnston to Hon. W.A. Watt, Acting Prime Minister of Australia, National Archives of Australia *'False accusations against Australian nurses serving in India'* series MP 367/1, item no. 527 27 501, 24 July 1918.
31. Decode of Cablegram received from the Viceroy of India from Simla, 25 May 1918, 8.15pm., National Archives of Australia *'False accusations against Australian nurses serving in India'* series MP 367/1, item no. 527 27 411, 25 May 1918; Minute Paper, Department of Defence, National Archives of Australia *'False accusations against Australian nurses serving in India'* series MP 367/1, item no. 527 27 411, 28 May 1918.
32. Letter from Principal Matron G.E.Davis to E.Tracy Richardson, Matron-in-Chief AANS, Victoria Barracks, National Archives of Australia *'False accusations against Australian nurses serving in India'* series MP 367/1, item no. 527 27 516, 26 May 1918.
33. Newspaper article, Sydney Bulletin dated 1 August 1918, National Archives of Australia *'False accusations against Australian nurses serving in India'* series MP 367/1, item no. 527 27 514, undated notation for General Fetherston and Defence stamp.

34. Narrative, Alma Bennett, Records of A.G.Butler, Historian of Australian Army Medical Services - Nurses' Narratives.
35. *Stawell News* 'An Exhibition of Dancing by the Misses Bate's Pupils', 17 November 1900; Correspondence, Dorothy King to Ruth Rae, 4 February 2005 in *Ruth Rae Collection*, National Nursing Archives, Canberra. The author gratefully acknowledges Dorothy King, Research Officer, Stawell Historical Society Inc, who provided background information on Emily Clare and her family.
36.Baptism Registry, St Patrick's Roman Catholic Church, Stawell, Victoria in Correspondence, Dorothy King to Ruth Rae, 4 February 2005 in *Ruth Rae Collection*, National Nursing Archives, Canberra.
37. *Stawell News* 'Died on Service — Nurse E Clare', 23 October 1918 in *Ruth Rae Collection,* National Nursing Archives, Canberra.
38. Emily Clare Military Forces of the Commonwealth Papers.
39.AWM Roll of Honour: http://www.awm.gov.au/database/roh.asp [on-line 18 August 2006]; Emily Clare Record, Central Army Records Office, Victoria Barracks, Melbourne.
40.Correspondence, Dorothy King to Ruth Rae, 4 February 2005 in *Ruth Rae Collection*, National Nursing Archives, Canberra.
41. Correspondence, Mrs J McNeece (C/ - Tatura State School) to officer-in-charge Base Records in Irene McPhail *Military Forces of the Commonwealth Papers*; H. Paterson *'5.30, Nurse!' The Story of the Alfred Nurses*, History Books, Melbourne, 1996, p.227.
42. Irene McPhail, *Military Forces of the Commonwealth Papers*, NAA, Canberra.

43. 'Confidential Proceedings of a Board of Medical Officers assembled at Poona on the 3rd May 1918' in Irene McPhail, *Military Forces of the Commonwealth Papers*.

44. Correspondence, Mrs J. McNeece to Major McLean (AIF), 12 August 1918 in Irene McPhail, *Military Forces of the Commonwealth Papers*.

45. 'Medical Report on an Invalid, 11 AGH, 10 March 1920' in Irene McPhail *Military Forces of the Commonwealth Papers*.

46. Narrative, Alma Bennett, Records of A.G.Butler, Historian of Australian Army Medical Services - Nurses' Narratives.
47. H.S. Gullett, *Official History of Australia in the War of 1914-18 Sinai and Palestine* (12th ed), vol.7, Angus and Robertson Ltd., Sydney, 1944, p.645.
48. Kathleen McAleer, *Military Forces of the Commonwealth Papers*.
49. Commonwealth War Graves website: http://www.cwgc.org/search/cemetery_details.[on-line 12 September 2006].

30 War is Over but Peace is Elusive

1. H. Strachan, *The First World War: A New Illustrated History*, Simon & Schuster, London, 2003, p.316.

2. Editorial 'The Last Post. 5000 Nurses in St Paul's. Women's Memorial Service' *The Australasian Trained Nurses' Journal*, The Journal of the Australasian Trained Nurses' Association, Vol XVI, no.7, 15 July 1918, pp.219-220. Nearly 200 British nurses died 1914-18. They were members of QAIMNS, QAIMNSR or VAD and additional deaths occurred in the Territorial Army Nursing Service (TANS) - J. Piggott *Queen Alexandra's Royal Army Nursing Corps,* Leo Cooper Ltd, London, 1975, p.62.

3. Strachan, *The First World War*, p.326.

4. Strachan, *The First World War*, pp.325-6; E.H. Carr, *The Interregnum 1923-1924*, MacMillan and Co., London, 1954, pp.188-9.

5. J. Bassett, *Guns and Brooches: Australian Army Nursing from the Boer War to the Gulf War*, Oxford University Press, Melbourne, 1992, pp.53-4.

6. Narrative, M.B. Donaldson, *Records of A.G. Butler, Official Historian of Australian Army Medical Services – Nurses' Narratives,* AWM, Canberra.

7. Narrative, E.S. Davidson, *Records of A.G. Butler, Official Historian of Australian Army Medical Services*

– *Nurses' Narratives*; P. Adam-Smith, *Australian Women at War*, Penguin Books Australia Ltd., Melbourne, 1996, pp.25-6.

8. Correspondence, O. Haynes, 9 August 1917 cited in M Young (ed) *We Are Here Too – Letters and Diaries of Sister Olive Haynes No. 2 AGH November 1914 to February, 1918*, Australian Down Syndrome Assoc Inc, Adelaide, 1991, p.223.

9. K. Holmes, 'Between the Lines: The Letters and Diaries of the WW1 Nurses', *Webbers*, Vol 2, May 1990, p.43.

10. A. Donnell, *Letters of An Australian Army Sister*, Angus and Robertson Ltd, Sydney, 1920, p.271.

11. Jean Nellie Miles Walker, *Military Forces of the Commonwealth Papers*, NAA, Canberra.

12. Donnell, *Letters of An Australian Army Sister*, p.273.

13. The service record of Jean Nellie Miles Walker includes official documents which list her mother as next-of-kin while others list her brother as next-of-kin; correspondence in Jean Nellie Miles Walker *Military Forces of the Commonwealth Papers*.

14. Correspondence, Jessie Tomlins to Margaretta Tomlins, 18 November 1917, copy in possession of author.

15. Edith Dina Jackson, *Military Forces of the Commonwealth Papers*, NAA, Canberra.

16. Elsie Tranter diary, 28 June 1917, in G.M. Gillings and J. Richards (eds), *...in all those lines: The diary of Sister Elsie Tranter 1916-1919*, s/p.2008, pp.62 & (*n*).

17. Y. McEwen, "*It's a Long Way to Tipperary*"*: British and Irish nurses in the Great War*, Cualann Press, Dunfermline, 2006, p.203.

18. Harries in G. Robinson, *The Forgotten Women*, s/p, Mt Gravatt, 1989, p.48.

19. Correspondence, Medical History File of the Official Medical Historian G.Butler, Box 41, AWM, 21 March 1917, AWM, Canberra; Michael Duffy (original material 2000-2007) 'On this day - 20 March 1917' http://www.firstworldwar.com/onthisday/1917_03_20.htm[online 26 February 2007; updated 28 July 2002]; www.qaranc.co.uk/qaimns.php (online 10 August 2014).

20. Correspondence, Colonel A.G. Butler to C.E.W. Bean, 21 March 1917, *Medical History File*, AWM, Canberra. Correspondence, Colonel A.G. Butler to Mr Balfour, 12 September 1938, *Medical History File*, AWM, Canberra. The 1917 letter claims J.J. Phillips was an Australian nurse but the 1938 letter states that the undermentioned quote is from the British Official Medical History (vol 1, General Appendix C p.370) 'HS 'Asturius' – Torpedoed on 21 March, 1917, at midnight, off Devonshire coast; no patients on board; Temporary Captain G.L. Atkinson, RAMC, Staff Nurse J.J. Phillips, and 12 RAMC orderlies were drowned; the ship was beached at Salcombe'. A.G. Butler writes that he was 'sorry it was overlooked before'. The rank of J.J. Phillips is unclear as she was listed as a 'sister' with the QAIMNS in McEwen,"*It's a Long Way to Tipperary*", pp.171 & 204. Note: p.171 incorrectly records the date of the torpedo attack as 3 March 1917. Michael Duffy (original material 2000-2007) 'On this day - 20 March 1917' [http://www.firstworldwar.com/onthisday/1917_03_20.htm [online 26 February 2007; updated 28 July 2002].

21. A troop transport of the same name was used in the Boer War but the construction of the First World War *Britannic* did not commence until November 1911 – Sheila M. Gray, *The South African War 1899-1902: Service Record of British and Colonial Women – A Record of theService in South Africa of Military and Civilian Nurses, Laywomen and Civilians*, s/p.Auckland, 1993, p.19; Website: http://www.webtitanic.net/frameBritannic.html [online 11 May 2005].

22. S.A. White (nee Furnifull), 'A World War One Nurse Remembers...', *Australian Woman's Weekly*, 31 October 1973, p.43.

23. Website: http://www.webtitanic.net/frameBritannic.html [online 11 May 2005].

24. White, 'A World War One Nurse Remembers...', p.43; Butler, *Special Problems and Services*, p.588.

25. A. Hill, *Soldier Boy: The True Story of Jim Martin the youngest Anzac*, Penguin Books Australia,

Melbourne, 2001, pp.121-2.

26. M. Cordia, *Nurses at Little Bay*, p.73; Edith Blake, *Military Forces of the Commonwealth Papers*, NAA, Canberra. Note: The name 'Enid Blake' is incorrectly used in a number of sources but her name was 'Edith Blake' as stated in correspondence from her family in her service record.

27. McEwen, *"It's a Long Way to Tipperary"*, pp.176, 202-03, 206. Note: The other seven nurses included six from the QAIMNS - K. Beaufoy (matron), J. Evans (sister), R.E. Kendall (sister) and Staff Nurses R.R. Beresford, E. Edgar, C.E. Henry and one from the Territorial Nursing Service - M. MacKinnon; correspondence, Solicitor to Officer-in-Charge Base Records, 16 October 1919 in Edith Blake, *Military Forces of the Commonwealth Papers*, Series No MT 1487/1, NAA, Melbourne [online 2 December 2004]. Website: http://www.union-castle-line.com/history/1900.htm [online November 2004] [update 2/12/2004].

28. Correspondence, Solicitor to Officer-in-Charge Base Records, 16 October 1919 in Edith Blake, *Military Forces of the Commonwealth Papers.*

29. AWM Commemorative Roll: http://www.awm.gov.au/database/[online 12 August 2006].

30. Cordia, *Nurses at Little Bay*, p.73. Note: The correct date was 26 February 1918.

31. J. McQuilton, *Rural Australia and the Great War: From Tarrawingee to Tangambalanga,* Melbourne University Press, Melbourne, 2001, pp.188-9; Correspondence, Jessie Tomlins to Margaretta Tomlins, 20 July 1918, copy in possession of author.

32. Correspondence, O. Haynes, 10 September 1916 cited in M Young (ed), *We Are Here Too - Letters and Diaries of Sister Olive Haynes No. 2 AGH November 1914 to February, 1918*, Australian Down Syndrome Assoc Inc, Adelaide, 1991, p.164.

33. R. Rae, 'Soldiers of the ANZAC Mounted Division and Nurses of the 14th Australian General Hospital - Desert Correspondents in World War One', *Australian Defence Force Journal,* 149:53, Canberra, 2001.

34. V. Brittain, *Testament of Youth*, Virago Press, London, 2006 (first published by Victor Gollancz Limited 1933), pp.404-5.

35. Correspondence, Fred Tomlins to Meg Tomlins, 15 November 1916, copy in possession of author.

36. C. Fallows, *Love and War: Stories of War Brides from the Great War to Vietnam*, Bantam Books, Sydney, 2002, pp.67, 69-70.

37. Correspondence, Jessie Tomlins to Nettie Tomlins, 27 June 1919, copy in possession of author.

38. Edith Kindred cited in Fallows, *Love and War*, p.82.

39. Jan Herivel, Research Librarian, Penrith City Council Website [online 8 September 2004]; M. Barker *Nightingales in the Mud: the Digger Sisters of the Great War 1914-1918*, Allen and Unwin, Sydney, 1989, p.166; Mary Rosa Harford, *Military Forces of the Commonwealth Papers*, NAA, Canberra.

40. Mary Rosa Harford, *Military Forces of the Commonwealth Papers.*

41. Catherine Adaway, *Military Forces of the Commonwealth Papers.*

42. Correspondence. Anthony T. Hendry to Secretary of Defence Department, 7 April 1920, Melbourne in Catherine Adaway *Military Forces of the Commonwealth Papers*; Mary Harford, *Military Forces of the Commonwealth Papers.*

43. Catherine Adaway, *Military Forces of the Commonwealth Papers*; Barker, *Nightingales in the Mud,* p.166.

44. R. Rae, 'An historical account of shell-shock during the First World War and reforms in mental health in Australia 1914-1939', *International Journal of Mental Health Nursing*, 2007, 16: 266-273; Ross McMullin, *Pompey Elliott*, Scribe Publications Pty Ltd, Melbourne, 2002, pp.655-6.

45. Barker, *Nightingales in the Mud,* p.169.

46. Bill Gammage, *The Broken Years: Australian Soldiers in the Great War,* Penguin Books Australia Ltd,

Sydney, 1974, p.166; D. Bungey, *Arthur Boyd: A Life*, Allen & Unwin, Sydney, 2007, p.12.

47. Brittain, *Testament of Youth*, p.455.

48. C.E.W. Bean, *Anzac to Amiens* (5th ed.), Australian War Memorial, Canberra, 1968, p.516.

49. Ruth Teale, 'Long, George Merrick (1874–1930)', Australian Dictionary of Biography, National Centre of Biography, Australian National University, https://adb.anu.edu.au/biography/long-george-merrick-610/text12505, published first in hardcopy 1986, accessed online 3 November 2025.

50. Bungey, *Arthur Boyd: A Life*, pp.4-5, 12.

51. Rose Creal, Record of non-military employment, Form D.29 in *Military Forces of the Commonwealth Papers.*

52. Moberly cited in Bassett, *Guns and Brooches,* p.93.

53. Donnell, *Letters of An Australian Army Sister*, p. 284.

54. Manning Clark, *A History of Australia: The Old Dead Tree and the Young Tree Green 1916-35*, Vol 6, Melbourne University Press, Melbourne, 1987, p.141.

55. Fallows, *Love and War,* p.108.

56. Diary entries, Fred Tomlins, 26 & 27 December 1918, copy in possession of author.

57. Clark, *The Old Dead Tree and the Young Tree Green 1916-35*, p.179.

58. M. Cannon, *The Human Face of the Great Depression*, Today's Australia Publishing Company, Mornington, 1996, p.119.

59. T. Whitford & D. Boadle, 'Remaking the Country: Australia's Rural Reconstruction Commission, 1943-46', *Journal of the Royal Australian Historical Society*, 95 (1), 2009, p.65.

60. Fallows, *Love and War,* p.108.

61. D. Morton & G. Wright, *Winning the second battle: Canadian veterans and the return to civilian life 1915-1930,* University of Toronto Press, Toronto, 1987, p.145.

62. R. Goodman, *Our War Nurses: The History of the Royal Australian Army Nursing Corps 1902-1988,* Boolarong Publications, Brisbane, 1988, p.46.

63. Electronic Correspondence, Selena Williams to Ruth Rae, 5 April 2005 in *Ruth Rae Collection,* National Nursing Archives, Canberra. The author gratefully acknowledges Selena Williams for information about Elizabeth Draper.

64. E.P. Wright, *Military Forces of the Commonwealth Papers*, NAA, Canberra.

65. Correspondence, Mr Wright to Base Records (AIF) in E.P. Wright, *Military Forces of the Commonwealth Papers.*

66. W. Newman & L. Green, *Tamworth: A Pictorial History*, Halbooks, Sydney, 1998, p.127 (photograph).

67. E.P. Wright, *Military Forces of the Commonwealth Papers; Sydney Morning Herald*, Obituary, 3 August 1985; electronic correspondence, Selena Williams to Ruth Rae, 5 April 2005. The author gratefully acknowledges Selena Williams for bringing the SMH article to my attention.

68. M .Tilton, *The Grey Battalion*, Angus and Robertson Ltd, Sydney, 1933, pp.208-9.

69. White (nee Furnifull), 'A World War One Nurse Remembers…', 31 October 1973.

70. Tilton, *The Grey Battalion*, p.292; Pearl Stella Goodman, *Military Forces of the Commonwealth Papers.*

71. Tilton, *The Grey Battalion*, pp.296-310.

72. Elsie Grant, *Military Forces of the Commonwealth Papers;* Tilton, *The Grey Battalion*, pp.306-7.

73. Donnell, *Letters of An Australian Army Sister*, pp.279, 289.

31 The Human Tragedy of Influenza

1. H. Strachan, *The First World War: A new Illustrated history*, Simon & Schuster, London, 2003, p.329.

2. Hunter New England Population Health NSW Health 'Communicable Disease Bulletin' Novel Influenza (H1N1 09), Vol 188, April 2009, p.1.

3. Geoff Speer in Department of Veterans' Affairs, *Simply Hell Let Loose: Stories of Australians at war*, ABC Books, Sydney, 2002, p.69.

4. N. Brennan, *Dr Mannix*, Rigby Limited, Adelaide, 1964, pp.167-8.; J.A. Williams & R.D. Goodman, *Jane Bell, O.B.E. (1873-1959): Lady Superintendent, The Royal Melbourne Hospital (1910-1934)*, Royal Melbourne Graduate Nurses' Association, Melbourne, 1988, p.40. Notes: Jane Bell was born in Scotland and regularly attended Scots Church in Collins Street, Melbourne

5. Worrall in Brennan, *Dr Mannix*, p.168.

6. C. Woodham-Smith, *Florence Nightingale 1820-1910*, Constable and Company Ltd, London, 1950, p.74.

7. Correspondence, O. Haynes, 6 January 1918 cited in M. Young (ed), *We Are Here Too – Letters and Diaries of Sister Olive Haynes No. 2 AGH November 1914 to February, 1918*, Australian Down Syndrome Assoc Inc, Adelaide, 1991, p.251.

8. AWM Honour and Awards: http://www.awm.gov.au/honours/[online 18 April 2008].

9. Merrilyn Lincoln 'Graham, Margaret (1860 - 1942)', *Australian Dictionary of Biography*, Volume 9, Melbourne University Press, Melbourne, 1983, p.68-69.

10. Diary, Susie Cone, 24 December 1918 in *S. Cone 1918-19 Diaries*, 2 vols, Royal Melbourne Hospital Archives, Melbourne, 1918-19 transcribed by author, with permission, and copy in *Ruth Rae Collection*, National Nursing Archives, Canberra. Note: The identity of Harriet Jackson's sister is not clear as she is not listed with the AWM Nominal Roll because she did not serve overseas nor is there reference to her with the NAA. Susie Cone makes mention of 'Jackson's sister'. Harriet Jackson (b. 1888) was from South Australia and had trained with Doris Ridgway. Before joining the *Wyreema* in Sydney she had served at 15 AGH and 7 AGH and was a shipboard companion to Susie Cone, Rosa O'Kane and Ada Thompson; Blanche May Morrison, *Military Forces of the Commonwealth Papers*, National Archives of Australia, Canberra; J. Durdin, *Eleven Thousand Nurses – A History of Nurse Education at the Royal Adelaide Hospital 1889-1993*, Royal Adelaide Hospital, 1999, pp.229-30; Nurses' Memorial Foundation of South Australia Incorporated, *Nursing –150 years of Caring in South Australia*, The South Australian Trained Nurses' Centenary Committee, Adelaide,1938 (Reprinted with 1939-1945 supplement in 1989), p.231.

11. Durdin, *Eleven Thousand Nurses*, p.31.

12. Blanche May Morrison, *Military Forces of the Commonwealth Papers*. Note: Her service record is a slim volume (2 pages) which tells the story of the 24-year-old nurse who trained at Wakefield Street Private Hospital, Adelaide, and had been an AANS member since June 1917. She had served at 15 AGH and volunteered to nurse influenza patients in 5 MD and left South Australia on 21 December 1918. She left the AANS when she married on 20 August 1919. As she did not serve overseas with the AANS she is not recorded on the AWM Nominal Roll.

13. Florence Hilda Watts, *Military Forces of the Commonwealth Papers* [online 19 March 2008].

14. Lily Nugent, NAA, Melbourne; ATNA Register, National Nursing Archives, Canberra; Lily Nugent, Roll of Honour cards, AWM, Canberra.

15. I. Darroch, *The Boonah Tragedy*, Access Press, Bassendean, 2004, pp.18, 21, 45.

16. R. Goodman, *Our War Nurses – The History of the Royal Australian Army Nursing Corps*, Boolarong Publications, Brisbane, 1988, p.105.

17. Correspondence from Mrs M.J. Hall (aunt) cited in Darroch, *The Boonah Tragedy*, p.159; Rosa

O'Kane, *Military Forces of the Commonwealth Papers* NAA, Canberra.

18. Attestation paper in Rosa O'Kane, *Military Forces of the Commonwealth Papers.*

19. Diary, Susie Cone, 5 December & 10 December 1918 1918 in *S. Cone 1918-19 Diaries.*

20. L. Potter (Pres), *A Passion to Care: Nursing and Nurses Western Suburbs Hospital 1984-1982,* The Western Suburbs Hospital Graduate Nurses' Association, Sydney, 2008, pp.129-30.

21. Diary, Susie Cone, 11 December 1918 in *S. Cone 1918-19 Diaries*; R. Rae, 'Infection Control Nursing circa 1918-19 - Woodman's Point Quarantine Station' *nursing.aust* Journal of The College of Nursing, vol 4, no 2, 2003, pp.23-4.

22. Diary, Susie Cone, 21 December 1918 in *S. Cone 1918-19 Diaries.*

23. Darroch, *The Boonah Tragedy,* p.159.

24. Correspondence, Mrs M. J. Hall (aunt) cited in Darroch, *The Boonah Tragedy,* p.159.

25. Darroch, *The Boonah Tragedy,* pp.123 &171.

26. Diary, Susie Cone, Multiple entries in *S. Cone 1918-19 Diaries.*

27. Darroch, *The Boonah Tragedy,* p.171.

28. Correspondence from 'Military Sisters, Quarantine Station, Woodman Point' to the editor, *West Australian*, 21 December 1918 cited in Darroch, *The Boonah Tragedy,* pp.171-3; R.Rae, *First World War Commemorative Nominal Roll,* ACN Trilogy, Canberra, 2015. Note: The exact number of nurses who became ill varies between sources. The diaries of Susie Cone - the only known primary source of the episode - names individual nurses who became ill and the date of the diary entry has been assigned in brackets next to the nurses. The author has not been able to identify the individual named K. (?H)ymer.

29. Correspondence from 'Military Sisters, Quarantine Station, Woodman Point' to the editor, *West Australian*, 21 December 1918 cited in Darroch, *The Boonah Tragedy,* pp.171-3.

30. Darroch, *The Boonah Tragedy,* pp.141-2.

31. Diary, Susie Cone, 24 & 25 December 1918 in *S. Cone 1918-19 Diaries.*

32. Record of death in Ada Mildred Thompson, *Military Forces of the Commonwealth Papers*; Diary, Susie Cone, 30 & 31 December 1918 in *S Cone 1918-19 Diaries*; Darroch, *The Boonah Tragedy,* p.176.

33. Diary, Susie Cone, 30 December 1918 & 2 January 1919 in *S. Cone 1918-19 Diaries.*

34. Telephone interview, Ruth Rae with John Sargent (nephew of Hilda Williams and son of Edith Lillian Sargent nee Williams), 27 November 2004, transcript in *Ruth Rae Collection*, National Nursing Archives, Canberra; Correspondence, John Sargent to Ruth Rae, 7 December 2004 in *Ruth Rae Collection*, National Nursing Archives, Canberra.

35. V. Hobbs, *But Westward Look - Nursing in Western Australia 1829-1979*, University of Western Australia Press for the Royal Australian Nursing Federation (WA Branch), Perth, 1980, p.207; Digger-Federation Index.Victoria 1889-1901 [18 August 2006].

36. Cited in electronic correspondence from Jane Dewing to Ruth Rae, 12 August 2006 in *Ruth Rae Collection,* National Nursing Archives, Canberra.

37. Helen Spanney (family member) was aware that Hilda's parents were not allowed to visit their daughter at Woodman's Point Quarantine Station; Correspondence, John Sargent to Ruth Rae, 27 June 2005 in *Ruth Rae Collection*, National Nursing Archives, Canberra; Diary, 30 December 1918 in *S. Cone 1918-19 Diaries.*

38. Diary, 4 & 5 January 1919 in *S. Cone 1918-19 Diaries.*

39. Doris Alice Ridgway, *Military Forces of the Commonwealth Papers* (Form D11); Royal Adelaide Hospital Nurses' Register, Royal Adelaide Hospital Heritage Office, Adelaide (reviewed by author February 2003).

40. Doris Alice Ridgway, *Military Forces of the Commonwealth Papers*; Blanche May Morrison, *Military Forces of the Commonwealth Papers.*

41. Diary, Susie Cone, 5 January 1919 in *S. Cone 1918-19 Diaries*; R. Rae 'Infection Control Nursing circa 1918-19 - Woodman's Point Quarantine Station', pp.23-4.

42. Several texts claim Doris Ridgway died on 1 January 1919 but given the comprehensive description of the date of her illness (5 January 1919), subsequent death on 6 January 1919 and burial the next day by her colleague, Susie Cone, the author considers 6 January 1919 to be correct - Diary, Susie Cone, 5-7 January 1919 in *S. Cone 1918-19 Diaries;* A.G. Butler, *The Official History of the Australian Army Medical Services in the war of 1914-1918: Special Problems and Services*, Vol 3, Australian War Memorial Canberra, 1943, p.588; Goodman, *Our War Nurses,* p.99.

43. Diary entries, Susie Cone, 5-7 January 1919 in *S. Cone 1918-19 Diaries*; Darroch, *The Boonah Tragedy,* p.98.

44. Doris Alice Ridgway, *Military Forces of the Commonwealth Papers.*

45. Darroch, *The Boonah Tragedy,* pp.96-7; Doris Alice Ridgway, *Military Forces of the Commonwealth Papers.*

46. B. Kingston, *My Wife, My Daughter and Poor Mary Ann*, Thomas Nelson Australia Pty Ltd, Melbourne, 1975, p.89.

47. Darroch, *The Boonah Tragedy,* p.247.

48. R. Rae, photograph, grave of Rosa O'Kane, 8 February 2003 in *Ruth Rae Collection*, National Nursing Archives, Canberra.

49. Darroch, *The Boonah Tragedy,* p.244; R. Pearce 'The Tragic destiny of Sister Rosa O'Kane', Bridgeheads of Northern Health, p.60.

50. Ada Mildred Thompson, *Military Forces of the Commonwealth Papers* (attestation papers); NSW Pioneer Index-Pioneer Series 1788-1888 [online 18 August 2006].

51. Ada Mildred Thompson, *Military Forces of the Commonwealth Papers* (copy of last will and testament).

52. Correspondence, Officer-in-Charge Base Records to Miss H.C. Thompson, in Ada Mildred Thompson *Military Forces of the Commonwealth Papers.*

53. Ada Mildred Thompson, *Military Forces of the Commonwealth Papers.*

54. R. Rae, photograph of the memorial plaque of Ada Mildred Thompson, Perth War Cemetery, Karrakatta, 8 February 2003 in *Ruth Rae Collection*, National Nursing Archives, Canberra.

55. CWGC website: http://www.cwgc.org/search/ [online 14 September 2006]; R. Rae, photograph of the grave of Ada Mildred Thompson, Fremantle Cemetery, 8 February 2003 in *Ruth Rae Collection*, National Nursing Archives, Canberra.

56. Author visited the Pallamallawa area in NSW in April 2005; R. Rae, photograph of King's Park Memorial, Perth, 7 February 2003 in *Ruth Rae Collection*, National Nursing Archives, Canberra.

57. Doris Alice Ridgway, *Military Forces of the Commonwealth Papers;* R. Rae, photograph of the Royal Adelaide Hospital Honour Board, Adelaide,February 2003 in *Ruth Rae Collection*, National Nursing Archives, Canberra.

58. Correspondence and photograph (taken by Dorothy Rowe) to Ruth Rae, 17 September 2003 in *Ruth Rae Collection*, National Nursing Archives,Canberra.

59. Narrative, Victor Mitton Ridgway (brother to Doris) dated 22 November 1970, copy given to author by Mr Ian Ridgway (nephew of Doris) in June 2005 in *Ruth Rae Collection*, National Nursing Archives, Canberra.

60. Ruth Rae photograph of Hilda Williams grave, February 2003 in *Ruth Rae Collection*, National Nursing Archives, Canberra.

61. Telephone interview, Ruth Rae with John Sargent, 27 November 2004, transcript in *Ruth Rae Collection,* National Nursing Archives, Canberra.

62. John Norton, Family History file of Elizabeth McGregor, copy sent to author in November 2007 in *Ruth Rae Collection*, National Nursing Archives, Canberra.

63. Telephone interview, Ruth Rae with Lady Jean Foley, 10 October 2007. The author gratefully acknowledges Lady Foley author of *'In Quarantine' – a history of the North Head Quarantine Station* – who provided an account of the plight of the soldiers aboard the *Medic* and the two nurses, Annie Egan and Elizabeth McGregor, who died caring for them.

64. Edith Kindred cited in C. Fallows, *Love and War: Stories of War Brides from the Great War to Vietnam*, Bantam Books, Sydney, 2002, p.101.

65. M/S Papers 'Anzac Fellowship of Women' M/S 2864, Box 14, File 9, National Library of Australia, Canberra. R. Rae, photograph of grave of Elizabeth McGregor, 19 October 2007 in *Ruth Rae Collection*, National Nursing Archives, Canberra.

66. AWM Embarkation Roll: http://www.awm.gov.au/nominalrolls/ww1/embarkation/results.asp [online 3 January 2008]. Note: There is no reference to Elizabeth McGregor being aboard the *Medic* at this site.

67. Correspondence, Mal Booth (Head Research Centre, AWM) to Mr John Norton (grand-nephew of Elizabeth McGregor), 14 May 2007; R. Rae, photographs of graves of Elizabeth McGregor and Annie Egan, 19 October 2007 in *Ruth Rae Collection*, National Nursing Archives, Canberra; ATNA Register, National Nursing Archives, Canberra.

68. John Norton, Family History file of Elizabeth McGregor in *Ruth Rae Collection*, National Nursing Archives, Canberra.

69. Potter, *A Passion to Care*, p.98.

70. Electronic correspondence, Helen Croll (archivist RPAH) to Ruth Rae, 23 October 2007 in *Ruth Rae Collection*, National Nursing Archives, Canberra.

71. R. Rae, photograph of the grave of Nurse Annie Egan, 19 October 2007 in *Ruth Rae Collection*, National Nursing Archives, Canberra.

72. Joanne Ewin, *Meet the Pioneers: Early Families of the Milton-Ulladulla District with Photographs* (ISBN 0 646 01711 X) 1991, p.177; R. Rae, 'The other Matron Porter' *The Milton-Ulladulla Times*, 8 January 2003.

73. A. McAndrew, *Milton-Ulludulla in the Wars*, s/p.(ISBN 0 9596744 6 2), Sydney, 1994, p.109; Photograph, taken by author, 24 October 2008 in *Ruth Rae Collection*, National Nursing Archives, Canberra.

74. Merrilyn Lincoln 'Graham, Margaret (1860 – 1942)', *Australian Dictionary of Biography*, pp.68-69.

75. R. Rae, photograph of Margaret Graham Building, February 2003 in *Ruth Rae Collection*, National Nursing Archives, Canberra.

32 Nursing and Medical Legacies

1. A.Maud Kellett interview (no. 11) L. Comber, AWM, Canberra, 1919.

2. A.G. Butler, *The Official History of the Australian Army Medical Services in the war of 1914-1918 Gallipoli, Palestine and New Guinea*, Vol 1, (2nd ed.), Australian War Memorial, Melbourne, 1938, pp.264-265, 265(*n*).

3. May Tilton, *The Grey Battalion*, Angus and Robertson Ltd, Sydney, 1933, p.103.

4. Butler, *Gallipoli, Palestine and New Guinea*, p.535.

5. R. Lynette Russell (ed.), *The Life and Times of Muriel Knox Doherty 1896-1988,* NSW College of

Nursing, Sydney, 1996, pp.4,7.

6. Narrative, E. Vickers Foote, *Records of A.G. Butler, Official Historian of Australian Army Medical Services – Nurses' Narratives,* AWM, Canberra.

7. Correspondence, N. Hobbes to 'My Dearest Smithkins', 26 July 1915 in AWM 2 DRL/162, AWM, Canberra.

8. J. Bassett, *Guns and Brooches: Australian Army Nursing from the Boer War to the Gulf War*, Oxford University Press Australia, Melbourne, 1992, pp.99-105.

9. R. Rae, 'Nursing Chauvel's Light Horsemen: Rose Creal and the Nurses of the 14 AGH, Egypt 1916-19', *Chauvel Lecture*, 31 August 2006, University of New England, Armidale.

10. Butler, *Gallipoli, Palestine and New Guinea*, pp.537-8.

11. Allan Tieu 'Battle for Graythwaite Estate not over' ABC, online 26 October 2009. 'In The Supreme Court Of New South Wales Equity Division Windeyer J Tuesday 14 August 2007 1994/06 Northern Sydney And Central Coast Area Health Service & Anor V Attorney-General For New South Wales & Ors Judgment'.

12. Butler, *Gallipoli, Palestine and New Guinea*, pp.535-6.

13. Annual Report 1917-18, NSW Division, Australian Red Cross Society, Sydney, 1916, p.20.

14. William Applegate Gullick 'Report of the Director-General of Public Health New South Wales for the Year Ended 31 December 1913', Government Printer, Sydney, 1915, pp.14-15.

15. William Applegate Gullick 'Report of the Director-General of Public Health New South Wales for the Year Ended 31 December 1913', Report upon the State Hospitals and Asylums under the Control of the Director-General of Public Health (Part IV), pp.162 & 185.

16. Butler, *Gallipoli, Palestine and New Guinea*, pp.535-6, 536(*n*).

17. A.G. Butler, *The Official History of the Australian Army Medical Services in the war of 1914-1918: Special Problems and Services*, Vol 3, Australian War Memorial Canberra, 1943, pp.77, 82-4,98.

18. Correspondence, Fred Tomlins, 27 January 1918, copy in possession of author.

19. Harries in G. Robinson, *The Forgotten Women*, s/p.Mt Gravatt, 1989, p.48. Note: A diary entry attributed to Sister Harries, 29 September 1916, indicates she later joined the AANS but there is no supporting evidence with the NAA or the AWM.

20. Ford in Butler, *Special Problems and Services,* p.88.

21. Manifold in Butler, *Special Problems and Services,* pp.111-2.

22. Butler, *Special Problems and Services,* p.85.

23. Butler, *Gallipoli, Palestine and New Guinea*, p.541.

24. Sinclair in Butler, *Special Problems and Services*, p.762; Narrative, Evelyn Vickers Foote, *Records of A.G. Butler: Official Historian of Australian Army Medical Services – Nurses' Narratives.*

25. Annual Report 1915-16, NSW Division, Australian Red Cross Society, Sydney, 1916, pp.18-9.

26. Bassett, *Guns and Brooches,* pp.96-102.

27. R. Goodman, *Our War Nurses – The History of the Royal Australian Army Nursing Corps*, Boolarong Publications, Brisbane, 1988, pp.51-2; Correspondence, Jessie Tomlins to Margaretta Tomlins, 8 June 1919, copy in possession of author.

28. Elizabeth Kenny, *Military Forces of the Commonwealth Papers.* Note: Elizabeth Kenny most likely enrolled in a course for infant welfare nurses at the private Norland Nursing School (circa 1911), Woollahra (NSW). The author gratefully acknowledges Kerry Highley for this additional information – Kerry Highley to Ruth Rae, electronic correspondence, 24 November 2008; Kerry Highley *"My Dear Miss Barron…" Letters from the Kenny Clinic in Townsville, 1934* at 'A Goldmine for Historians: The Archives', The College of Nursing. Sydney, 23 October 2008. There is no evidence Kenny completed a

prescribed ATNA training program at an ATNA recognised hospital.

29. S. De Vries, *Great Australian Women*, Harper Collins Publishers, Sydney, 2001, pp.253-5; J. Morris, 'The Trial of Elizabeth Kenny', *The Chronicle*, Toowoomba, 26 April 1997, p.14.

30. L.R.G. Crandon & A. Ehrenfred, *Surgical After-treatment: a Manual for the Conduct of Surgical Convalescence* (2nd ed), Saunders, Philadelphia, 1914, p.317.

31. L. Potter (Pres), *A Passion to Care: Nursing and Nurses Western Suburbs Hospital 1984-1982,* The Western Suburbs Hospital Graduate Nurses' Association, Sydney, 2008, p.39.

32. Editor, British Medical Journal, *War Wounds and Air Raid Casualties*, H.K. Lewis and Co. Ltd., London, 1939, xi-xii.

33. E.B. Clayton, *Electrotherapy and Actinotherapy,* Baillière Tindall and Cox, London, 1949, p.316.

34. H.E. Cuff & G.W.T. Pugh, *Practical Nursing including Hygiene and Dietetics* (7th ed), William Blackwood & Sons Ltd, London, 1928, p.621.

35. Clayton, *Electrotherapy and Actinotherapy,* pp.150, 320-1.

36. A. Gregory, *The Ever Open Door: A history of the Royal Melbourne Hospital 1848-1998,* Hyland House, Melbourne, 1998, p.298; J. Frederick Watson, *The History of the Sydney Hospital from 1811 to 1911,* Government Printer, Sydney, 1911, p.178.

37. Gregory, *The Ever Open Door,* p.298.

38. Butler, *Special Problems and Services,* p.275; Gregory, *The Ever Open Door,* p.152.

39. R. Rae, 'Ellen Julia Gould: a civilian nurse and founder of the military nursing tradition in Australia (1860-1941)' *Journal of the Royal Australian Historical Society,* 92(2), 2006, pp.172-3.

40. Butler, *Gallipoli, Palestine and New Guinea,* p.419.

41. Butler, *Special Problems and Services,* p.601 (*n*).

42. P. Adam-Smith, *Australian Women at War,* Penguin Books Australia Ltd, Melbourne, 1996, p.30.

43. C.E.W. Bean, *Anzac to Amiens* (5th ed.), Australian War Memorial, Canberra, 1968, p.532 (*table*).

44. Correspondence, Jessie Tomlins to Margaretta Tomlins, 8 June1919, copy in possession of author.

45. C. Woodham-Smith, *Florence Nightingale 1820-1910,* Constable and Company Ltd, London, 1950, pp.126-8.

46. A.Maud Kellett interviews, C. Donnelly (no. 18), F.M. Howitt (no. 41), AWM, Canberra.

47. Elsie Tranter diary, 27 October 1917, in G. M. Gillings and J. Richards (eds), *...in all those lines: The diary of Sister Elsie Tranter 1916-1919,* s/p.2008, p.81.

48. Anne Donnell, *Letters of an Australian Army Sister,* Angus and Robertson Ltd, Sydney, 1920, pp.59, 75.

49. Narrative, Blodwyn E. Williams, *Records of A.G. Butler, Official Historian of Australian Army Medical Services - Nurses' Narratives.*

50. Narrative, Gertrude Davis, *Records of A.G. Butler, Official Historian of Australian Army Medical Services - Nurses' Narratives.*

51. Narrative, Jessie McHardy White, *Records of A.G. Butler, Official Historian of Australian Army Medical Services - Nurses' Narratives,* p.2.

52. J.A. Williams & R.D. Goodman, *Jane Bell, O.B.E. (1873-1959): Lady Superintendent, The Royal Melbourne Hospital (1910-1934),* Royal Melbourne Graduate Nurses' Association, Melbourne, 1988, pp.63-5.

53. Potter, *A Passion to Care,* pp.44-5.

54. Tilton, *The Grey Battalion,* p.40.

55. Donnell, *Letters of an Australian Army Sister*, pp.59-60.

56. Narrative, Emma Cuthbert, *Records of A.G. Butler, Official Historian of Australian Army Medical Services - Nurses' Narratives*.

57. Matron's Report, 2 AAH, Southall, July 1918 cited in M. Barker, *Nightingales in the Mud,* Allen & Unwin, Sydney, 1989, p.163.

58. Narrative, Mabel Brown, *Records of A.G. Butler, Official Historian of Australian Army Medical Services - Nurses' Narratives.*

59. Annual Report 1915-16, NSW Division, Australian Red Cross Society, Sydney, 1916, pp.15-16.

60. Potter, *A Passion to Care,* pp.56-7, p.127.

61. Armidale and New England Hospital Board, 'House Committee Report', 30 September 1915, Newling Archives, University of New England, Armidale, p.330.

62. Armidale and New England Hospital Board, 'Special Meeting of the General Committee', 7 March 1916, Newling Archives, University of New England, Armidale.

63. A. Hyslop, *Sovereign Remedies: A History of Ballarat Base Hospital 1850s to 1980s,* Allen and Unwin Australia Pty Ltd, Sydney, 1989, p.214.

64. Armidale and New England Hospital Board, 'Board Report 1916', Newling Archives, Armidale.

65. Butler, *Special Problems and Services,* p.588.

66. Rose Creal, Discharge Summary in *Military Forces of the Commonwealth Papers.*

67. B.F. Cape, *Baillière's Nurses' Dictionary* (14th ed), London, 1957, p.6.

68. Correspondence, Alisha Baird Omar (previous Deputy Matron Bridgman of Sydney Hospital), 19 January 1961, 53 Carcoar Street, Blayney, Lucy Osburn - Nightingale Foundation, Sydney Hospital & Sydney Eye Hospital, Sydney copy in *Ruth Rae Collection*, National Nursing Archives, Canberra.

69. Rose Ann Creal, Death Certificate (No 1921/009915), Creal, *Births, Deaths and Marriages Registration Act 1995* copy in *Ruth Rae Collection*, National Nursing Archives, Canberra.

70. Cape, *Baillière's Nurses' Dictionary*, pp.67-8, 259, 284.

71. Freda MacDonnell 'Creal, Rose Ann (1865 - 1921)', *Australian Dictionary of Biography,* National Centre of Biography, Australian National University,Volume 8, Melbourne University Press, Melbourne, 1981, pp.142-3.

72. Ann M. Mitchell 'Maitland, Sir Herbert Lethington (1868 - 1923)', *Australian Dictionary of Biography,* National Centre of Biography, Australian National University,Volume 10, Melbourne University Press, Melbourne, 1986, pp.387-388.

73. Freda MacDonnell 'Creal, Rose Ann (1865 - 1921)', *Australian Dictionary of Biography,* pp.142-3.

74. W.S.T. 'Farewell Matron Creal - Mother Chief of Hospital - Friend of Broken Humanity' (n/d) in Lucy Osburn - Nightingale Foundation copy in *Ruth Rae Collection*, National Nursing Archives, Canberra.

75. Correspondence Miss E. Pidgeon (Matron, Nightingale Wing, Sydney Hospital) to F. Arnold, Monumental Sculptors, 53 Regent Street, Sydney, 14 May 1948 in historical file, Lucy Osburn - Nightingale Foundation, copy in *Ruth Rae Collection*, National Nursing Archives, Canberra.

76. Last will and testament of Rose Ann Creal dated 18 August 1916 in Probate file of Rose Ann Creal, copy in *Ruth Rae Collection*, National Nursing Archives, Canberra. The author gratefully acknowledges Selena Williams for providing probate details of Rose Creal.

77.This change occurred in the late 1960s.When the '*NSW Nurses' Registration Board changed to a new system of electronically generated and marked, multiple-choice format for examinations, hospital-based examinations were abandoned*' and the '*Rose Creal prize was awarded to the Sydney Hospital nurse who gained the highest marks in the State examinations*' - Late Judith Cornell, 'Sydney Hospital Special

Nursing Awards', in historical file, Lucy Osburn - Nightingale Foundation in *Ruth Rae Collection*, National Nursing Archives, Canberra.

33 Professional and Personal Legacies

1. M Tilton, *The Grey Battalion*, Angus and Robertson Ltd, Sydney, 1933, foreword.

2. Mark Day, 'Gallant girls under fire', *The Weekend Australian (Inquirer)*, 30-31 August 2008, p.29.

3. Correspondence, Private Records Collections (PR 00596) AWM, Canberra; Correspondence, Katherine Pawley (assistant curator) to Ruth Rae, 1 June 2005, Official Records, AWM, Canberra in *Ruth Rae Collection*, National Nursing Archives, Canberra. Note: The Central Army Records Office, Victoria Barracks, Melbourne recorded the date of death of Elsie Grant as 12 August 1918 (reviewed by author 25 February 2003). The author gratefully acknowledges Katherine Pawley who provided background information on Sister Elsie Rose Grant; Mark Day, 'Gallant girls under fire' *The Week-End Australian (Inquirer)*, 30-31 August 2008, p.29.

4. J. Bassett, *Guns and Brooches: Australian Army Nursing from the Boer War to the Gulf War*, Oxford University Press, Melbourne, 1992, p.99.

5. Returned Sailors and Soldiers' Imperial League of Australia 'Official Year Book 1937', R.S. and S.I.L.A. (NSW Branch), Anzac Memorial, Hyde Park, Sydney, p.193; R.Rae, *First World War Commemorative Nominal Roll*, ACN Trilogy, Canberra, 2015.

6. Telephone interview, Ruth Rae with John Sargent (nephew of Hilda Williams and son of Edith Lillian Sargent nee Williams), 27 November 2004; Correspondence, John Sargent to Ruth Rae, 7 December 2004 in *Ruth Rae Collection*, National Nursing Archives, Canberra.

7. C. Fallows, *Love and War: Stories of War Brides from the Great War to Vietnam*, Bantam Books, Sydney, 2002, p.109.

8. Telephone interview, Ruth Rae with John Sargent, 27 November 2004; Correspondence, John Sargent to Ruth Rae, 7 December 2004 in *Ruth Rae Collection*, National Nursing Archives, Canberra.

9. V. Brittain, *Testament of Youth*, Virago Press, London, 2006 (first published by Victor Gollancz Limited 1933), p.172.

10. Narrative, Victor Mitton Ridgway (brother to Doris) dated 22 November 1970, copy given to author by Mr Ian Ridgway (nephew of Doris) in June 2005 in *Ruth Rae Collection*, National Nursing Archives, Canberra.

11. J.Durdin, *Eleven Thousand Nurses – A History of Nurse Education at the Royal Adelaide Hospital 1889-1993*, Royal Adelaide Hospital, 1999, p.236.

12. Narrative, Victor Mitton Ridgway, 22 November 1970 in *Ruth Rae Collection*, National Nursing Archives, Canberra.

13.Durdin, *Eleven Thousand Nurses*, p.230.

14. Narrative, Victor Mitton Ridgway, 22 November 1970 in *Ruth Rae Collection*, National Nursing Archives, Canberra.

15. Durdin, *Eleven Thousand Nurses*, p.237.

16. AWM Nominal Roll: http://www.awm.gov.au/database/[online 6 March 2008]; Nurses' Memorial Foundation of South Australia Incorporated, *Nursing –150 years of Caring in South Australia*, The South Australian Trained Nurses' Centenary Committee, Adelaide,1938 (Reprinted with 1939-1945 supplement in 1989).

17. AWM Nominal Roll: http://www.awm.gov.au/database/[online 6 March 2008].

18. E.I. Uren, 'Thousands of Miles' in Lieutenant Colonel Edith DK Eadie (nee Butler) (ed) *With the AANS 1939-1945*, (ISBN 0 646 23629 6) no page numbers, circa 1995.

19. Dorothy Mary Armstrong, *The First Fifty Years: A history of nursing at the Royal Prince Alfred Hospital, Sydney from 1882 to 1932,* The Royal Prince Alfred Hospital Graduate Nurses' Association, Sydney, 1965, p.89.

20. Brittain, *Testament of Youth*, p.568.

21. A.Maud Kellett interview (no.119) of Sister J. Tomlins, AWM, Canberra, 1919; Bassett, *Guns and Brooches*, p.83.

22. R. Goodman, *Our War Nurses: The History of the Royal Australian Army Nursing Corps 1902-1988,* Boolarong Publications, Brisbane, 1988, p.118.

23. V. Hobbs, *But Westward Look – Nursing in Western Australia 1829-1979,* University of Western Australia Press for the Royal Australian Nursing Federation (WA Branch), Perth, 1980, p.115.

24. Ann M. Mitchell, 'Kellett, Adelaide Maud (1873 - 1945)', *Australian Dictionary of Biography,* National Centre of Biography, Australian National University, Volume 9, Melbourne University Press, Melbourne, 1983, pp.549-550.

25. '200 Years of Nursing – A Bicentennial Photographic History' in *The Lamp*.Journal of the NSW Nurses Association, April 1988, p.22.

26. Betty Jeffrey, *White Coolies,* Angus and Robertson, Sydney, 1954; Lynette Ramsay Silver, *Sister Bullwinkel: The untold, uncensored story,* Sally Milner Publishing, 2025.

27. R. Lynette Russell (ed.), *The Life and Times of Muriel Knox Doherty 1896-1988,* NSW College of Nursing, Sydney, 1996, p.7; Armstrong, *The First Fifty Years,* p.15.

28. M.K. Doherty, M.B. Sirl, & O.I. Ring, *Modern Practical Nursing Procedures,* Dymocks Book Arcade Ltd., Sydney, 1944, p.478.

29. Hobbs, *But Westward Look,* pp.72-3.

30. Minnie Jane Lightbody, *Military Forces of the Commonwealth Papers,* NAA, Canberra.

31. Kings Park Memorial, Perth, WA (viewed by author February 2003).

32. Narrative, Evelyn Vickers Foote, *Records of A.G. Butler, Official Historian of Australian Army Medical Services – Nurses' Narratives,* AWM, Canberra.

33. Death certificate in Mary Florence Stafford, *Military Forces of the Commonwealth Papers,* NAA, Canberra.

34. Correspondence, Mrs Ivey (sister) in Mary Florence Stafford, *Military Forces of the Commonwealth Papers.*

35. Correspondence, Officer-in-Charge, Victoria Barracks, Melbourne to Headquarters, Keswick, SA, 11 July 1925 in Mary Florence Stafford *Military Forces of the Commonwealth Papers;* Photograph, The Royal Adelaide Hospital Honour Board, Adelaide, taken by author February 2003 (*Ruth Rae Collection,* National Nursing Archives, Sydney).

36. Nurses' Memorial Foundation of South Australia Incorporated, *Nursing –150 years of Caring in South Australia,* p.208.

37. A.G. Butler, *The Official History of the Australian Army Medical Services in the war of 1914-1918: Special Problems and Service*s, Vol 3, Australian War Memorial Canberra, 1943, p.455.

38. C. Coulthard-Clark, *Soldiers in Politics: The Impact of the Military on Australian Political Life and Institutions,* Allen & Unwin Pty Ltd., Sydney, 1996, pp.123-4.

39. Bassett, *Guns and Brooches,* pp.96-7.

40. Hobbs, *But Westward Look,* p.61.

41. Edith Jackson, *Military Forces of the Commonwealth Papers.*

42. 'Edith Cavell file' F 940.394/5, Mitchell Library of the State Library of NSW, Sydney.

43. 'Medical Report on an Invalid, 11 AGH, 10 March 1920' in Irene McPhail, *Military Forces of the Commonwealth Papers.*

44. Returned Sailors' and Soldiers' Imperial League of Australia 'Official Year Book 1937', RS&SILA (NSW Branch), Anzac Memorial, Hyde Park, Sydney, p.246.

45. Irene McPhail, *Military Forces of the Commonwealth Papers.*

46. 'ATNA Rules and Regulations & Schedule of Study, clause (iv)' reprinted in Hobbs, *But Westward Look,* p.231.

47. Rose Creal, *Military Forces of the Commonwealth Papers.*

48. Mary Dickenson, 'Nowland, Evelyn Grace Ione (1887 - 1974)', *Australian Dictionary of Biography,* National Centre of Biography, Australian National University, Supplementary Volume, Melbourne University Press, Melbourne, 2005, p.308.

49. Durdin, *Eleven Thousand Nurses,* pp.49-51.

50. E. Burchill, *Australian Nurses since Nightingale 1860-1990,* Spectrum Publications Pty Ltd, Melbourne, 1992, pp.48,79.

51. A. Gregory, *The Ever Open Door – A History of the Royal Melbourne Hospital 1848-1998,* Hyland House, Melbourne, 1998, pp.201-2.

52. Burchill, *Australian Nurses since Nightingale 1860-1990,* pp.35-6.

53. Gregory, *The Ever Open Door,* p.111.

54. Correspondence, Jessie Tomlins to Margaretta Tomlins, 28 July 1917, copy in possession of author.

55. Mary Dickenson, 'Nowland, Evelyn Grace Ione (1887 - 1974)', *Australian Dictionary of Biography,* p.308.

56. Research relating to this topic has been previously published in R. Rae 'An historical account of shell-shock during the First World War and reforms in mental health in Australia 1914-1939', *International Journal of Mental Health Nursing,* 2007, 16: 266-273; R. McMullin, *Pompey Elliott,* Scribe Publications Pty Ltd, Melbourne, 2002, pp.655-6.

57. E.S. Conklin, *Principles of Abnormal Psychology,* George Allen & Unwin Ltd, London, 1928, p.79.

58. W.M. O'Neil, 'Lovell, Henry Tasman (1878 - 1958)', *Australian Dictionary of Biography,* National Centre of Biography, Australian National University, Volume 10, Melbourne University Press, Melbourne, 1986, pp.155-6.

59. Butler, *Special Problems and Services,* pp.57-8.

60. S. Ebury, *Weary: The life of Sir Edward Dunlop* Penguin Books, Melbourne, 1994, pp.258-9.

61. Stephen Garton, 'Winn, Roy Coupland (1890 - 1963)', *Australian Dictionary of Biography,* National Centre of Biography, Australian National University, Volume 12, Melbourne University Press, Melbourne, 1990, pp.540-1.

62. Electronic correspondence, Mary Ann Hamilton (NSW Heritage Office) to Ruth Rae, 7 July 2005; Perdita M McCarthy, 'Pocock, Mary Anne (Bessie) (1863 - 1946)', *Australian Dictionary of Biography,* National Centre of Biography, Australian National University, Volume 11, Melbourne University Press, Melbourne, 1988, p.251-2; Perdita M. McCarthy, 'Gould, Ellen Julia (1860 - 1941)', *Australian Dictionary of Biography,* National Centre of Biography, Australian National University, Volume 9, Melbourne University Press, Melbourne, 1983, pp.59-60.

63. Oral history interview, Joan Durdin with Enid Cherry, Royal Adelaide Hospital Heritage Office, Adelaide.

64. R. Goodman, *Queensland Nurses: Boer War to Vietnam,* Boolarong Publications, Brisbane, 1985, p.32.

65. Janice McCarthy 'Wilson, Grace Margaret (1879-1957)', *Australian Dictionary of Biography,* National Centre of Biography, Australian National University, Volume 12, Melbourne University Press, 1990,

pp.522-3.

66. Goodman, *Our War Nurses*, p.68.

67. H. Paterson, *'5:30, Nurse!': The story of the Alfred Nurses*, History Books, Melbourne, 1996, p.102.

68. J.A. Williams & R.D. Goodman, *Jane Bell, O.B.E. 1873-1959*, The Royal Melbourne Hospital Graduate Nurses' Association, Melbourne, 1988, pp.7-8; H. Gregory & C. Brazil, *Bearers of the Tradition: Nurses of the Royal Brisbane Hospital 1888-1993*, Boolarong Publications, Brisbane, 1993, p.222; Paterson, *'5:30, Nurse!'*, p.106.

69. Armstrong, *The First Fifty Years*, p.15.

70. Paterson, *'5:30, Nurse!'*, pp.104, 109.

71. Goodman, *Our War Nurses*, p.119.

72. Janice McCarthy 'Wilson, Grace Margaret (1879-1957)', *Australian Dictionary of Biography*, National Centre of Biography, Australian National University, Volume 12, Melbourne University Press, 1990, pp.522-3.

73. Ruth Henderson cited in Paterson, *'5:30, Nurse!'*, p.110.

74. Janice McCarthy, 'Wilson, Grace Margaret (1879-1957)', *Australian Dictionary of Biography*, pp.522-3.

75. *ibid;* Grace Wilson, *Military Forces of the Commonwealth Papers*, NAA, Canberra. Note: The Australian Dictionary of Biography entry states that she resigned in August 1941 and her AANS Service Record states that the date was 8 October 1941.

76. Grace Wilson, *Military Forces of the Commonwealth Papers.*

77. Janice McCarthy, 'Wilson, Grace Margaret (1879-1957)', *Australian Dictionary of Biography*, pp.522-3.

78. D. Bungey, *Arthur Boyd: A Life*, Allen & Unwin, Sydney, 2007, pp.123, 532, 568-9.

79. Janice McCarthy, 'Wilson, Grace Margaret (1879-1957)', *Australian Dictionary of Biography*, pp.522-3.

80. 'An Angel Honoured', *North-West News*, Wednesday 4 July 2007, Brisbane circulation.

81. Obituary, Miss Jane Bell, *Una*, Nursing Journal, 1959, cited in Williams & Goodman, *Jane Bell, O.B.E. 1873-1959*, p.168.

34 The Final Word

1. R. Brooke, '1914: The Soldier' in G. Walter (ed), *The Penguin Book of First World War Poetry*, Penguin Classics, London, 2004, p.108.

2. V. Brittain, *Testament of Youth*, Virago Press, London, 2006 (first published by Victor Gollancz Limited 1933), p.416.

3. J. Caligari cited in 'Model of a Modern Digger' by Cynthia Banham, *Sydney Morning Herald, Weekend Edition,* March 15-16, 2008, p.31.

4. J. Bassett, *Guns and Brooches: Australian Army Nursing from the Boer War to the Gulf War*, Oxford University Press, Melbourne, 1992, p.8.

5. K.S. Inglis, *Sacred Places: War Memorials in the Australian Landscape*, Melbourne University Press, Melbourne, 1998, p.172.

6. B.H. Liddell Hart, *History of the First World War*, Cassell and Co. Ltd., London, 1970, p.17; B. Jones, *Dictionary of World Biography*, Information Australia, Melbourne, 1994, p.268; H. Strachan, *The First World War,* Simon & Schuster, London, 2003, p.3.

7. P. Singer, *Pushing Time Away*, Harper Perennial, Sydney, 2003, pp.285-6.

8. C. Fallows, *Love and War: Stories of War Brides from the Great War to Vietnam*, Bantam Books, Sydney, 2002, p.20.

9. Ludwig Feuerbach, 'The Essence of Christianity', 1843, edited and abridged by E.Graham Waring and F.W. Strothmann, New York, 1989, p.53.

10. Brittain, *Testament of Youth*, p.134.

11. Plato, *The Trial and Death of Socrates: Four Dialogues* (unabridged), Dover Publications Inc, New York, 1992, p.114.

Appendices

Appendix 1: List of nurses from the Australian colonies who served in the South African (Boer) War (1899-1902)

Name (award/date)	Colony of Origin
E. Nixon *RRC (27.09.1901) MID (04.09.1901)*	NSW
*M. A. (Bessie) Pocock *MID (23.06.1902)*	NSW
*A. Austin	NSW
*P. Frater	NSW
A. G. Garden	NSW
*E. J. (Nellie) Gould	NSW
*E. Hoadley	NSW
*J. B. Johnston	NSW
E. W. Lister	NSW
**M. P. Martin	NSW
A. J. Matchett	NSW
N. Newtown	NSW
Wilcox	NSW
T. E. Woodward	NSW
M. Rawson *RRC(22.08.1902) MID (23.06.1902)*	Victoria
I. Ivey *MID (23.06.02)*	Victoria
J. B. Anderson	Victoria

Name (award/date)	Colony of Origin
F. E. Hines	Victoria
*J. M. Lempriere	Victoria
A. McCready	Victoria
Villiers	Victoria
E. Walter	Victoria
A. M. Chatfield	Queensland
R. A. Hinton	Queensland
B. Huston	Queensland
L. H. M. O'Ryan	Tasmania
M. M. A. Robertson	Tasmania
*A. M. H. Thomson	Tasmania
M. G. A. Warner	Tasmania
K. O. White	Tasmania
M. S. Bidmead *RRC (29.11.1900) MID (23.06.1902) Devoted Service Cross*	South Australia
B. Brooks	South Australia
A. G. Cocks	South Australia
M. A. Glenie *Devoted Service Cross*	South Australia
N. B. Harris	South Australia
M. A. O'Shanahan	South Australia

Name (award/date)	**Colony of Origin**
Samuels	South Australia
A. Teesdale	South Australia
*E. A. Watts	South Australia
*S Armstrong	Western Australia
*E. A. Bole	Western Australia
A. Emmins	Western Australia
B. Milne	Western Australia
L. A. Naylor	Western Australia
M. Nicolay	Western Australia
M. Plover	Western Australia
L. E. Rogers	Western Australia
I. Tchan	Western Australia
Speers	Western Australia
R. L. Shappere *MID (02.12.1899)*	Unknown
D. Burgess	Unknown
A. R. Chutt	Unknown
L. Dawson	Unknown
*G. Fletcher	Unknown
M. A. Grace	Unknown

Name (award/date)	**Colony of Origin**
R. Gwyer	Unknown
B. Kennedy	Unknown
E. Langlands	Unknown
L. Mansfield	Unknown
**E. Marsh	Unknown
**D. Smith	Unknown
**E Smith	Unknown
**M. Steele	Unknown
A. B. Stephenson	Unknown
T. Tiddy	Unknown

*Indicates also served overseas during the First World War.

**Indicates may have served overseas during the First World War.

Appendix 2: First AIF contingent of AANS nurses including rank on enlistment (highest rank), awards received (date gazetted) and name of ship

Name	Rank on enlistment (highest rank)	Awards (dates of Commonwealth Government Gazette Australia)	Ship
Bertha Mary Williams	Sister (HS)	ARRC (25.7.17)	*Omrah*
Constance Mabel Keys	Sister (HS)	MID (19.4.17) ARRC (29.6.17) MID (23.5.19) RRC (3.6.19) Gold Medaille des Epidemies (17.6.19)	*Omrah*
Eunice Muriel Paten	Sister (Acting M)	ARRC (27.11.18)	*Omrah*
Alice Kidd Hart	Sister (HS)	MID (23.5.19)	*Omrah*
(M. A.) Bessie Pocock	Sister (HS)	MID (21.9.16) MID (21.9.16) RRC (21.9.16)	*Argylshire*
Clementina Hay Marshall	Sister (Matron)	ARRC (25.7.17)	*Argylshire*
Nellie Gould	Principal Matron	RRC (6.4.16)	*Euripides*
Julia Bligh Johnston	Sister	ARRC (21.9.16) MID (21.9.16)	*Euripides*
Adelaide Maud Kellett	Sister (Matron)	MID (21.9.16) RRC (25.7.17) CBE (6.10.19) MID (30.10.19)	*Euripides*
Nellie Miles Walker	Sister (Matron)	MID (19.4.17) RRC (29.6.17)	*Euripides*
Alice Joan Twynam	Sister (HS)	MID (21.9.16) RRC (15.9.19)	*Euripides*
Penelope Frater	Sister	N/A	*Euripides*
Mary Mackenzie Finlay	Matron	RRC (29.6.17)	*Shropshire*
Evelyn Augusta Conyers	Sister (Matron-in-Chief)	MID (21.9.16) RRC (21.9.16) CBE (17.6.19) Bar to RRC (25.3.20)	*Shropshire*
Ethel Sarah Davidson	Sister (Matron)	MID (21.9.16) ARRC (21.9.16) RRC (18.4.18) CBE (6.10.19) MID (1.4.20)	*Shropshire*

Appendix 2 (continued)

Name	**Rank on enlistment (highest rank)**	**Awards (dates of Commonwealth Government Gazette Australia)**	**Ship**
Jessie McHardy White	Matron (Principal Matron)	MID (21.9.16) RRC (21.9.16) MID (7.11.18) MBE (23.7.19) Order of St Sava (5th Class – Serbia)Greek Medal of Military Merit (1.4.20)	*Benalla*
Janey M. Lempriere	Sister	N/A	*Benalla*
Hilda Theresa Samsing	Sister	N/A	*Benalla*
Alice E. Kitchen	Sister	N/A	*Benalla*
Margaret Graham	Matron	MID (19.4.17) RRC (29.6.17)	*Asconius*
Louise Ellen White	Sister	MID (18.4.18)	*Asconius*
Annie Heath	Sister	N/A	*Asconius*
Tessa Eleanor Rogers	Sister	N/A	*Asconius*
Alice Gordon King	Sister	MID (21.9.16)	*Geelong*
Janet Radcliffe	Sister	MID (21.9.16)	*Geelong*

Photographs

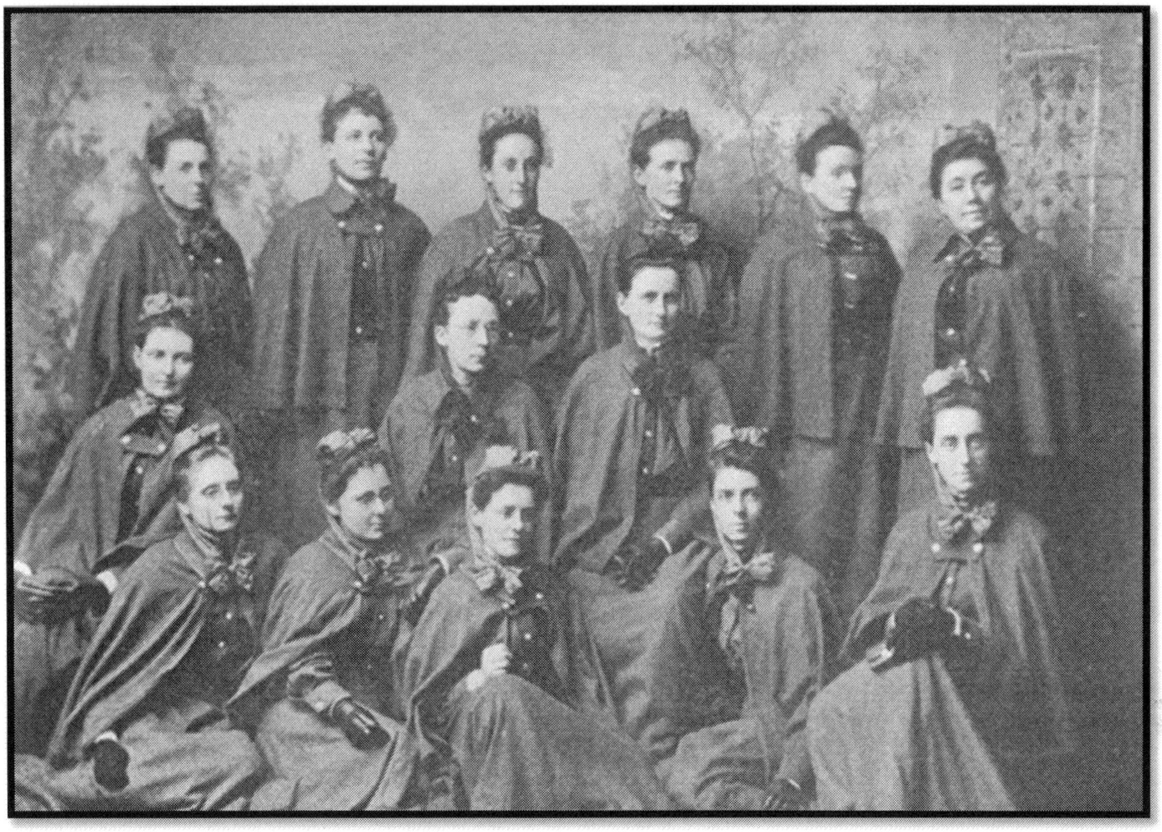

Members of the New South Wales Army Nursing Service Reserve who served in the South African War.
Back row, left to right: Sister Annie Austin, Sister Elizabeth Ward Lister, Sister Mabel Steele, Sister Emily Hoadley, Sister Bessie Pocock, Sister Marion Martin.
Middle row: Sister Annie Matchett, Sister Julia Bligh Johnston, Matron Nellie Gould.
Front row: Sister Elizabeth Nixon, Sister Penelope Frater, Sister Anna Garden, Sister Nancy Newton, Sister Therese Woodward.
(Photograph and information courtesy AWM A02766)

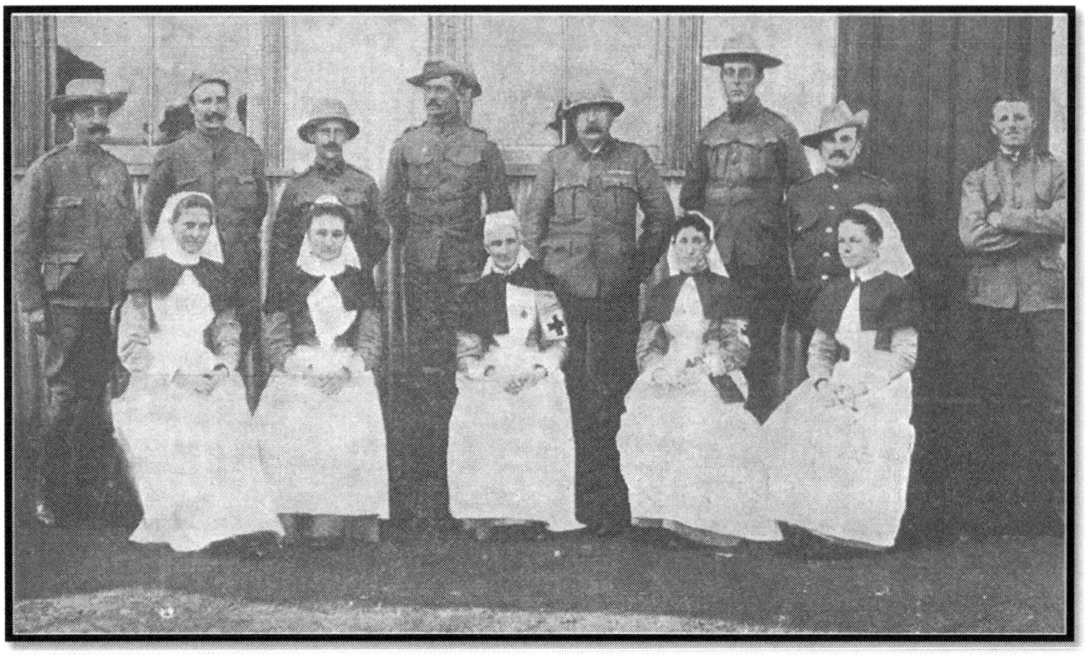

Sister Frances 'Fanny' Hines, **seated on left**, photographed with General Sir Frederick Carrington and medical staff in Rhodesia, died on active service during the Boer War. From Victoria, Hines left for South Africa with the Third Victorian Contingent in March 1900. Posted to Enkeldoorn, she was left alone to care for more than twenty patients; by August she was dead from pneumonia. She was buried with military honours in the cemetery at Bulawayo. NLA, The Australasian, 7 July 1900. (Photograph and caption courtesy AWM)

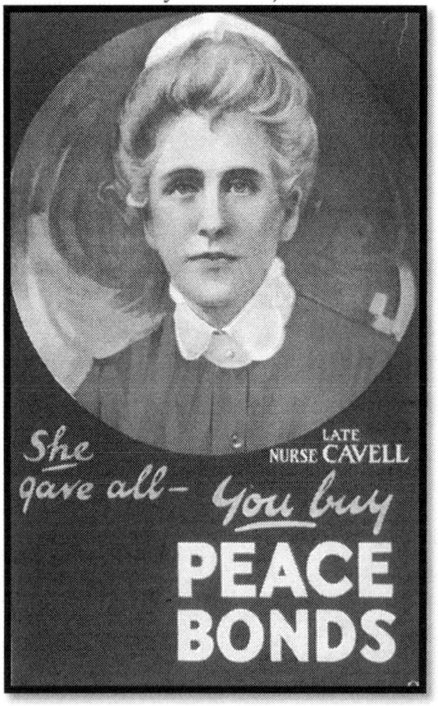

The execution of Edith Cavell created an effective allied propaganda program. (Image courtesy AWM ARTV0002)

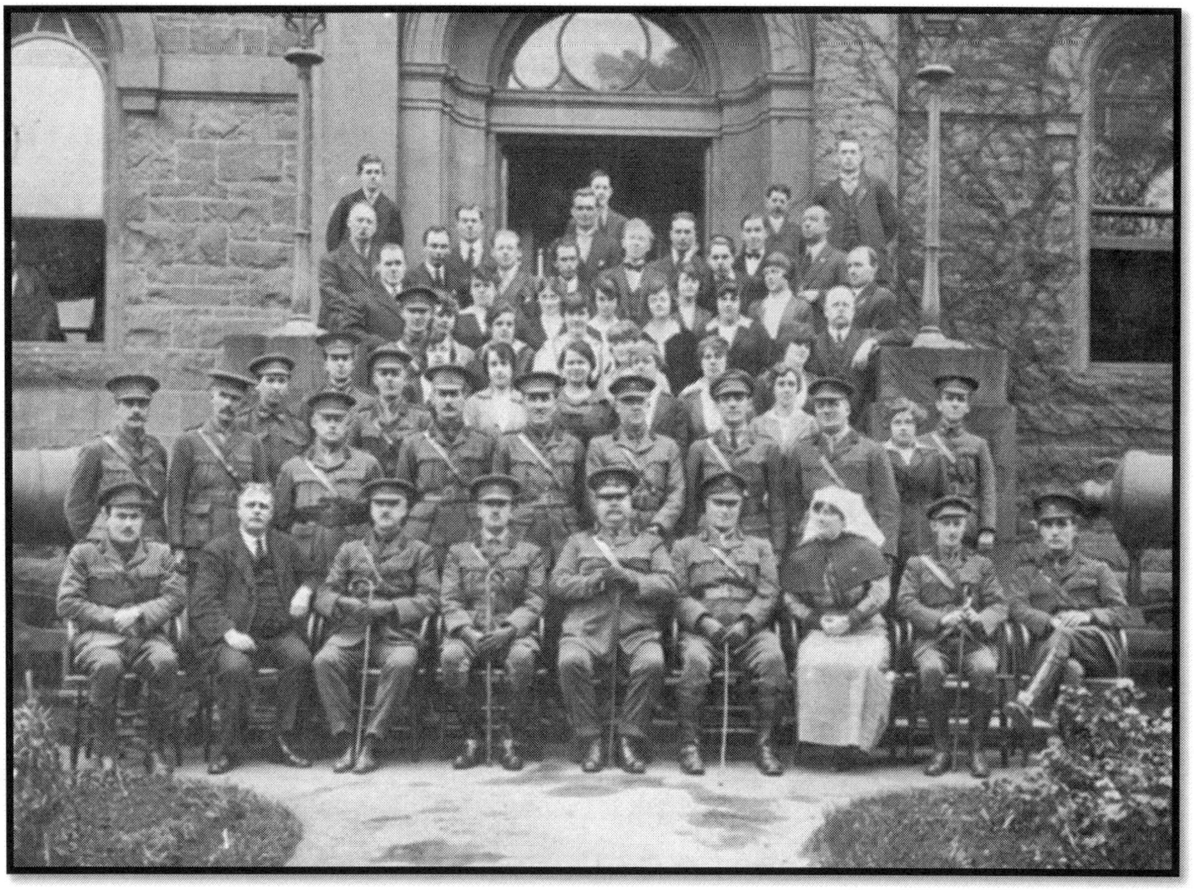

Group portrait taken outside the main entrance of Victoria Barracks, St Kilda Road, Melbourne. In 1901, following Federation, Victoira Barracks became HQ for Department of Defence. Australian based AANS Matron-in-Chief E. Tracey Richardson is seated in front row **(3rd from R)**. There were seventeen female staff members in the Department of Defence. **Below**: Studio portrait E.Tracey Richardson. (Photgraphs and details courtesy AWM P04293002 and below H06179)

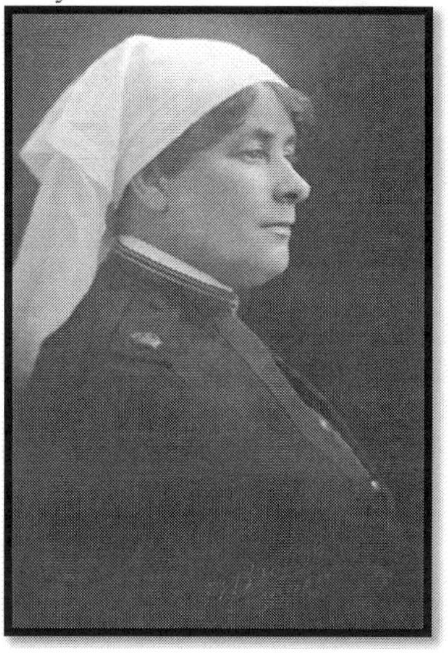

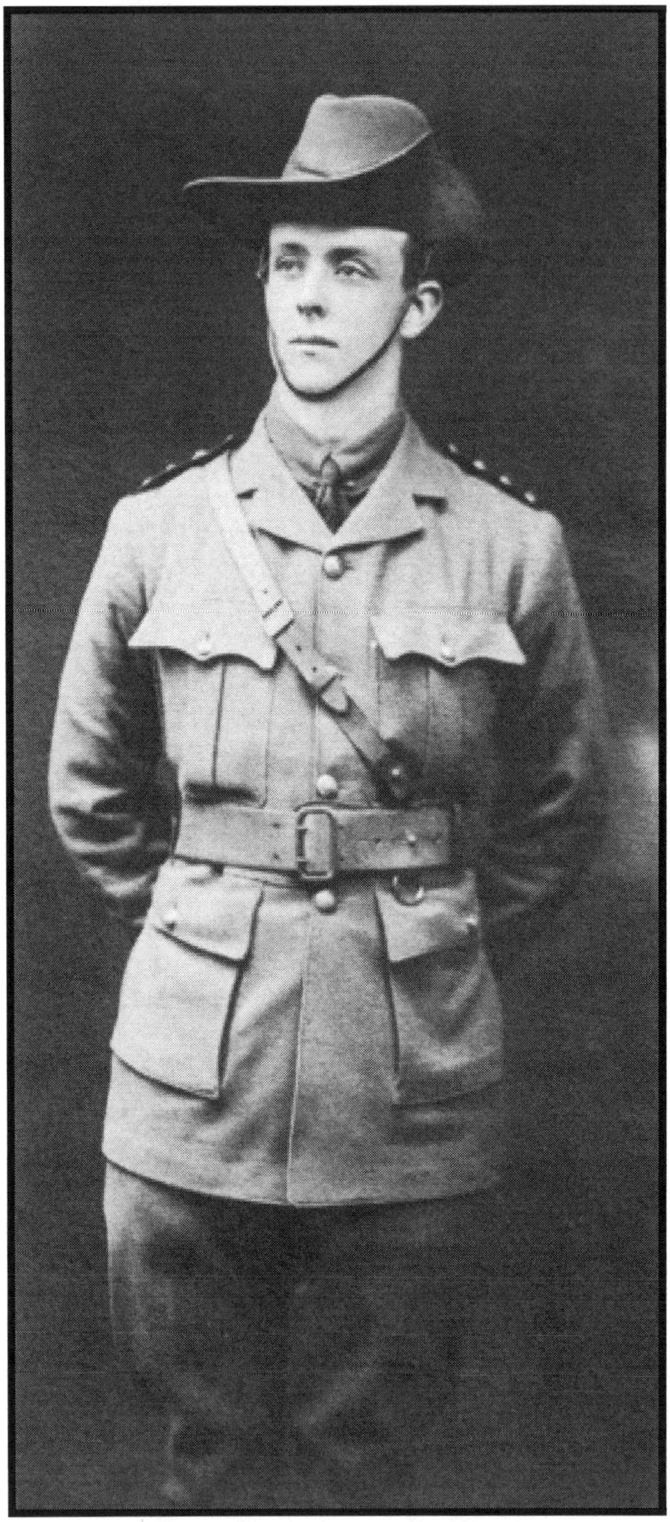

Dr Brian Pockley, AAMC

(Photograph courtesy AWM H19316)

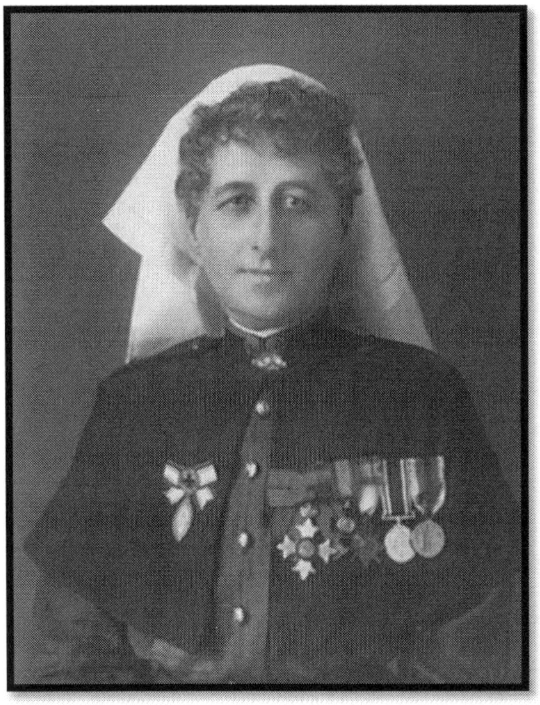

Portrait photograh of Matron-in-Chief (overseas) Evelyn Conyers

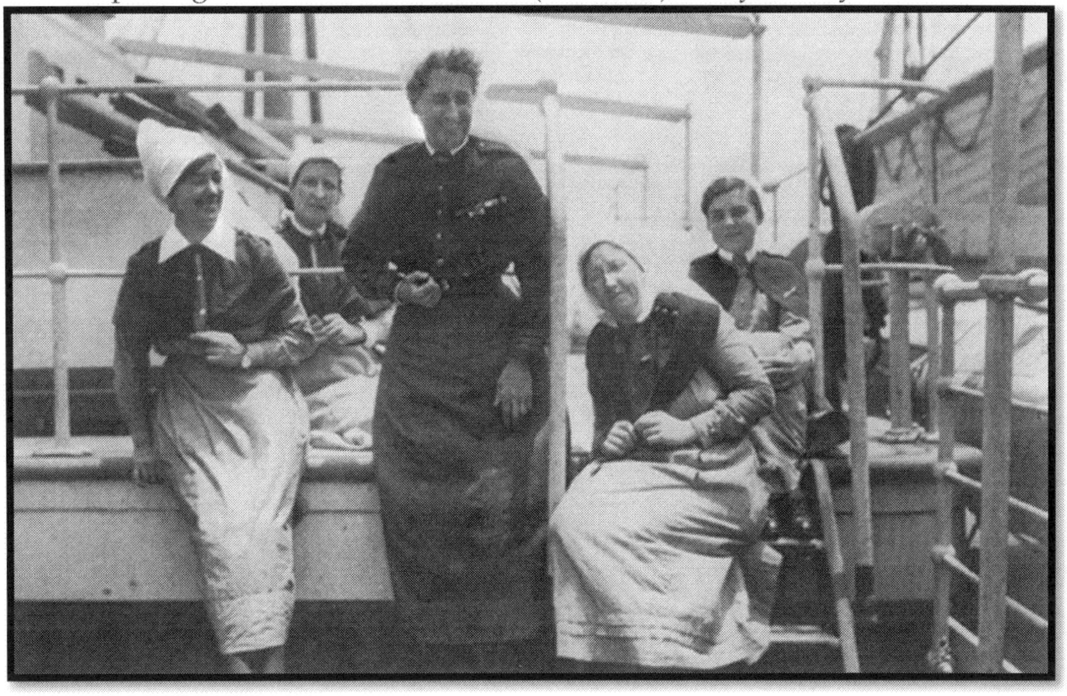

Matron-in-Chief Evelyn Conyers, **centre front**, standing with four unnamed nurses returning to Australia 1919.
(Photographs courtesy AWM M13175 (top) and H06813

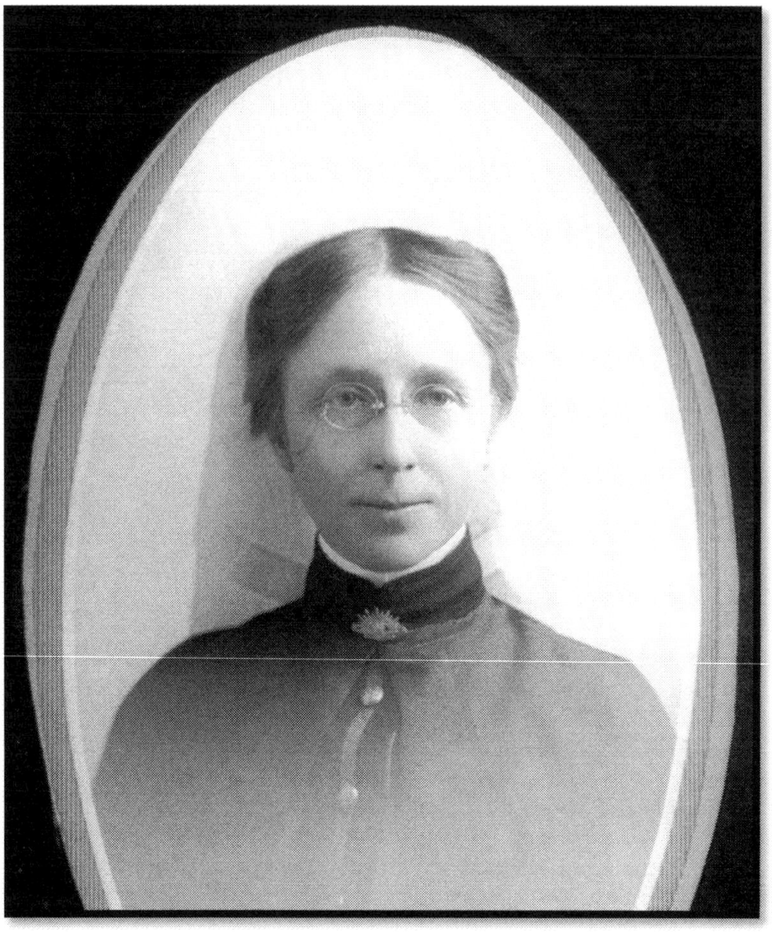

Principal Matron Jane Bell, AANS.
(Photograph courtesy Royal Melbourne Hospital Archives)

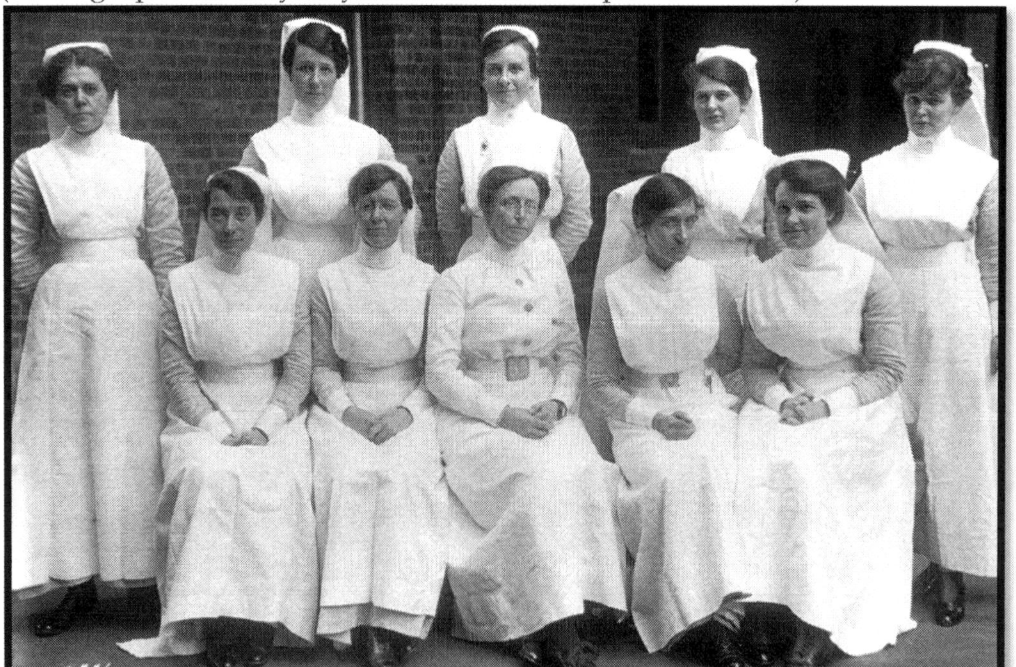

Principal Matron Jane Bell (**centre, seated**) and nurses at 1AGH, Egypt, circa 1915.
(Photograph Courtesy AWM)

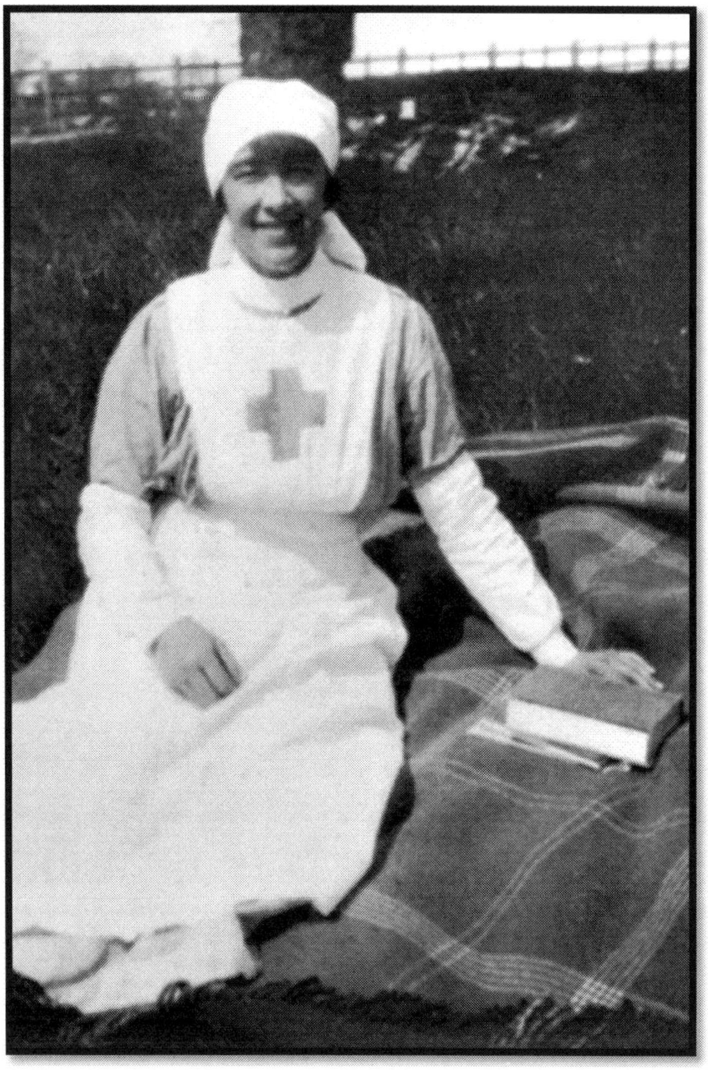

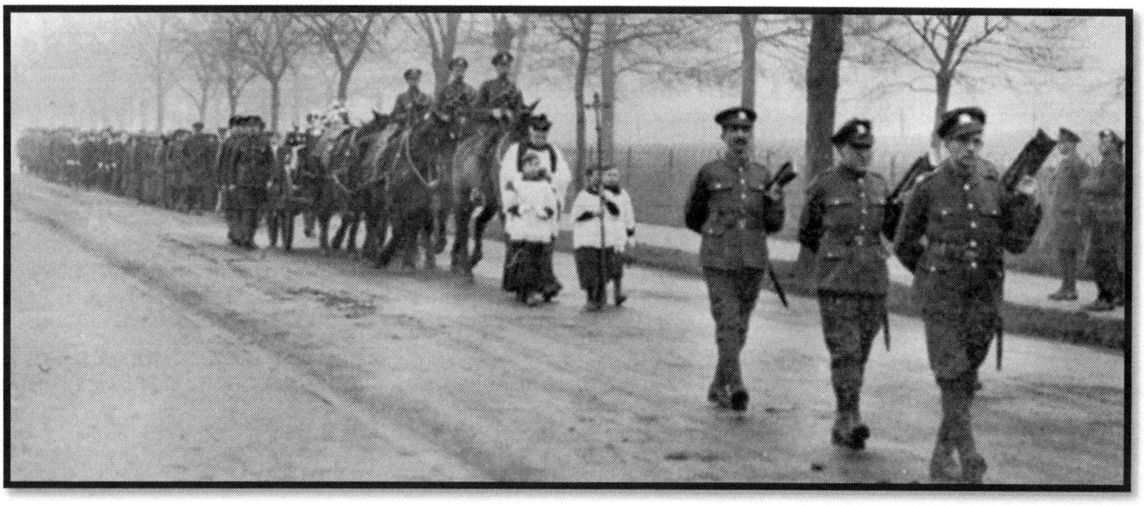

Top: Australian VAD nurse, Adele Brennan, England.
Bottom: Adele Brennan funeral procession.
(**P**hotographs courtesy AWM P05074.002 and AWM P5074.004)

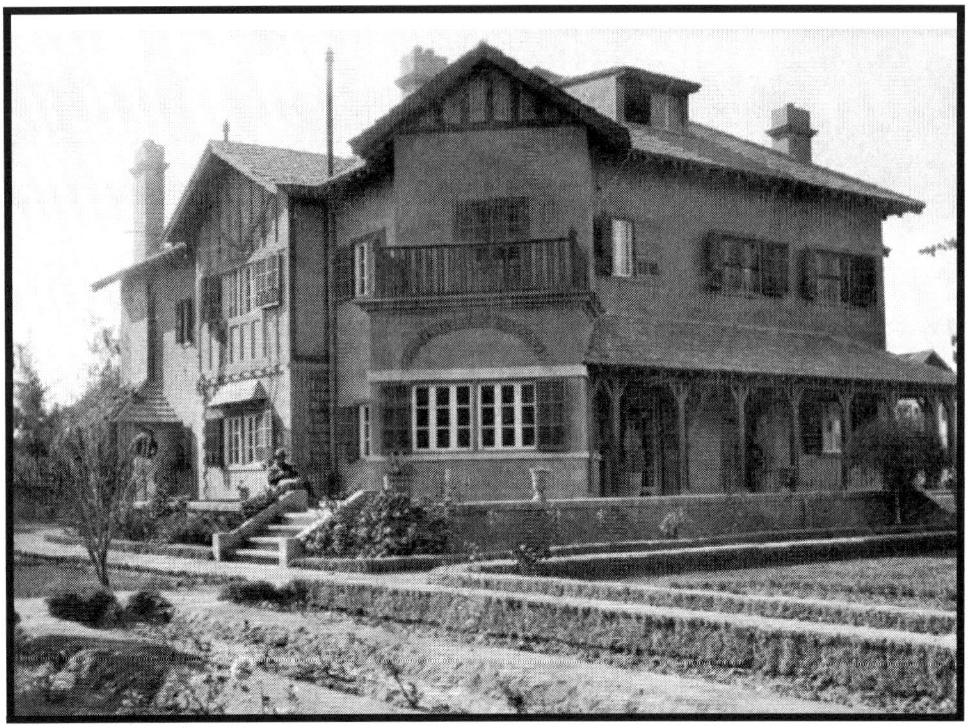

1 ASH, Ismalia, Egypt
(Photograph courtesy AWM P0139.024)

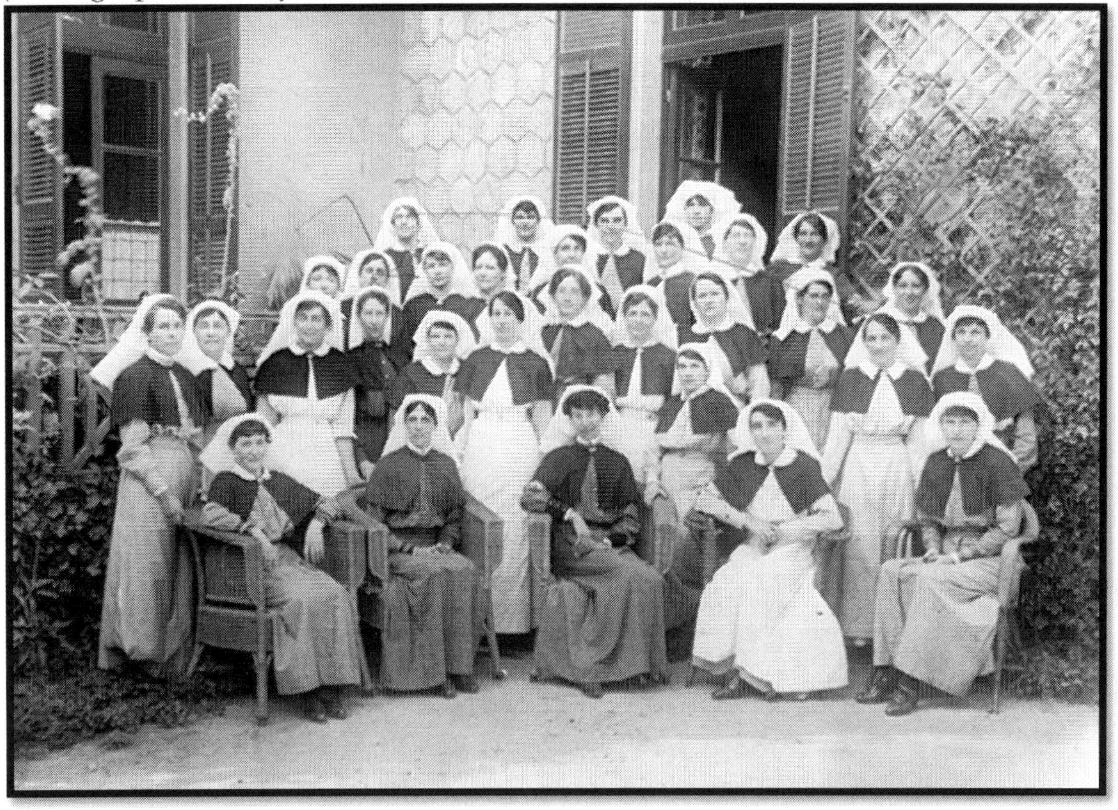

Matron Nellie Miles Walker **(front, seated, third from left)** and staff of 1ASH, Ismailia, Egypt
(Photograph courtesy AWM C02305)

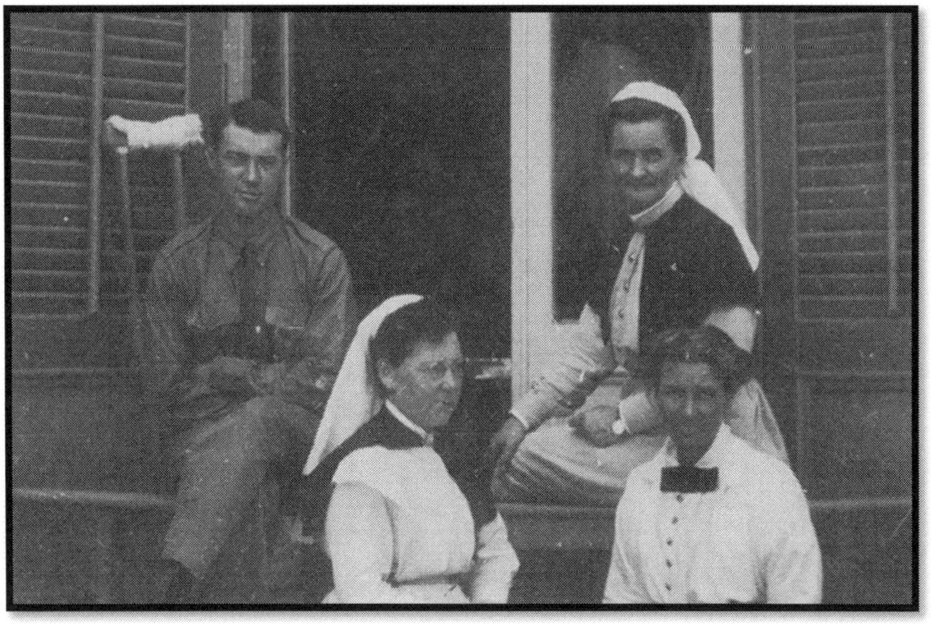

Matron Nellie Gould (**back right**) with Captain Fletcher. Sister Penelope Frater (**front left**) with unidentified Red Cross Nurse at 2AGH, Ghezireh Palace, Egypt, circa 1915 (Photograph P10871.002 courtesy AWM)

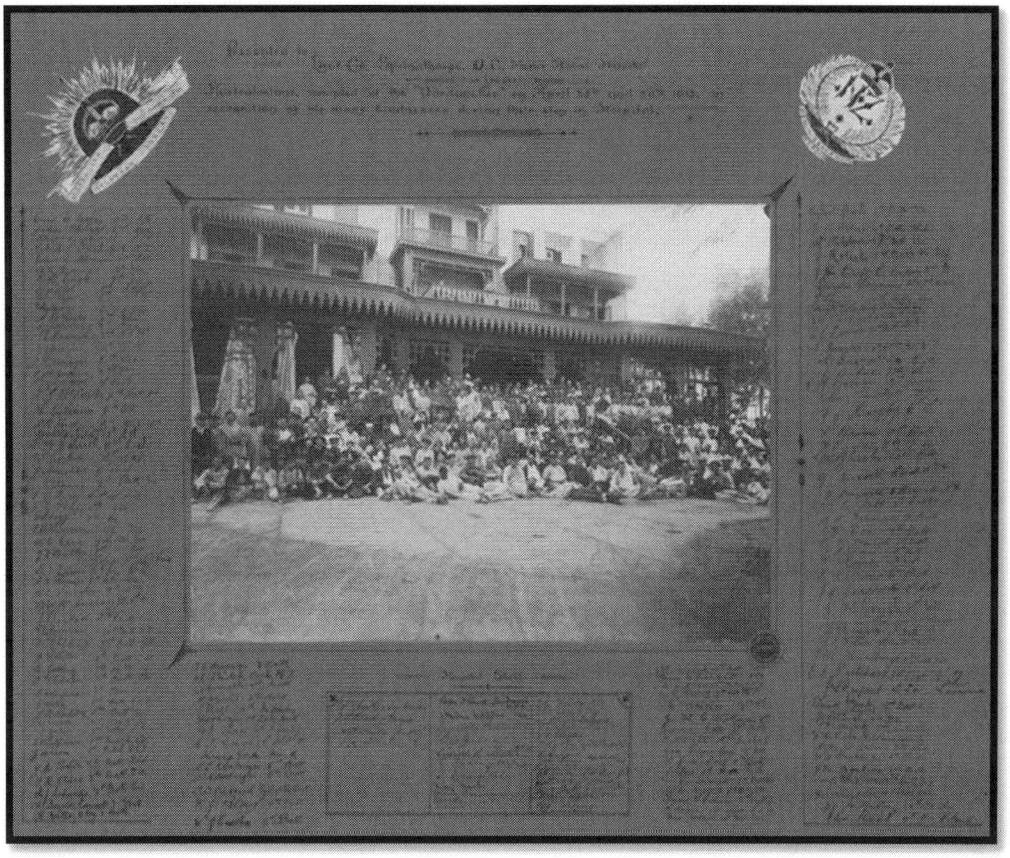

Group portrait with signatures of hospital staff at Mena House Hotel, 2AGH. Presented to Lt Col Springthorpe,OC, '…in recognition of his many kindnesses…' to the Australasians wounded at the Dardanelles. 1915. (Photograph and details courtesy AWM P03291.001)

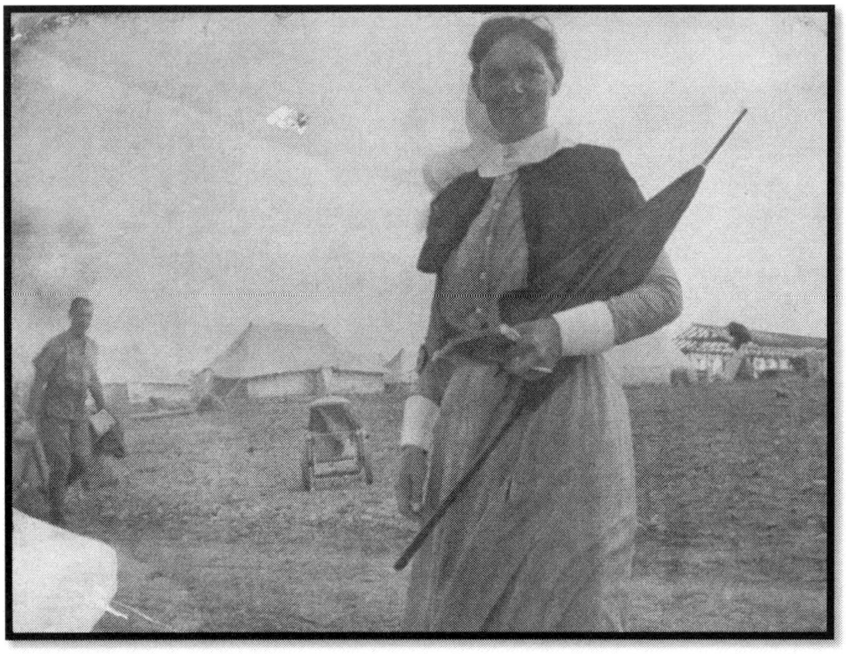

Matron Grace Wilson doing her rounds at her tented hospital, 3AGH on the Greek island of Lemnos during the Gallipoli campaign, 1915.
(Photograph courtesy AWM A05332)

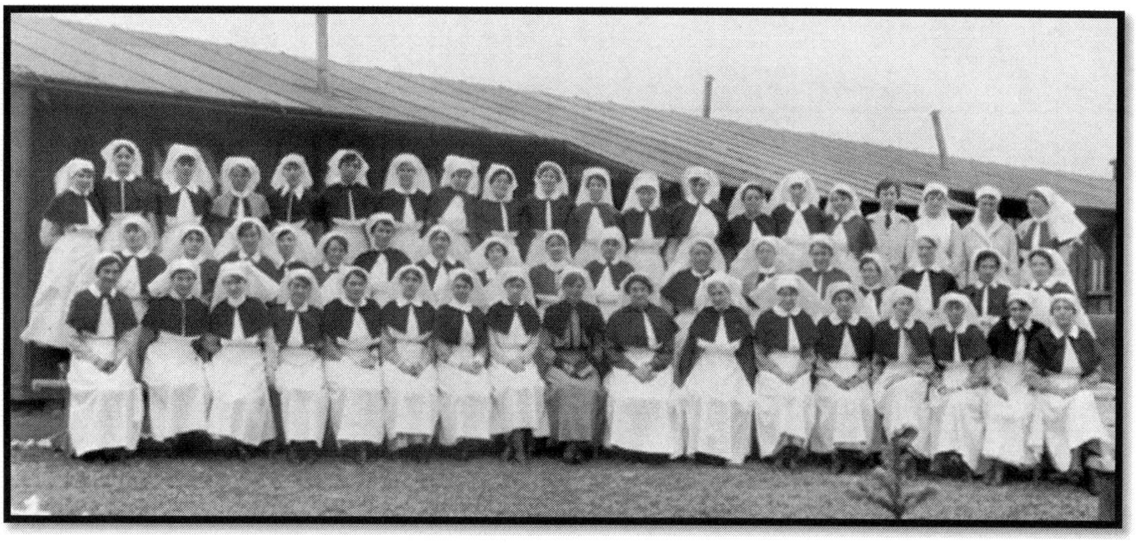

Group portrait of Matron Grace Wilson (**seated middle front row**) and nursing staff 3 AGH, Abbeville, France. 23 June 1918.
Back Row(L-R):Sister Hazelton-Heard;Sister Huxley; SN P.Marsh;Sister Charter (QAIMNSR);Sister Skelly; SN Vicars Foote; Sister Ethel Smith;Sister Callander;Sister D.Thompson;Sister M.Thompson;Sister Gallagher;Sister Linehan;Sister Slater;SN Marquardt;SN Adams; Sister Warne;Miss Bell; Miss Birdwood(VAD);Miss Murdoch(VAD);Sister Fisher (TFNS).
Middle Row(L-R): Sister Cavanagh;Sister Soden;SN Everard;Sister Eulalie Margaret Hamersley;Sister Malster; Sister Sweeney;Sister J.Hall;SN Lindsay;Sister Willock;Sister Elsie Clare Pidgeon;Sister Pierre Humbert;Sister Foxall(TFNS);Sister McFadyen;Sister Winter;Sister M.K.Brown;Sister L.McIntosh;SN M.D.Smith.
Front Row(L-R):SN G.Trebilco;SN M.M.McKay;Sister A.Linklater;Sister V.Drewitt;Sister Chataway;SN Webb;Sister Burbury;Sister Elsie Stewart Greig; Matron Grace Wilson (in dark uniform);Sister Andrews;Sister De Mestre;Sister Fitzgibbon;Sister Steele;Sister Duddy;Sister Belstead;Sister Leslie Smith;Sister Moir.

(Photograph and caption details courtesy AWM E02578)

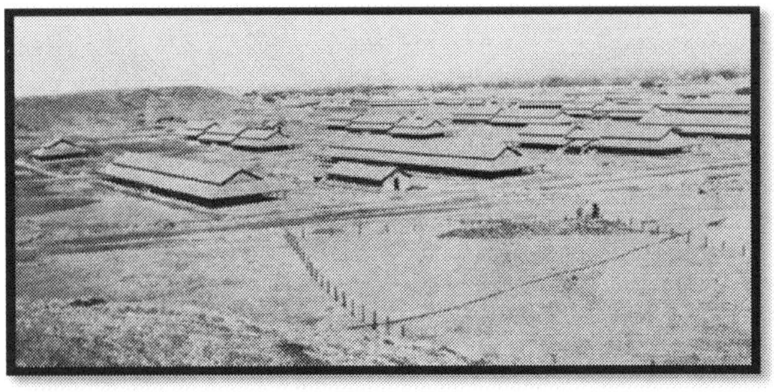

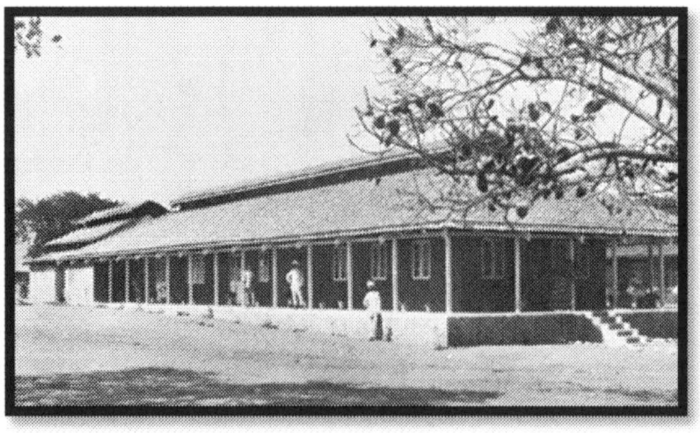

Photographs of 34 WGH, Maharashta, Deolali, India.
(Photographs courtesy AWM P00562.1757 and H12551)

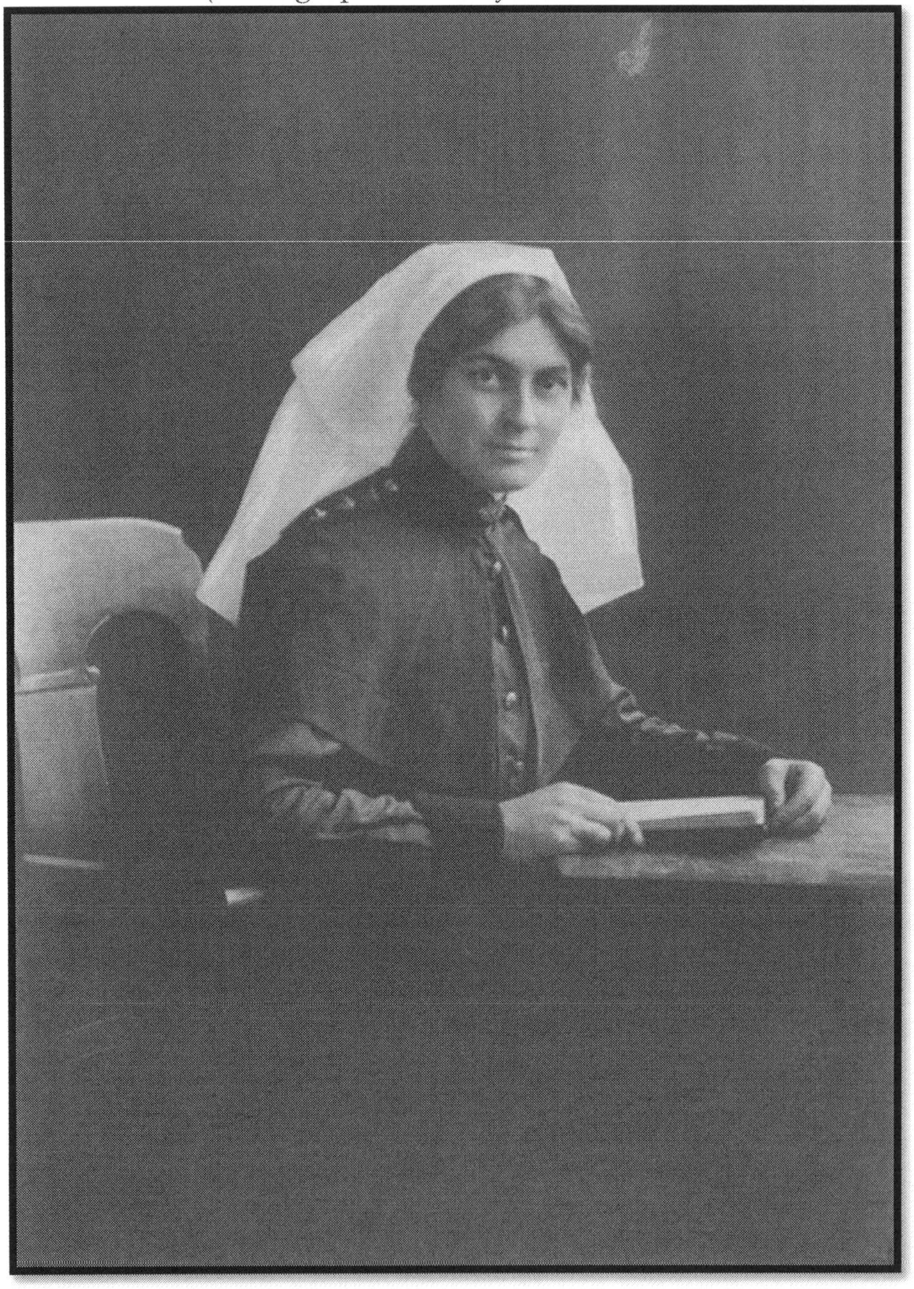

Principal Matron, India, Gertrude Davis.
(Photograph courtesy AWM H15352)

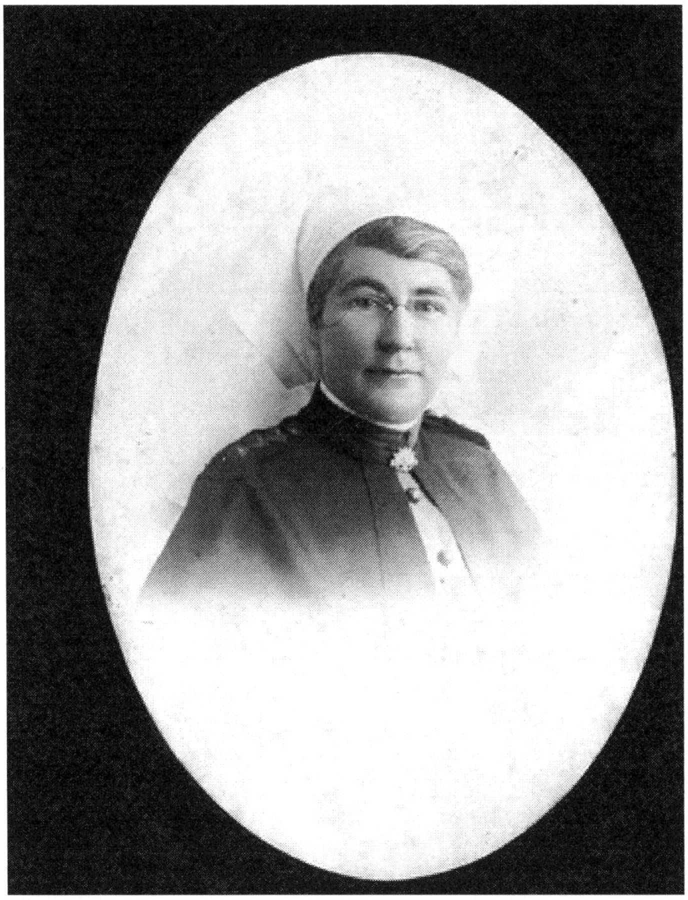

Matron Rose Creal, AANS, circa 1916.
(Reprinted with permission Lucy Osburn-Nightingale Foundation, Sydney Hospital).

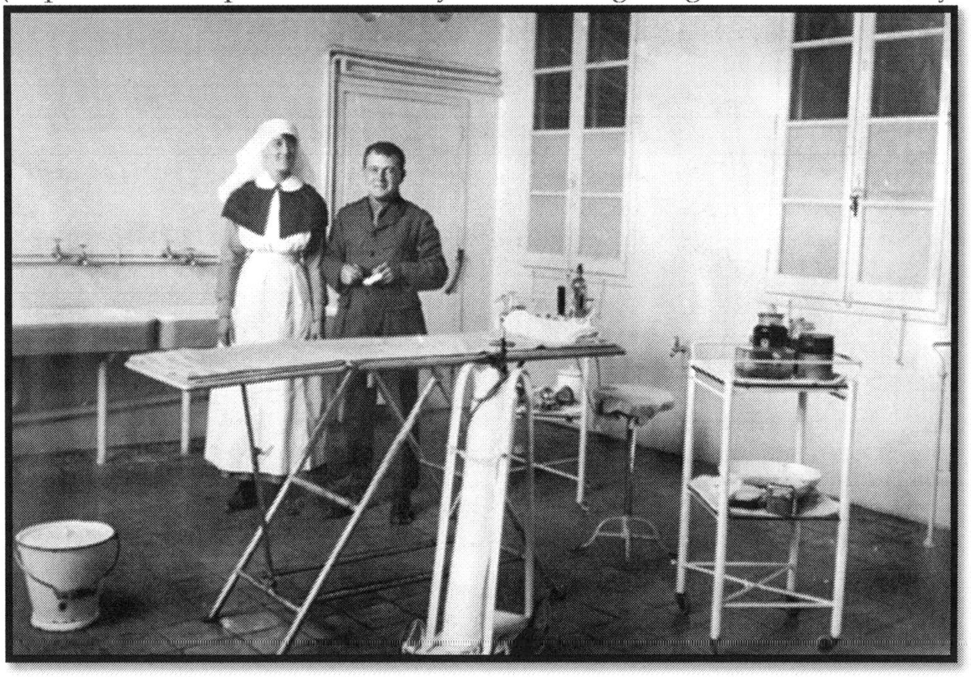

Operating Theatre 14AGH, Abbassia Army Barracks, Egypt
(Photograph courtesy AWM P00812.003)

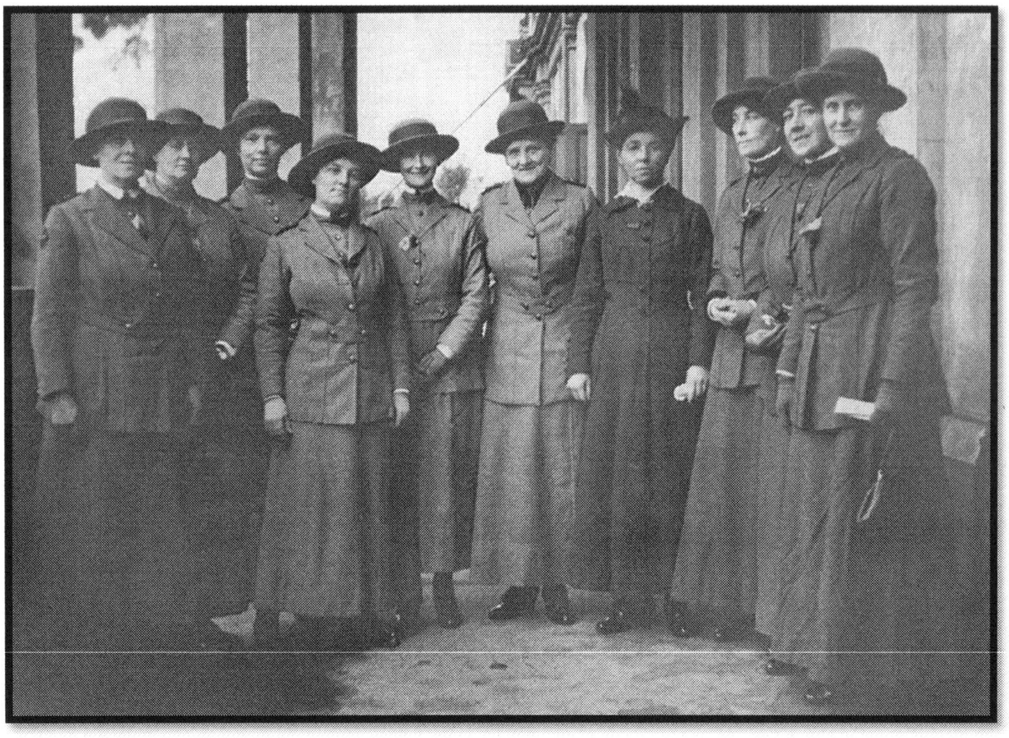

14 June 1917: Group of nurses leave Australia for Salonika with Principal Matron Jessie McHardy White **(5th from right)**. (Photograph courtesy AWM H16005)

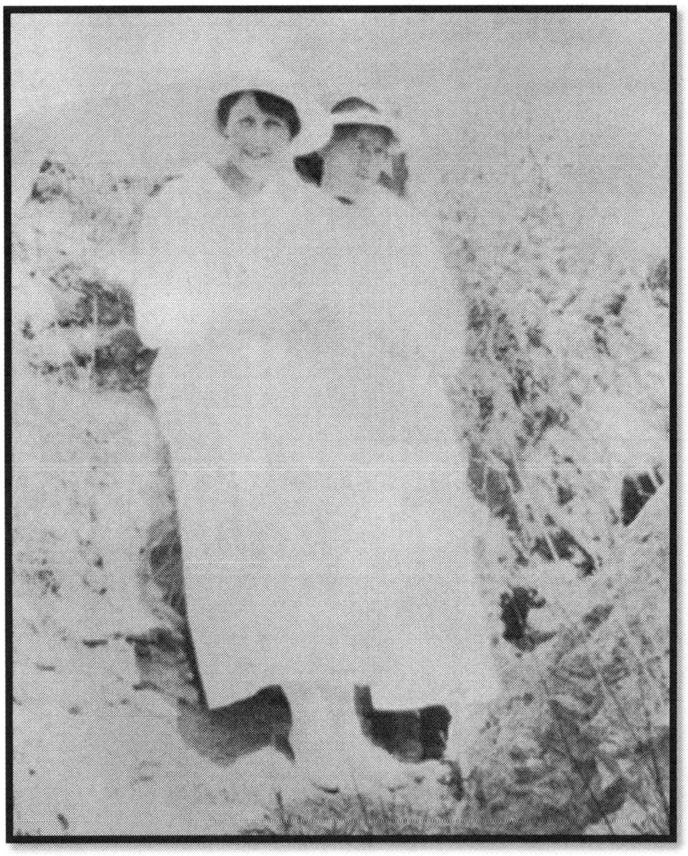

Sisters Gertrude Munro and Amy Christie, Salonika.
(Photograph courtesy AWM; Donor Mrs E.Munro)

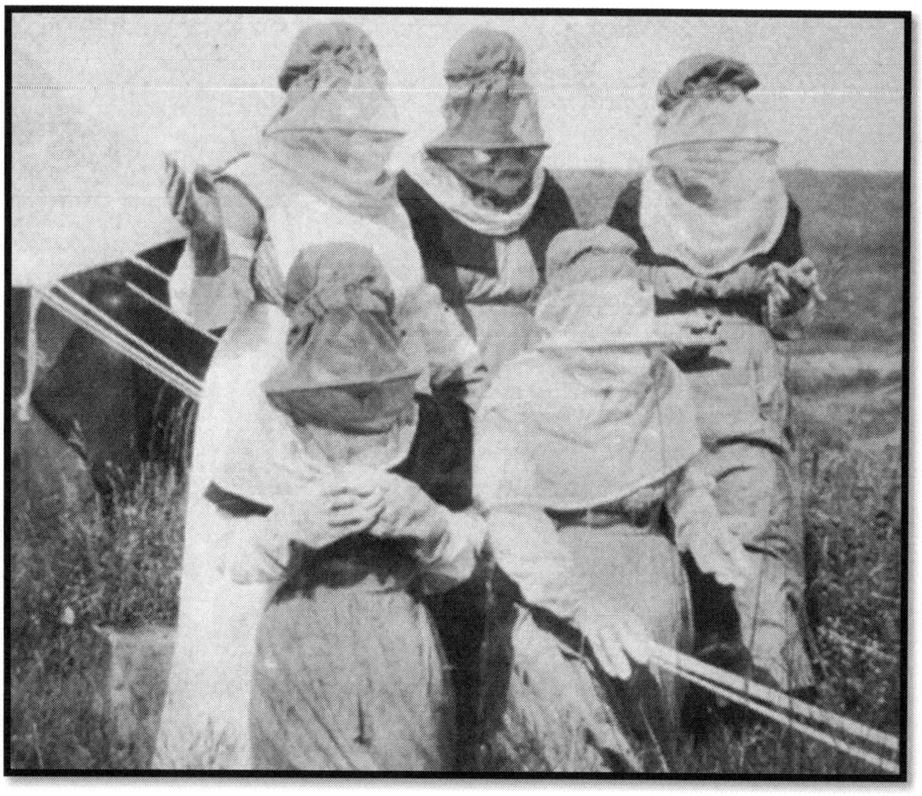

Salonika, Greece c.1918. A group of AANS nurses, 52 BGH, Kalamaria, ready for night duty wearing mosquito protective headdress.
(Photograph courtesy AWM. Donated by PM Jessie McHardy White)

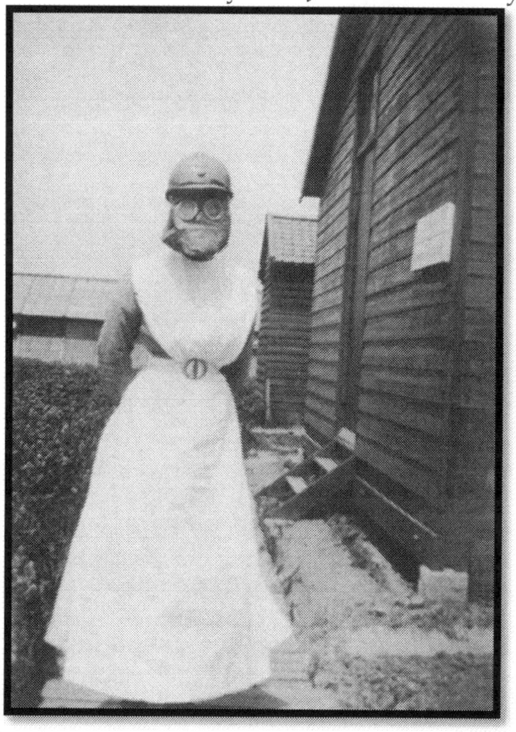

Australian Sister Winifred Hough with her gas mask. Winifred worked with her colleagues, Sisters Hilda Loxton, Annie Jamieson, Helen Wallace and Lynette Crozier, all of whom were sent to France by the Australian Red Cross in 1916. When close to the front line, they were frequently subjected to gas attacks.

(Photograph and caption courtesy AWM P01908.017)

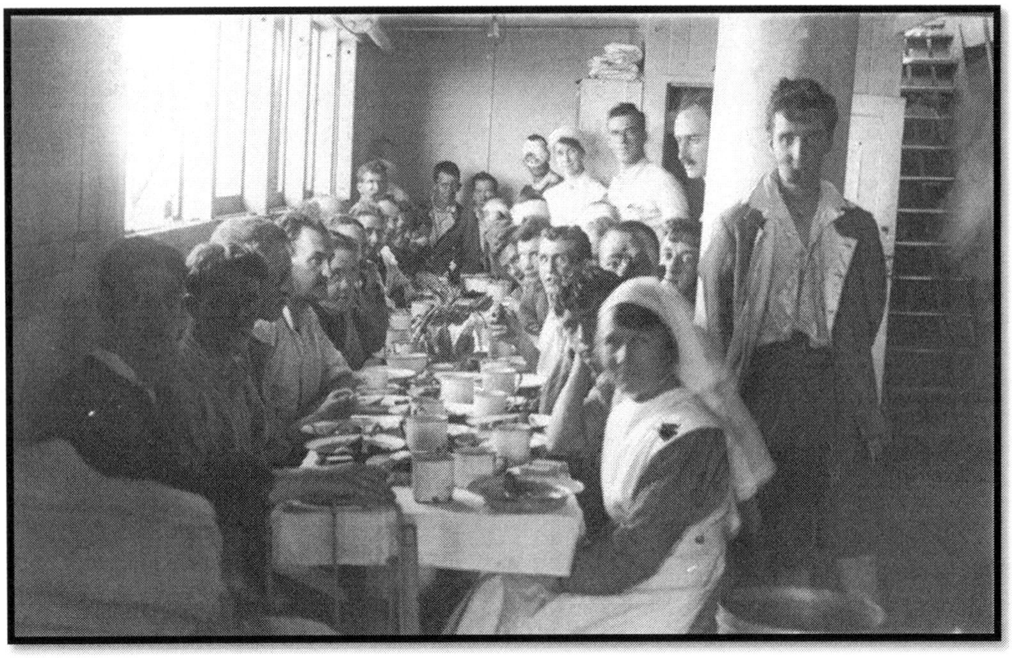

Interior of Karoola Hospital Transport.
(Photograph courtesy of AWM)

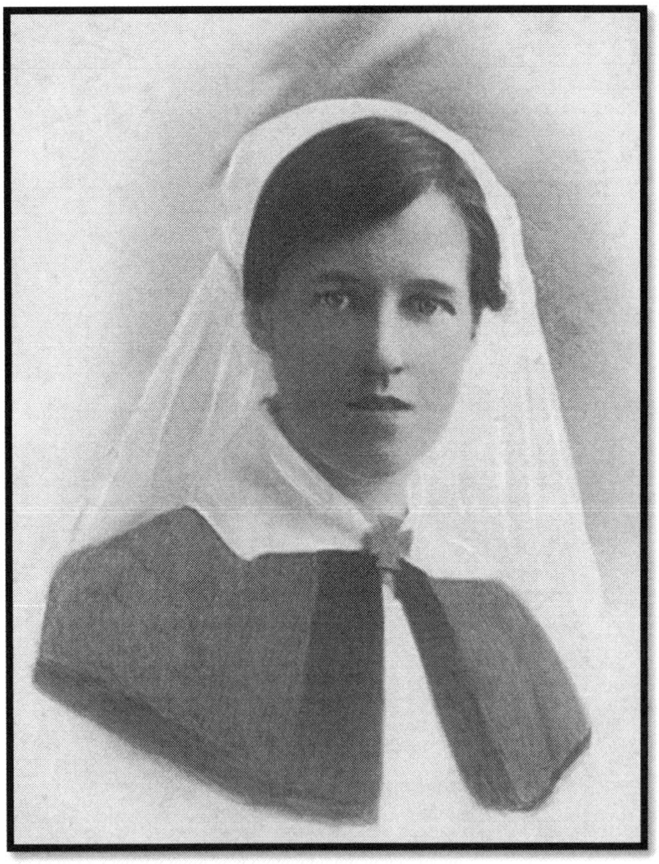

ATNA qualified Australian nure, Edith Blake, QAIMNSR, who died at sea.
(Photograph courtesy AWM P1193.004)

About the Author

Dr Ruth Rae (FACN) registered as a nurse in 1978 and has worked as a freelance researcher and writer for more than forty years. Her PhD thesis *Jessie Tomlins: An Australian Army Nurse - World War One* (2001) highlighted a dearth of historical material about the contribution of Australian nurses who served overseas during this period.

Ruth Rae has recently re-edited the first of book of the ACN Trilogy *From Narromine to the Nile* which was re-edited and published in 2017 as an ebook. A dramatic review was undertaken which included the diaries of Jessie Tomlins. The book was renamed *The biography of an Australian First World War army nurse: Jessie Tomlins* and is now available as an ebook and a paperback (2025).

Ruth continued her research for another three years and The NSW College of Nursing published *Scarlet Poppies: The Army Experience of Australian Nurses during World War One* (2004) which gives a history of a number of Australian nurses who served in all theatres of the 1914-18 war. Dr Rae followed this up with a further five years of study into the social histories of Australian war nurses which led to the publication of *Veiled Lives: Threading Australian Nursing History into the Fabric of the First World War* (The College of Nursing, 2009). The first edition of *Veiled Lives* was published in 2009 by The College of Nursing and formed the third book of the trilogy in 2015.

This edition of *Veiled Lives* has been renamed *Unveiling the History of Australian Nursing in the First World War* and dramatically re-edited. It will also ensure the book can be purchased as a stand alone ebook and/or print book. Her next project will be a light re-edit of *Scarlet Poppies* and include a comprehensive nominal roll in the next edition.

Dr Rae has also recently published the biography of Jessie's brother, Fred Tomlins, *The Biography of an Australian Light Horseman: Fred Tomlins.* Jessie's training matron at Sydney Hospital was the remarkable leader, Rose Creal, who, by chance, was also her matron at the 14 AGH, Egypt. Ruth Rae completed the biography of Rose in 2023 (see *Rose Creal: the biography of an Australian nurse leader 1865-1921*).

Acknowledgements

I reiterate my appreciation to those who assisted me with my initial research. Wendy Kleyn, Roger Bacon, Peter Edwell and Bronwyn Hyde have provided friendship, encouragement and most importantly editorial comments on this edition. I am indebted but take full responsibility for the re-editing of this edition.

Many families of the now deceased First World War nurses provided anecdotes, photographs and shared memories with me; I am indebted to them. I also acknowledge Ken Bascombe, John Holman, (late) Dorothy Rowe, Ian Darroch, John Sargent, Ian Ridgway and Joan Wheeler.

The First World War nurses who provided narratives, interviews and diaries to official historians, colleagues or their families have given me wonderful source material and I am indebted to them, as well as to the custodians of their material at the Australian War Memorial (AWM) – in particular, Joanne Smedley. I acknowledge the co-operation and assistance of the staff at the National Archives of Australia, in particular Yvonne Wise, who provided prompt access to the service records of many nurses prior to digitalization. Local public libraries throughout Australia, especially the State Library of NSW and the Battye Library (WA), have created comprehensive repositories of primary sources and I am indebted to the staff for their assistance.

Emeritus Professor R. Lynette Russell AO taught me how to write history and I am forever in her debt. The late Judith Cornell AM has given me a strong appreciation of the importance of maintaining archival material for which I am forever grateful. I have missed her support and never ending encouragement in the importance of telling the story of the nurses and ensuring their contribution is recorded as accurately as possible.

I am grateful for the co-operation and assistance always given to me by archivists and local historians whose names appear throughout the endnotes. Local historical societies, family history groups, local councils and their associated libraries are a genuine asset to the communities they serve and I gratefully acknowledge the many volunteers and local researchers who were generous with their time and research skills. In particular I thank David Cotton (Bendigo), Greg Kirk (Benalla), Heather Rendle (Echuca Historical Society Inc), Pearl Collins (Echuca/Moama Family History Group Inc), David Endacott (Daylesford Historical Society), Ellen Porter (Malvern Archives), David Lloyd (Goldfields Library Corp), Alan Kitchen, Craig Laffin, Eric Barton (Myrtleford and District Historical Society), Joanne Ewin (Milton, NSW), Dorothy King (Stawell Historical Society Inc), Helen Kindt (Mareeba History Society) Jan Wegert (Bundaberg Genealogical Association Inc), Peta Kinch (Bundaberg Library), Mike Moore (Fitzroy History Society) and Katherine Pawley (AWM). To those I have inadvertently omitted I apologise. I also acknowledge Emeritus Professor David Kent, Professor Frank Bongiorno and Janet Uhr.

I also acknowledge the support of the Australian Department of Veterans' Affairs, which provided a grant to assist in the first edition of the publication under the Australian Government's commemorations program, *Saluting Their Service.* The Department has not participated in the research or production or exercised editorial control over the work's contents and the views expressed and conclusions reached herein do not necessarily represent those of the Commonwealth, which expressly disclaims any responsibility for the content or accuracy of the work.

My heartfelt thanks to my husband, Rick Young, without whose support the process of research and writing would lose much of its satisfaction. My children and their partners – Alison Carter, Jenna and Julian Young, Caitlin and Phillip Lois – sustain me while my grandchildren – Audrey Young, Hudson Carter, Alex Lois, Asha Carter, Theo Lois and Archer Young – are a constant source of joy.

Made in the USA
Monee, IL
05 November 2026

67815671R00265